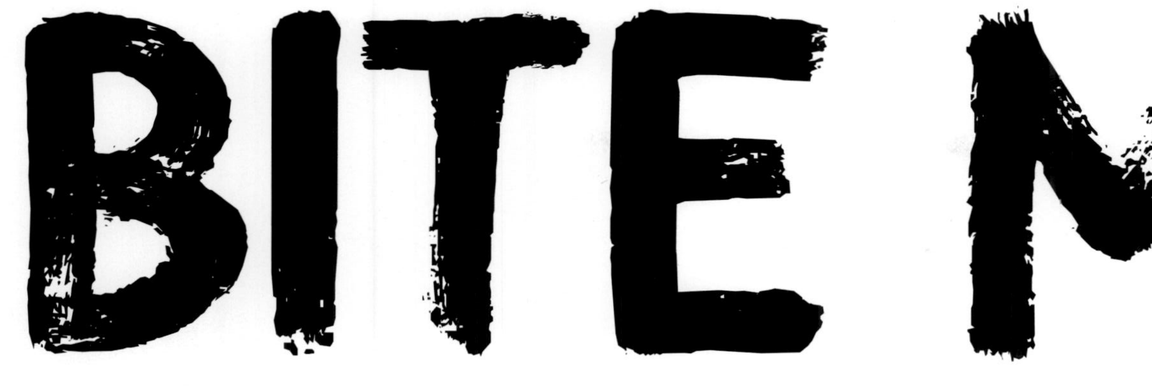
BITE
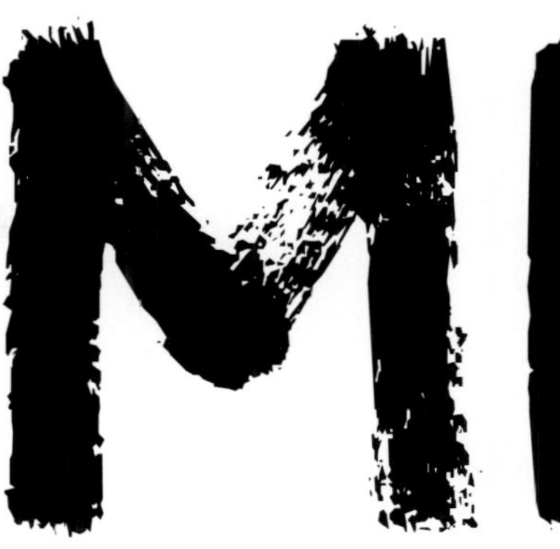
M
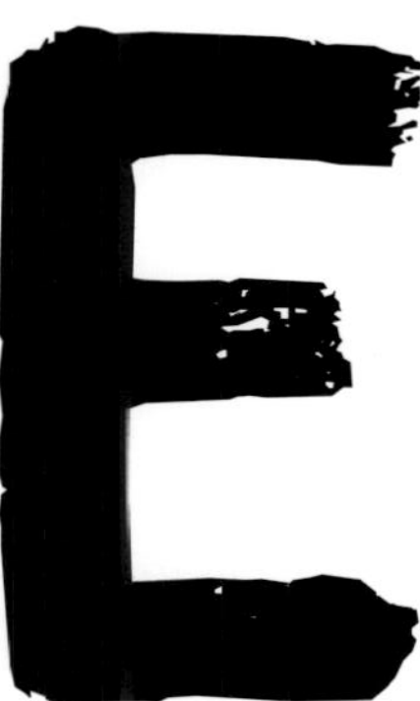
E

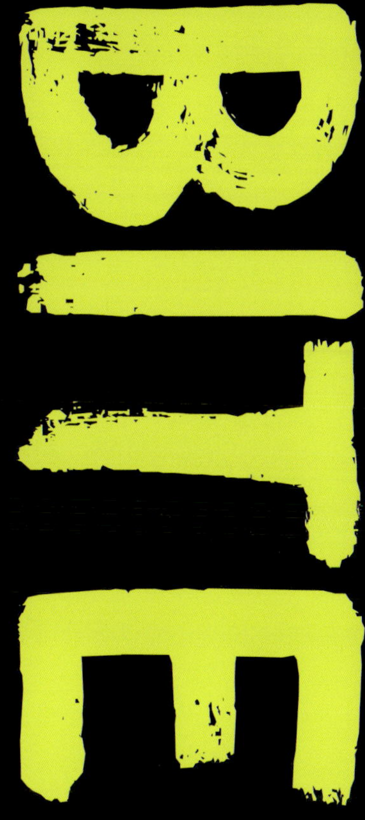
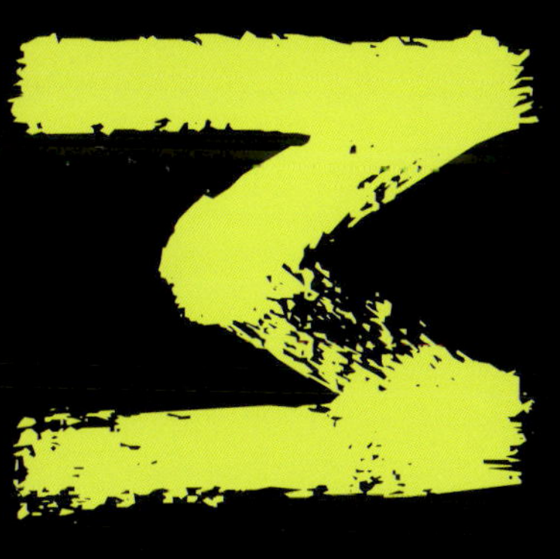
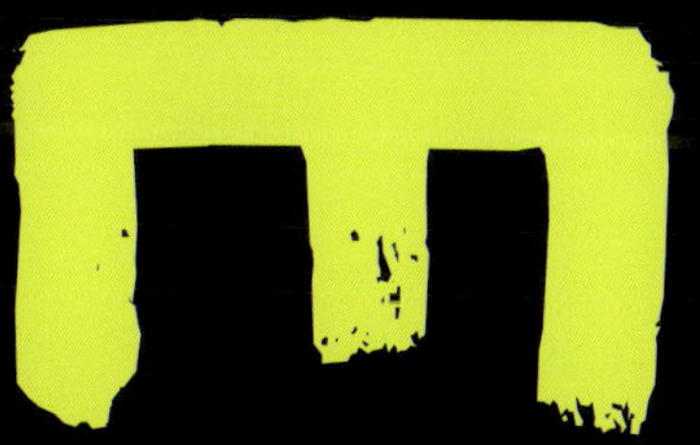
BITE ME
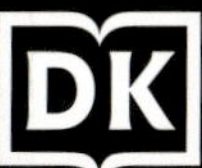
DK

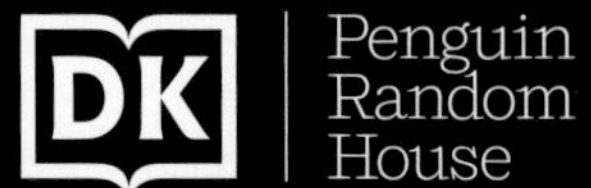

Publisher Mike Sanders
Art & Design Director William Thomas
Editorial Director Ann Barton
Editor Anna Wostenberg
Food Photographer Leonora Brebner | LRB Creative
Cover & Lifestyle Photographer Yianni Demetriadis and Patrick Leung
Illustrator Clemence Langevin
Proofreader Lisa Himes
Indexer Celia McCoy

First American Edition, 2025
Published in the United States by DK Publishing
1745 Broadway, 20th Floor, New York, NY 10019

The authorized representative in the EEA is Dorling Kindersley Verlag GmbH. Arnulfstr. 124, 80636 Munich, Germany

25 26 27 28 29 10 9 8 7 6 5 4 3 2 1
001-352614-DEC2025

A catalog record for this book is available from the Library of Congress.
ISBN 979-8-2171-3084-9

DK books are available at special discounts when purchased in bulk for sales promotions, premiums, fund-raising, or educational use. For details, contact SpecialSales@dk.com

Printed and bound in China

www.dk.com

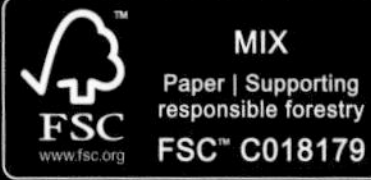

This book was made with Forest Stewardship Council™ certified paper – one small step in DK's commitment to a sustainable future.
Learn more at
www.dk.com/uk/information/sustainability

For Ollie

CONTENTS

Mum's Foreword 8
Introduction 11
Favorite Ingredients 12
Meal Prep 101 14
A Quick Note about Ingredients and Measurements 16
Kitchen Equipment Essentials 18
Cooking Conversion Chart 20

CHAPTER 1: WAKE AND BAKE:
BREAKFAST BAKES 23
Will's Favorite Exercises for Each Muscle Group 24
Ham and Cheddar Omelet Roll Up 26
Breakfast Stuffed Peppers 29
Savory Oats with Tempeh "Bacon" 30
Italian Baked Eggs 33
Healthy Fried Chicken and Waffles with Mustard Syrup 34
Turkey-Sausage Breakfast Casserole 37
Breakfast Pizza 38
Savory Quinoa Egg Breakfast Muffins 41
Egg Turkey-Bacon Muffins 42
Shredded Potato-Wrapped Quiches 45
Egg-White Vegetable Frittata 46
Protein Coffee Muffins 49
Chocolate-Chip Protein Muffins 50
Cottage-Cheese Protein Bagels 53
French Toast Protein Bagels 54
Protein Banana Bread 57

CHAPTER 2: MORNING QUICKIES:
TRADITIONAL BREKKIES 59
An Ode to Coffee 60
Breakfast Quesadilla 62
Vegan Maca Bowl 65
PB&J Protein Pancake 66
Lemon-Ricotta Protein Crepes 69
Breakfast Burritos with Homemade Sweet-Potato Wraps 70
Healthy Sausage and Egg McWills 73
Zucchini Hashbrowns 74
Chocolate Protein Pancake 77
3-Minute Breakfast Sandwich 78
Protein Waffles 81
Microwave Breakfast Bowl 82
Chocolate Peanut Butter No-Bake Energy Balls 85
PB&J Protein Roll Up 86
Breakfast Toast 3 Ways 88

CHAPTER 3: AFTERNOON DELIGHTS:
LUNCHTIME INDULGENCES 91
Will's Favorite Eats around the GTA (Greater Toronto Area) 92
Spicy Crispy Chicken Sandwiches 94
Curried Chicken Lettuce Wraps 97
Pecan Chicken Salad 98
Asian Mango Chicken Pita 101
Grilled Vegetable Salad 102
Savory Sweet-Potato Chicken and Waffle 105
BBQ Pulled Chicken Sliders 106
Ricotta-Stuffed Healthy Peppers 109
Tuna Burger with Pineapple Bun 110
Steak Taco Salad 113
Turkey Meatball Subs 114
White Bean and Artichoke Flatbread 117
Shawarma Chicken 118
Tofu Veggie Scramble 121

CHAPTER 4: BITE ME, BABY:
APPETIZERS 122
YouTube Q&A with Will 124
Zucchini Boats 126
Butternut Squash Fritters 129
Quick-Bake Falafel 130
Mexican Twice-Baked Stuffed Sweet Potato 133
Cauliflower and Leek Soup 134
Enhanced Twice-Baked Potato 137
Chicken Summer Rolls 138
Buffalo Cauliflower Bites 141
Warm Root-Vegetable Salad 142
Healthy Caesar Salad 145
Tuna-Stuffed Avocados 146
Anabolic Spinach Artichoke Dip with Pita Chips 149
Pineapple Salsa 150
Chicken Potstickers 153

CHAPTER 5: FEEDING THE FAMILY:
MAINS 154
Khichri and Air-Fried Tofu 158
Cabbage and Chicken Stir Fry 161
One-Pot Hearty Vegetable Chicken Stew 162
One-Pot Deconstructed Lasagna 165
Stuffed Chicken Breast with Spinach, Sun-Dried Tomato, and Ricotta Filling 166
Mexican Lasagna 169
Chicken Parmesan Bake with Quinoa 170
Budget-Friendly Chili 173
Coconut Chicken Curry 174
Chicken Cauliflower Fried Rice 177
Cauliflower-Rice Arancini with Turkey Sausage 178
Healthy Pad Thai 181
Cottage-Cheese Fettuccini Alfredo 182
Creamy Tarragon Shrimp Pasta 185

CHAPTER 6: CHEAT CODES:
FAKE THE TAKEOUT 187
Ollie "The Goat" Tennyson 188
Anabolic Pizza 190
Anabolic Shepherd's Pie 193
Cheeseburger Spring Rolls with Thousand Island Dip 194
Chicken Nuggies 197
Animal-Style Fries 198
Crispy Cheese Chicken Cups 201
Healthier Baked Mac and Cheese 202
Protein Scalloped Potatoes 205
Fried Zucchini Chips with Marinara Dip 206
Crispy Fried PB&J Sandwich 209
Pizza Casserole 210
Curry Chicken Tenders with Greek-Yogurt Dip 213
Blended Creamy Vanilla-Protein Iced Coffee 214

CHAPTER 7: HAPPY ENDINGS:
DELECTABLE DESSERTS 217
Will's Favorite Movies 218
Greek Yogurt Ice Pops 220
Handheld Apple Pies 223
Microwave Apple Pie 224
Protein Apple Fritters 227
Chocolate Peanut-Butter Protein Bark 228
S'mores Protein Cookies 231
Pumpkin Protein Mousse Cake 232
Dark Desire Chocolate Oat Cake 235
Anabolic "Spreadaroo" Cookies 236
Protein Crispy Rice Squares 239
Blueberry Cottage-Cheese Protein Cheesecake Bowl 240
No-Churn Vanilla-Protein Ice Cream 243
Raspberry Chocolate Protein Blondies 244
Chocolate-Chip Protein Cheesecake 247
Protein Whoopie Pie 248

Dietary Considerations 250
Acknowledgments 251
Index 254
About the Author 256

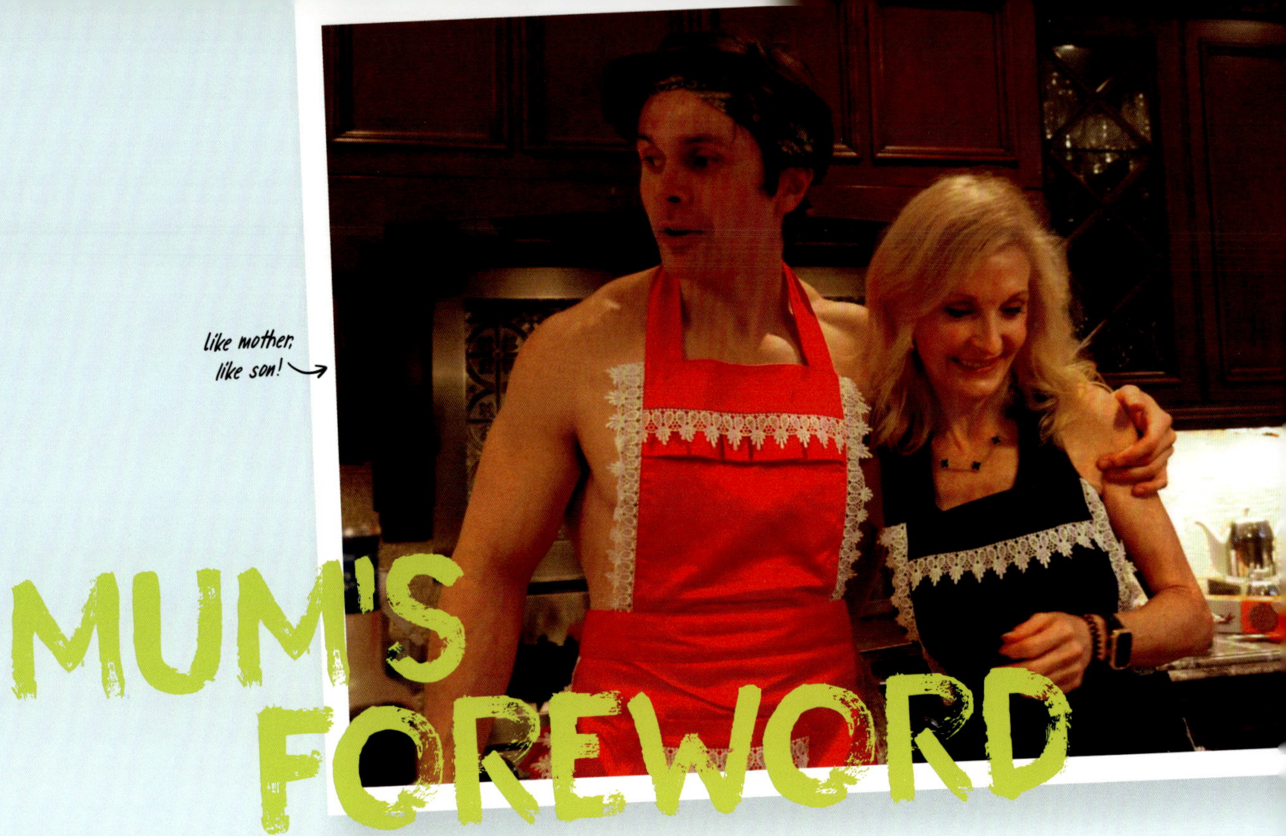

like mother, like son!

MUM'S FOREWORD

When the phone rang just after noon, and the call display showed the little Montessori school Will and his sister, Victoria, attended, I had that brief moment of mom panic. Was everything okay? Why were they calling me? I was home with baby Elizabeth, and Will had started going to school with Victoria that fall. The school principal was on the phone with young William (as he was known until high school) in her office. Will, who was four years old, had gone to the principal with a major problem and was insistent that his mother be called. He didn't like his lunch!

Will had suddenly developed an aversion to tuna sandwiches. I assured the principal that he loved tuna, but I could hear little William protesting in the background. He did not like *this* tuna! The principal was concerned that the poor little fellow was hungry, but his next sentence revealed all . . . "Couldn't she just go to McDonald's and pick me up a Happy Meal, like my friend's mom did today? I'd be fine with that." His four-year-old brain saw an opportunity and gave it a try. It didn't work that time, but he was just getting started.

Will has always been a food guy—a "good" food guy. His eating was not indiscriminate. He was not wolfing down chips and chocolate bars! He loved trying new foods (though there was one particularly hilarious time that we attempted to get him to eat escargot in a restaurant . . . We've never been back there).

My husband's mom—Will's grandma—was born in India, and all the kids have loved spicy Indian food since they were toddlers—keema with peas was a huge favorite, along with hot chicken tikka masala, chana masala (Victoria's fave), and butter chicken with fresh roti. As for the ultra-sweet Indian desserts, not so much! The savory side of Will's palate definitely had the upper hand, and there were no Boston creams!

As a family, we traveled often, and food played a huge part in our experiences. Cruising was a favorite, and we were able to take the kids to see the Berlin Wall, the Hermitage Museum, the Sistine Chapel, the Mona Lisa, and the statue of the Little Mermaid. We strolled Las Ramblas, watched whales in the Pacific, and marveled at the crown jewels at the Tower of London. No excursion was complete without the food to go with it. Pizza in Italy, pelmeni in Russia, tapas in Spain, smoked fish in Alaska, meatballs in Sweden—though there were no takers on the pickled herring!

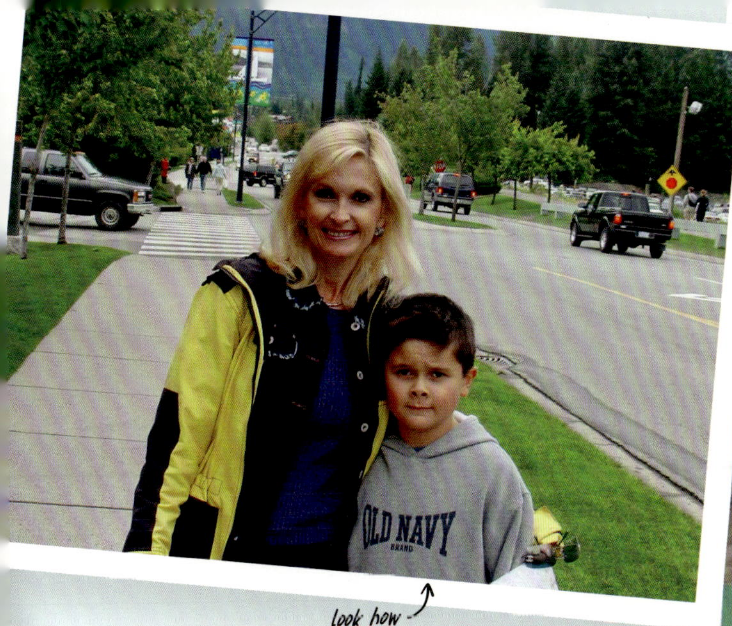

look how cute he was!

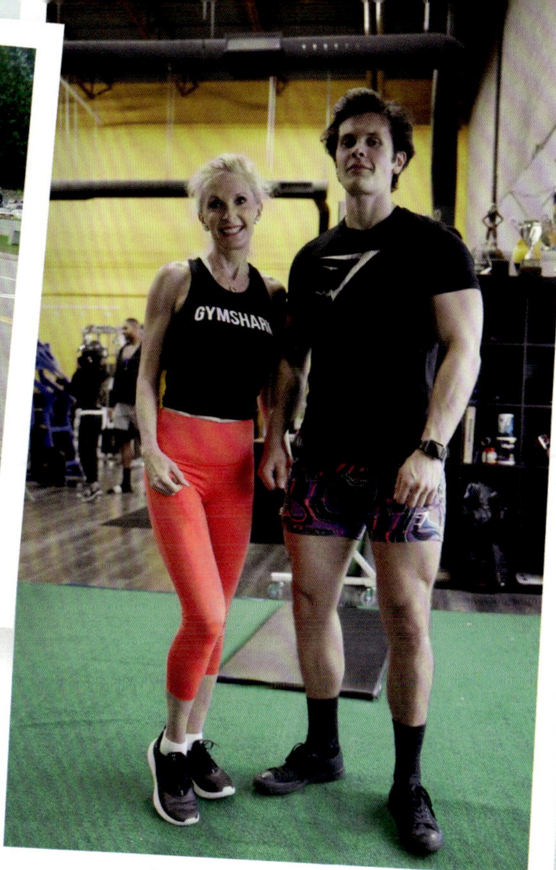

gym buddies for life!

Will certainly loved food, but he also became interested in the presentation and other components of the meal. When I entertained at home, Will became my sous chef. When we hosted dinner parties, I relied on Will as my free labor. He was an integral part of menu planning and grocery shopping. (I'd still rather send eight-year-old Will shopping than my husband, Paul!) He cooked alongside me, and I often left him to his own devices on a particular dish—garnishing the plates and helping to serve. His presentation skills were spot on. It seemed that Will had found his passion.

Many of you may be surprised to know that Will was particularly shy growing up. He was a boy of few words outside the house, but inside, he was quite the storyteller! I remember one time in particular, we were on a family trip, driving to Florida, and Will just started telling a story. It was about "Jimmy the Pig," and it was completely and spontaneously made up, weaving the most ridiculous, hilarious, out-of-nowhere adventures of this little pig. Tears were streaming down our faces, we were laughing so hard. I remember asking myself, "How does he come up with this stuff?" But this was not the Will he allowed the world to see, until YouTube. All of a sudden, the funny, crazy, witty, and outlandish Will was revealed.

As Will was wrapping up his undergraduate degree at the University of Guelph, the idea of him pursuing his cooking passion at the Le Cordon Bleu school in Ottawa became more and more of a possibility. The problem? Will was now a fitness fanatic, to put it mildly. He was tracking calories and macros like a Wall Street trader tracks the stock market. Will didn't want to cook with copious amounts of butter; thick, creamy sauces; ganache; or foie gras. Nor was he going to sweat through his days eating oatmeal, chicken breast, and yogurt (at least not all the time!). He wanted tasty, delicious, approachable food that would fit into his newfound passion for fitness—and this is what he hopes to share with you in this cookbook.

As a fitness enthusiast myself, I'm in awe of what Will has accomplished both personally and professionally. I have seen firsthand the letters and testimonials people have sent to him about their own experiences. His ability to relate and motivate, be funny and yet serious when speaking from the heart, is unrivaled. Will is talented in so many ways, and as his mother, I am immensely proud of him. This book is a reflection of Will and the man he has become. You are going to love it—enjoy!

—Nancy <3

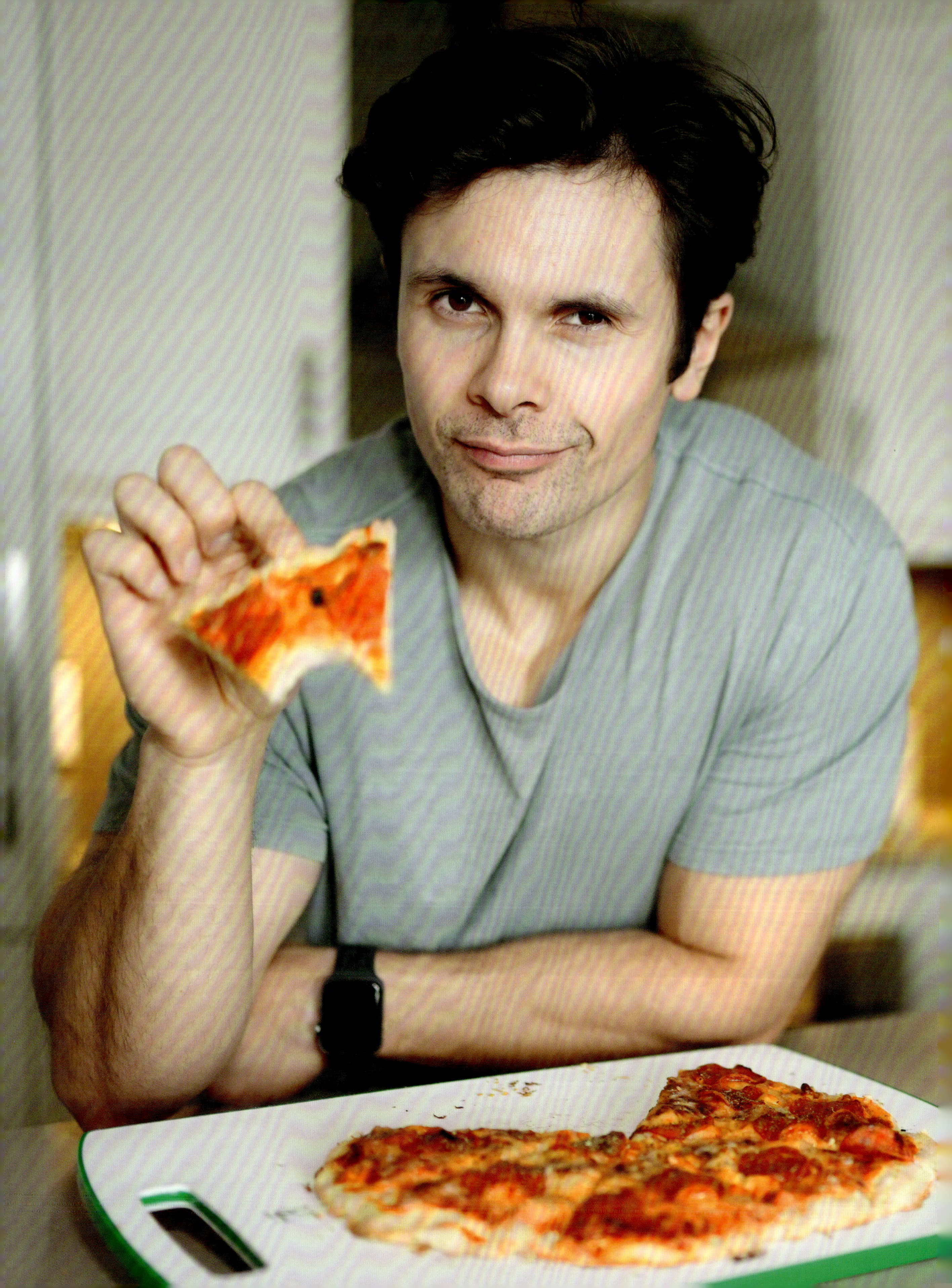

INTRODUCTION

What's up, guys? Will here. I wanted to take some time to thank you all for being part of the most supportive community on YouTube for the past few years. Without you following me, this cookbook would have just stayed a dream of mine—but here we are!

As much as I dedicate my life to being strong and active, my number one passion and joy has always been food. Eating it? Of course. But also creating fresh recipes, experimenting with different ingredients, learning new techniques, and sharing it all with my loved ones. From a young age, I was glued to the Food Network, with Jamie Oliver being a personal favorite for his rustic, approachable, and often healthy dishes, and his relatable sense of humor. Strangely enough, my other food god was Guy Fieri. I could never get enough of *Diners, Drive-Ins, and Dives* and all the outrageous, mouth-watering food that definitely wouldn't fit into anyone's macros . . . but that's okay. Be good most of the time, right?

I began cooking with my mom, studying her every move as she chopped and sautéed and broiled. Together, we made everything from seafood pasta to chicken shumai to cheddar shortbread topped with red-pepper jelly. Eventually, I was confident enough to tackle the kitchen on my own, and making dinner for my family became my form of meditation, helping me unwind and relax. My weekends were full of grocery shopping and menu planning, and I spent my weeknights perfecting sauces and marinades when I should have been doing my homework. I had found my calling.

Then, I got really into lifting, and along with that came tracking macros and a shift in my approach to cooking—though not in the way you might think. Sure, I began to create dishes that were more protein forward and lighter on the carbs, and yes, I used butters and oils sparingly. Okay, lots of sugar-free ingredients and low-calorie alternatives too. However, what has never changed is my love of getting creative in the kitchen. I continue to challenge myself to create healthy, satiating meals that don't compromise on the bold, complex flavors I love. For me, having fun with cooking is huge, and this is something I'd like to share with all of you.

With this cookbook, I hope to bridge the gap between strict macro-focused cooking and cooking as a (tasty) art form. The recipes in this book are things you can impress your friends and family with and that can also fit in your macros. I want to spread my passion for cooking, and I promise you all that it is possible to make healthy dishes that are so delicious, every day will feel like a cheat day. Enjoy!

—Will

FAVORITE INGREDIENTS

ALWAYS IN MY PANTRY

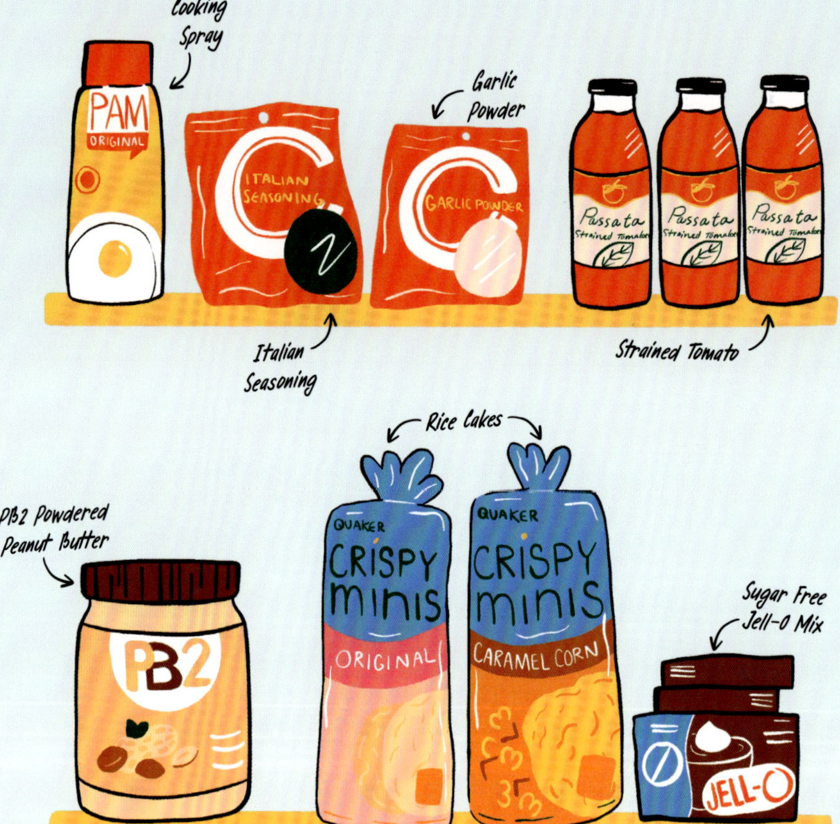

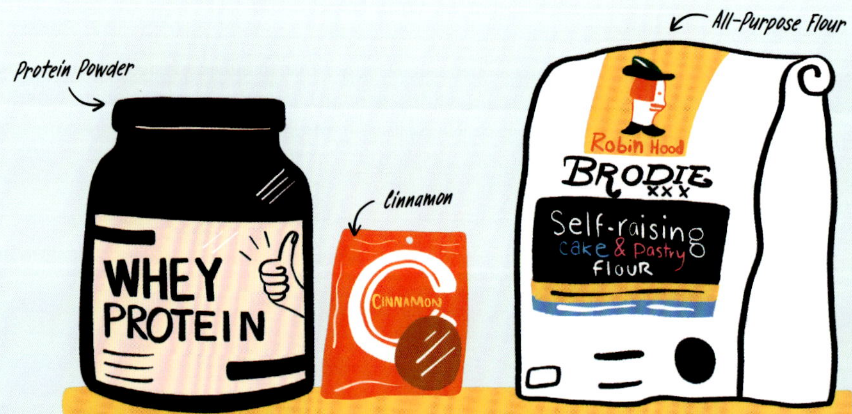

ALWAYS IN MY FRIDGE

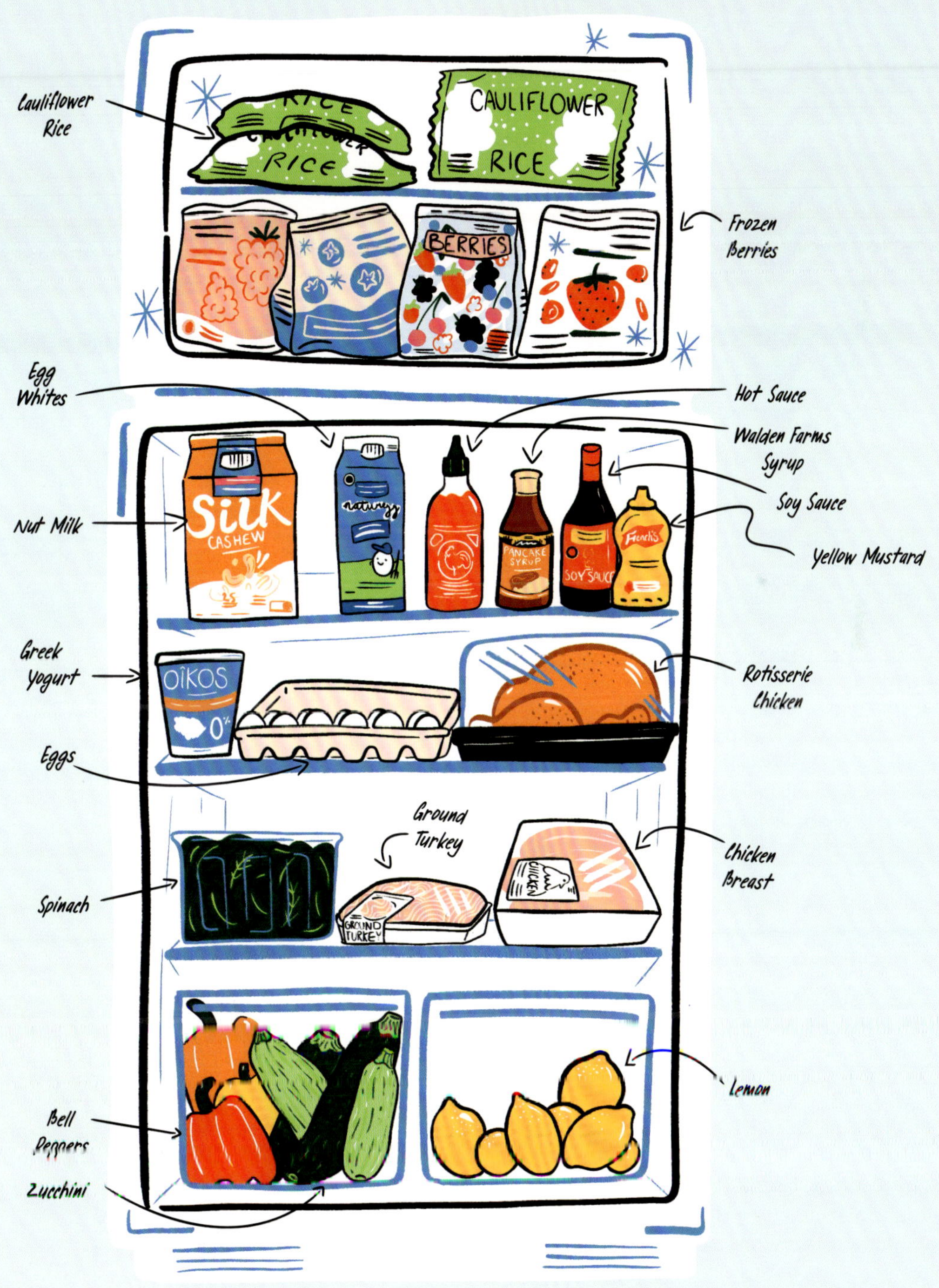

MEAL PREP 101

MASTERING THE BASICS WITHOUT LOSING YOUR SOUL

Meal prep doesn't have to feel like a chore. You're not signing up for a week of bland chicken and soggy vegetables unless you want to (and if you do, we need to have a serious talk). To me, meal prepping is less about turning your kitchen into a food factory and more about setting yourself up for a week of wins—while still leaving room for spontaneity.

Here's the plan: Master a few basics, keep it flexible, and always give yourself options. Think of meal prep as controlled chaos. Just enough structure to keep you on track, but enough freedom to avoid getting bored. Let's break it down.

1. COOK YOUR PROTEINS IN BULK.

Chicken breast, ground turkey, tofu, shrimp—pick your building block of gains, season it like you care about flavor, and cook it all at once. Air fry it, grill it, bake it—you do you. I like to mix up the seasonings so I'm not stuck eating the same flavors all week. Lemon and pepper for one batch, garlic and paprika in another, and maybe some taco seasoning in the last one. Now, you've got options: Wrap it in a tortilla, toss it on a salad, or throw it into a stir-fry. You've got range now.

Pro tip: A number of recipes in this book call for cooked chicken breast, so prepping it ahead of time will save you major time and effort throughout the week. My go-to method to cook chicken breast is to pop it in a 425°F (220°C) oven for 18 to 20 minutes, until it reaches an internal temperature of 165°F (74°C). Make sure you store it properly in a sealed container in the fridge for no more than 4 days—or freeze portions if you're prepping way ahead.

A Quick Note on Over-Prepping (aka the Meal Prep Trap)

It's easy to get hyped up and prep every single meal, snack, and side for the entire week, but don't overdo it. Cooking should be enjoyable, not a marathon that burns you out. Start with a couple of basics (like a protein, a carb, and a veg), and leave room to cook fresh meals when you feel like it. Think of meal prep as a safety net—not a prison sentence. You can always cook something new midweek if inspiration strikes.

At the end of the day, meal prep is about making your life easier. Keep it simple, stay flexible, and remember:

Healthy eating isn't about restriction—it's about balance. Now go forth and meal prep like the legend you are.

2. DON'T BE LAZY WITH VEGGIES.

I get it—chopping veggies can feel like cruel and unusual punishment, but no pain, no gain. Roasting a big tray of them while your protein cooks is a time saver you'll thank yourself for later. Broccoli, carrots, zucchini, bell peppers—you name it, you can roast it. Toss them in a little olive oil, salt, pepper, and a bit of garlic powder, and suddenly your veggies aren't just edible—they're satisfying.

And since a lot of recipes in this book use chopped veggies, having them prepped ahead of time will save you from midweek "I don't feel like cooking" moments. Like your proteins, store them properly in sealed containers, and don't leave them too long, or the only thing you'll be prepping is regret.

3. CARBS ARE YOUR FRIEND, NOT THE VILLAIN.

I don't want to hear any carb-phobic nonsense. Prepping carbs ahead of time is a lifesaver. Cook a batch of rice, quinoa, or sweet potatoes—you can even rotate through them each week if you're the "I need variety, or I'll self-combust" type.

Pro tip: Flavor your carbs as you cook them. Throw some cilantro and lime in your rice, or roast your sweet potatoes with cinnamon and a touch of chili powder. If you're on a low-carb kick, no worries—cauliflower rice or zucchini noodles can step in like your mom's new boyfriend.

4. HAVE A FLAVOR ARSENAL READY.

You know what makes meal-prep meals feel less like meal-prep meals? Sauces, dips, and seasonings. A drizzle of sriracha, a tahini dressing, or a squirt of mustard can change the game. I keep hot sauce, salsa, soy sauce, and balsamic glaze on hand at all times, because life's too short to eat bland food. Experiment, and you might stumble on your new go-to.

5. PORTION AND STORE.

Glass containers, reusable plastic, bento boxes—whatever works for you. Just make sure they seal well and keep things organized. You can either preassemble full meals or store everything separately so you can mix and match. Feeling spicy on Thursday? Combine taco-seasoned chicken with lime rice and roasted peppers. Need something basic on Monday? Go with lemon-pepper chicken and broccoli. Future you is already smiling.

6. DON'T FORGET THE "FUN" FOODS.

Meal prep doesn't mean you're locked into "clean eating" 24-7. I always leave room for a couple of treats—whether it's a few squares of chocolate, a protein dessert, or a bag of popcorn. You're allowed to have fun with food, and trust me, a little indulgence won't wreck your progress. You're in it for the long haul.

7. FIND RECIPES MADE FOR MEAL PREPPING.

If you're wondering which recipes in this book are perfect for meal prepping, don't worry—I've got you. Any recipe that makes multiple portions can easily be added to your weekly plan. To make it even easier, I've included a sticker next to the ones that are ideal for meal prep. So, whether you're making a big batch of protein-packed muffins or a meal prep-friendly casserole, you'll know exactly which recipes will help you crush the week ahead.

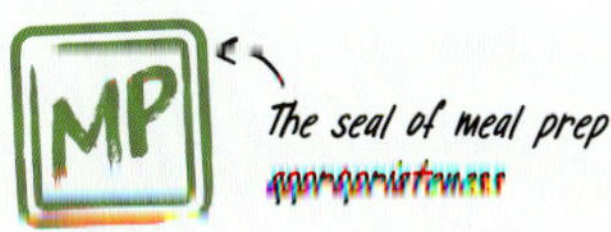

A QUICK NOTE ABOUT INGREDIENTS AND MEASUREMENTS

BEFORE YOU GET INTO THE NITTY GRITTY OF MY RECIPES, I WANT TO LEAVE YOU WITH SOME WORDS OF WISDOM.

I'm a big believer that cooking and eating healthy is more of an art than a science. The ingredients I use are guidelines, not rules, and my recipes are often a result of me foraging through my fridge and using whatever isn't covered in mold. What I'm trying to say is feel free to swap out ingredients and use what you have (or what you like). If you don't have fresh herbs, use dried instead. If you don't have turkey sausage, use ground turkey seasoned the way you like, or any other ground meat for that matter. I use some seasonings that might be specific to the grocery stores in my city, such as the Parmesan-and-herb seasoning featured in many of my recipes. If you don't have it, use a sprinkle of Parmesan cheese instead. Many of the recipes use various dried herbs and seasoning blends, but don't feel tied down. If you hate oregano, don't use Italian seasoning! Love spice? Add some chili powder or cayenne pepper. I have no doubt that as a result of your experimentation with ingredients, some of you will come up with even better versions of these recipes. Just note that differences in ingredients (even brands of ingredients) can alter the macros, so please use the macros in this book merely as a guide. They're accurate to the ingredients we used to create these recipes, but based on what you have on hand or what's available in your grocery store, they may differ. Also note that optional ingredients, ingredient swaps, and ingredient additions change the macros too. Use your preferred tracker to count your macros, and enjoy the recipes with your own flair.

Another thing that needs to be addressed is the fact that, yes, I realize my measurements are all over the place. Art, not science, remember? Sometimes, I'll provide an exact amount of a veggie, for example, and other times, I'll just give you the size of that veggie. The important thing to know here is that it'll all work out. The macros will be so close that it won't make a noticeable difference, and where precision actually matters—like baking or protein content—I've got you covered with exact measurements. So don't stress. Just cook, eat, and be merry.

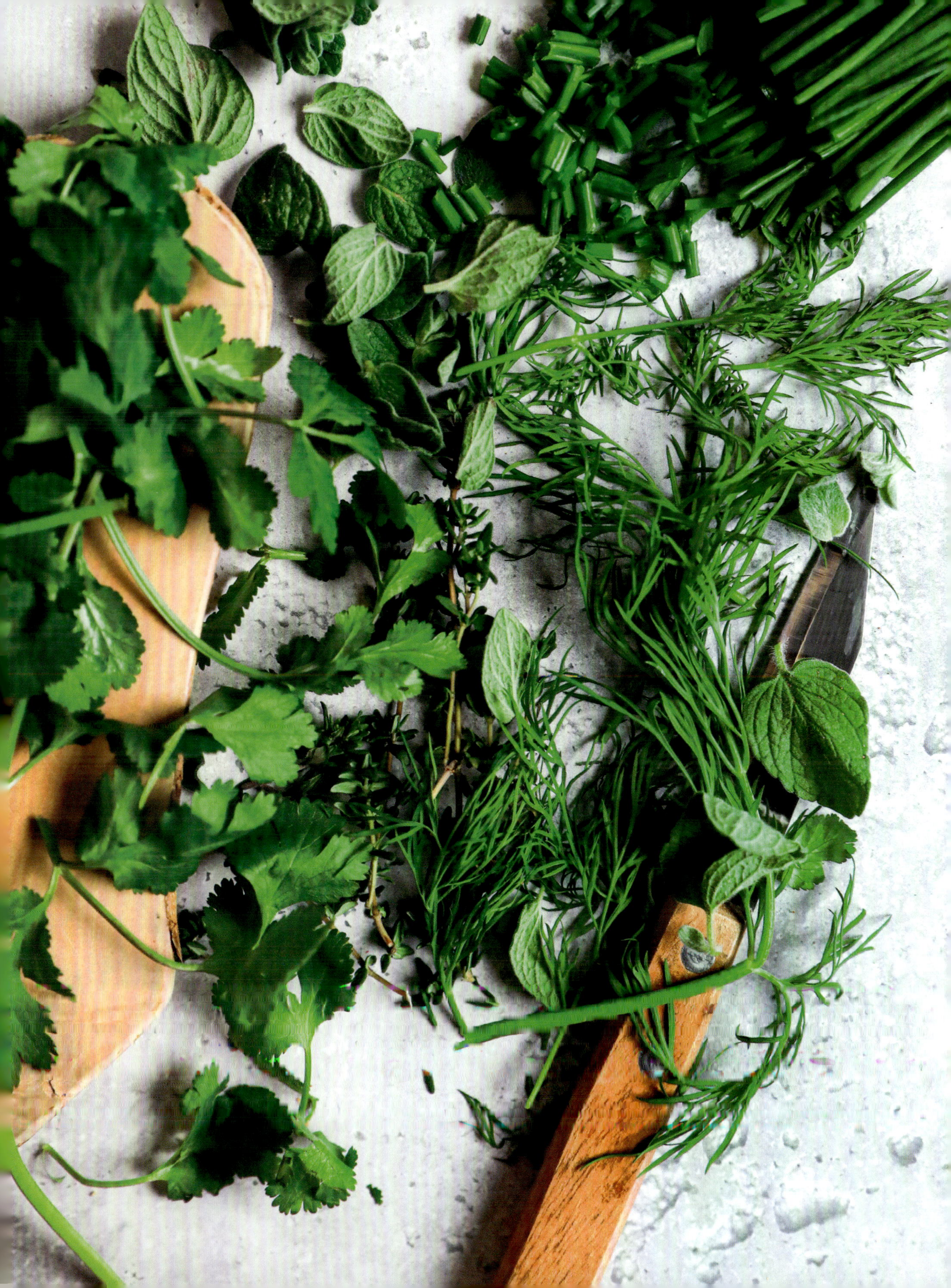

KITCHEN EQUIPMENT ESSENTIALS

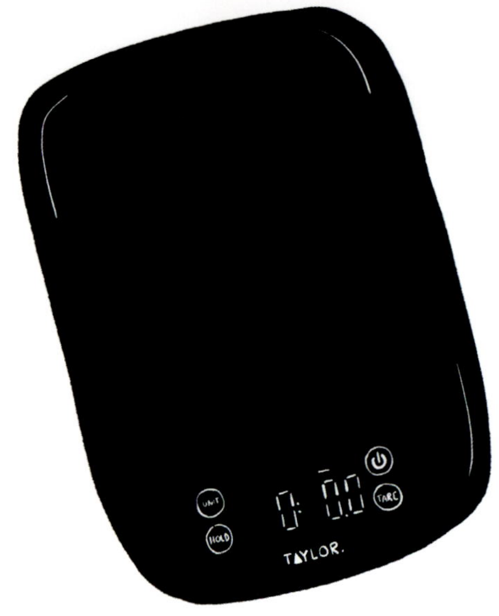

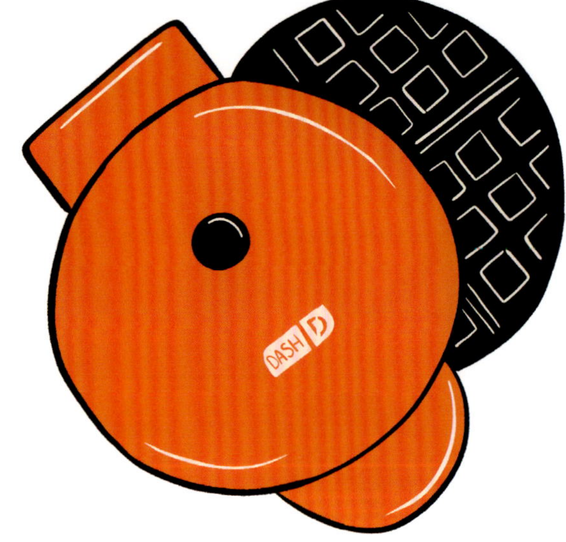

FOOD SCALE

If you take one thing away from this section, please grab a kitchen food scale. On top of the fact that a lot of my suggested measurements in this cookbook are by weight, I think it's extremely important to teach yourself what different serving sizes look like. This way, you will eventually be able to estimate your calorie intake with confidence. When looking for a food scale, some things to keep in mind are its size, accuracy, ease of use, and maximum weight it can hold. I use the Taylor Waterproof Digital Kitchen Scale that I got from Costco, which works great for me and is very affordable.

WAFFLE IRON

I love a good waffle in the morning . . . or in the afternoon or evening for that matter. You'll see I have a number of waffle recipes in this cookbook, both sweet and savory, and between you and me—they're some of my best. When looking for a waffle iron, it doesn't need to be anything fancy. I use the Dash Express Waffle Maker from Amazon, which has held up over time and fits in my condo's small kitchen. Find a waffle maker that's perfect for you in terms of shape, size, and cost, and you'll be all set.

While you shouldn't turn to me for advice on day trading, you can trust that I have your best interests in mind with these four kitchen investments—which are guaranteed to bring your anabolic cooking game to the next level.

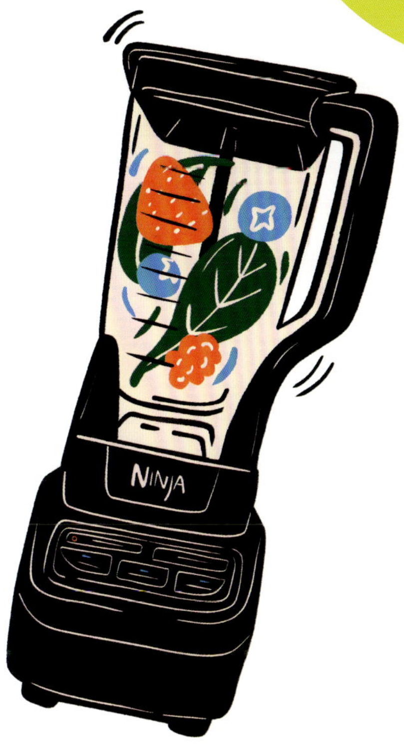

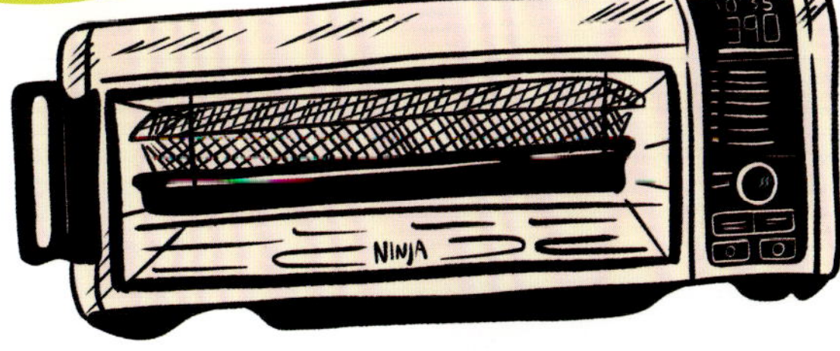

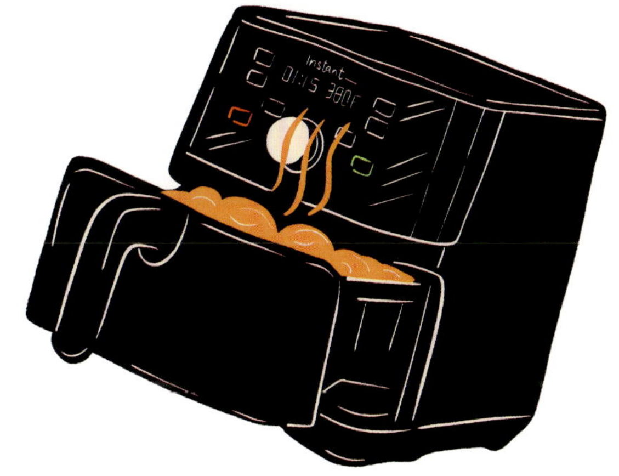

BLENDER

Whether you're looking to make Coach Greg's anabolic ice cream or one of my cookbook recipes, you're going to need a blender. I can't comment on the age-old Vitamix versus Ninja debate, but I do have to say that the Ninja Professional Blender 1000 has never let me down (and neither has my Vitamix stick). In my opinion, the most important things to look for in a blender are its level of power and the settings offered. Determine the size you're looking for and your budget, and get blending.

AIR FRYER

The popularity of air fryers has gone through the roof, and it's easy to see why. You can crisp up just about anything without submerging it in pools of oil and adding tons of unnecessary calories. They're also incredibly versatile, and depending on your air fryer model, you can also bake, broil, roast, or toast without using your conventional oven. I use the Instant Pot Vortex 6QT Large Air Fryer Oven Combo at my condo, and the Ninja Foodi 8 in 1 Digital Air Fry Oven at my parents' house—which my mom uses every day. Just get an air fryer, and thank me later.

COOKING CONVERSION CHART

WEIGHT

Imperial	Metric
½oz	15g
1oz	30g
2oz	60g
3oz	85g
4oz	115g
5oz	140g
6oz	175g
7oz	200g
8oz	225g
9oz	250g
10oz	300g
11oz	325g
12oz	350g
13oz	375g
14oz	400g
15oz	425g
1lb	450g

MEASUREMENTS

Cups	Milliliters	Ounces	Tablespoons
1⁄16 cup	15ml	½oz	1 tbsp
⅛ cup	30ml	1oz	2 tbsp
¼ cup	60ml	2oz	4 tbsp
⅓ cup	80ml	2½oz	5½ tbsp
⅜ cup	90ml	3oz	6 tbsp
½ cup	120ml	4oz	8 tbsp
⅔ cup	160ml	5oz	11 tbsp
¾ cup	180ml	6oz	12 tbsp
1 cup	240ml	8oz	16 tbsp

TEMPERATURE

Fahrenheit	300°F	325°F	350°F	375°F	400°F	425°F	450°F	475°F	500°F
Celsius	150°C	160°C	180°C	190°C	200°C	220°C	230°C	240°F	260°C

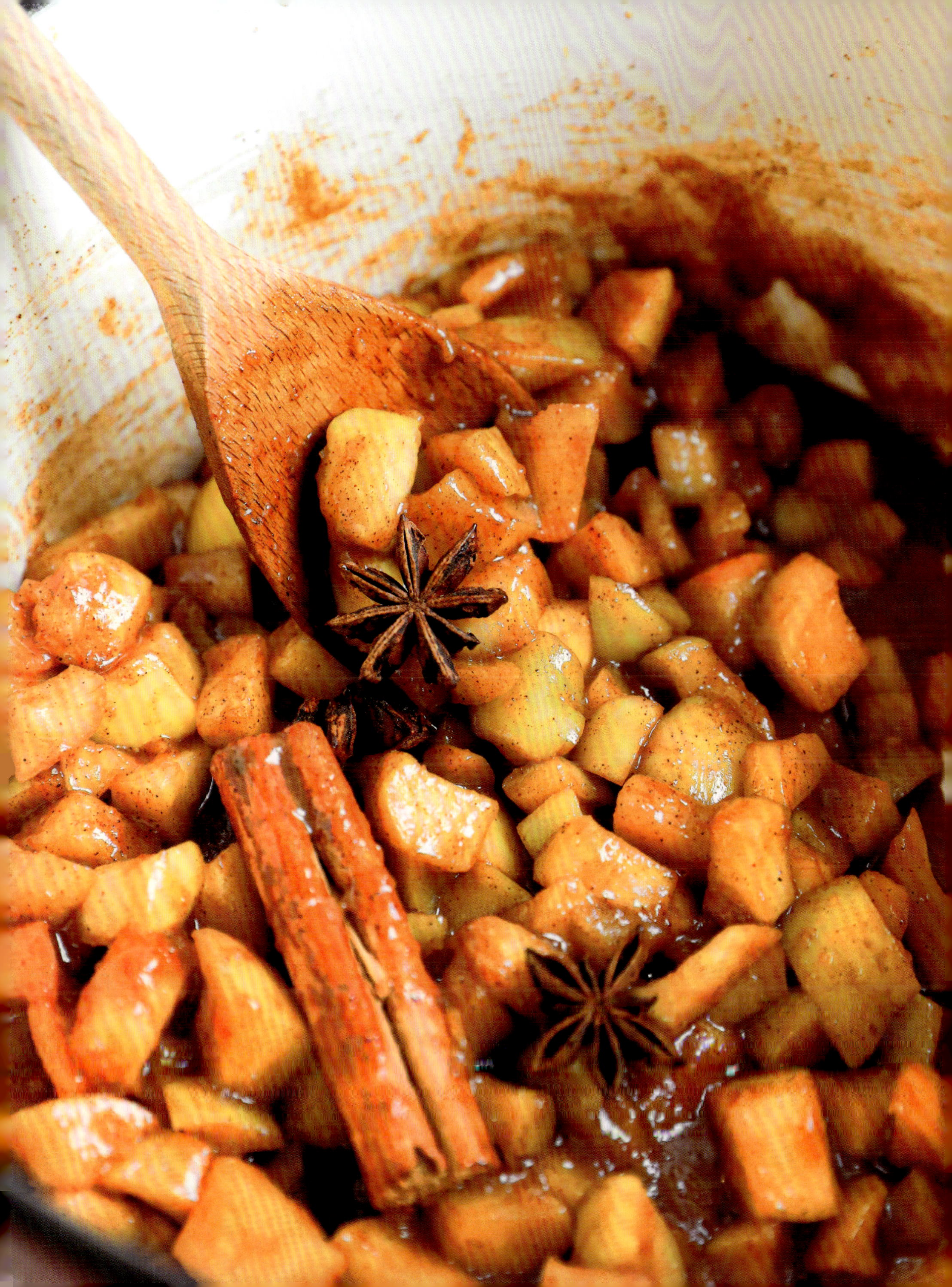

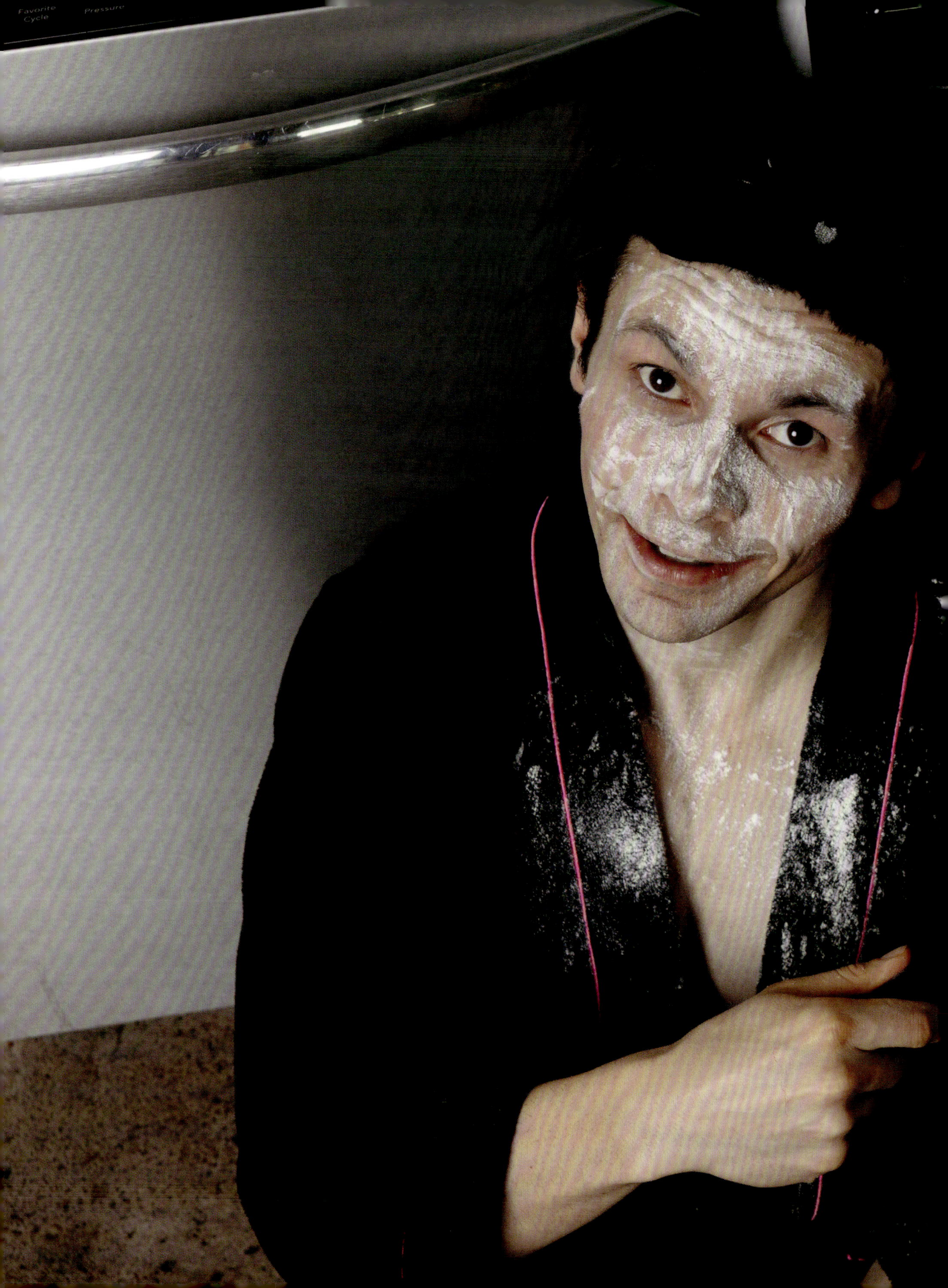
Favorite
Cycle
Pressure

CHAPTER 1

WAKE AND BAKE

BREAKFAST BAKES

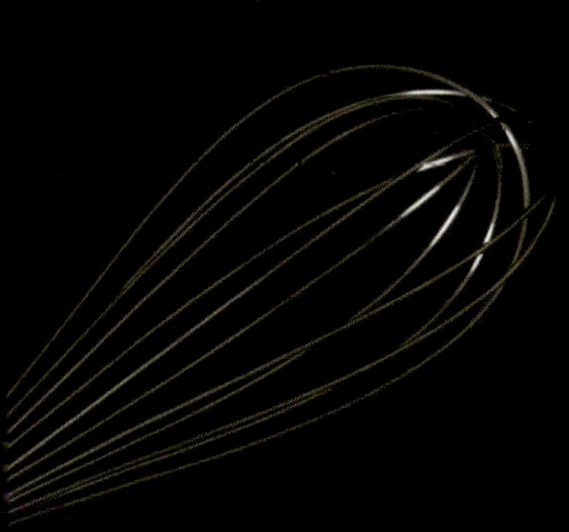

WILL'S FAVORITE EXERCISES

FOR EACH MUSCLE GROUP

I can safely say that I've spent more time in the gym than a Canadian spends apologizing. While I've made lots of changes to the way I train over the years, these exercises have always been my go-tos. Now, I'm sharing them with you in the hopes that they'll help you level up your training too.

CHEST

- Incline Dumbbell Press
- Machine Chest Press

BACK

- Incline Bench 2 Arm Dumbbell Row
- Machine High Row

SHOULDERS

- Standing Cable Lateral Raise
- Cable Y Raise

BICEPS

- Dumbbell Spider Curl
- Cable EZ Barbell Curl

TRICEPS

- Overhead Cable Rope Tricep Extension
- Dumbbell Skull Crusher

QUADS

- Hack Squat
- Leg Extension

HAMSTRINGS

- Seated Hamstring Curl
- Toes Elevated Dumbbell Romanian Deadlift

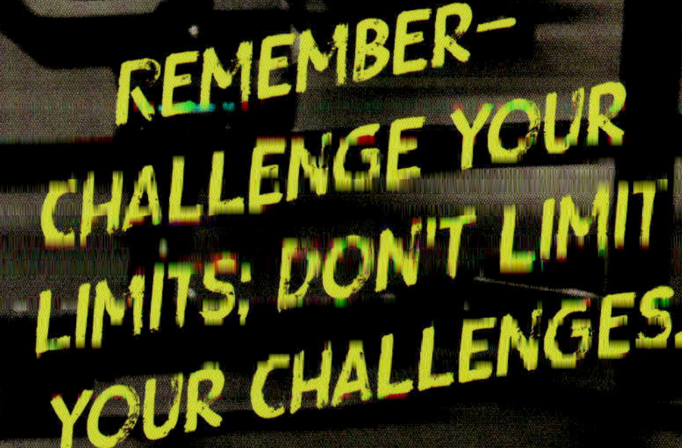

HAM AND CHEDDAR OMELET ROLL UP

6 eggs
1 cup (240ml) Silk unsweetened cashew milk
½ cup (60g) all-purpose flour
Salt and pepper, to taste
8 slices (145g) Black Forest ham
¾ cup (90g) shredded low-fat cheddar cheese
4 tsp (20g) green onion, diced

Switching to a vape doesn't mean you can't still roll up in the morning. This high-protein wake 'n bake recipe is a perfectly girthy solution to those morning munchies. It's easy to swap out the filling ingredients based on what you need to get rid of in your fridge—if you can roll it, you can fill it. If you're on a veggie kick, throw some spinach and caramelized onions in there. Feeling carnivorous? Bacon works, too. If you want to save some for later, store it in the fridge for up to 4 days, and to reheat, microwave on high for 1½ minutes.

1. Preheat the oven to 450°F (230°C). Line the bottom and sides of an 11 x 17-inch (28 x 43cm) rimmed baking sheet with parchment paper.
2. In a large bowl, combine the eggs and cashew milk and whisk until frothy, about 20 seconds.
3. Slowly add the flour, season with salt and pepper, and whisk for 1 to 2 minutes, until the mixture has a smooth consistency with no clumps.
4. To the prepared baking sheet, pour the egg mixture, making sure it is evenly distributed.
5. Bake for 10 minutes, until the eggs are firm and fluffy.
6. Remove the baking sheet from the oven and lay the ham slices evenly spaced across the surface of the eggs. Sprinkle the cheese and green onions on top.
7. Bake for an additional 5 minutes. The cheese should be melted and the ham warmed through.
8. Roll the omelet tightly into a long log and slice into 8 even slices.

makes 1 omelet / 8 servings

NUTRITION (PER SERVING)

116 calories	**6.5g** fat
11g protein	**3.6g** net carbs

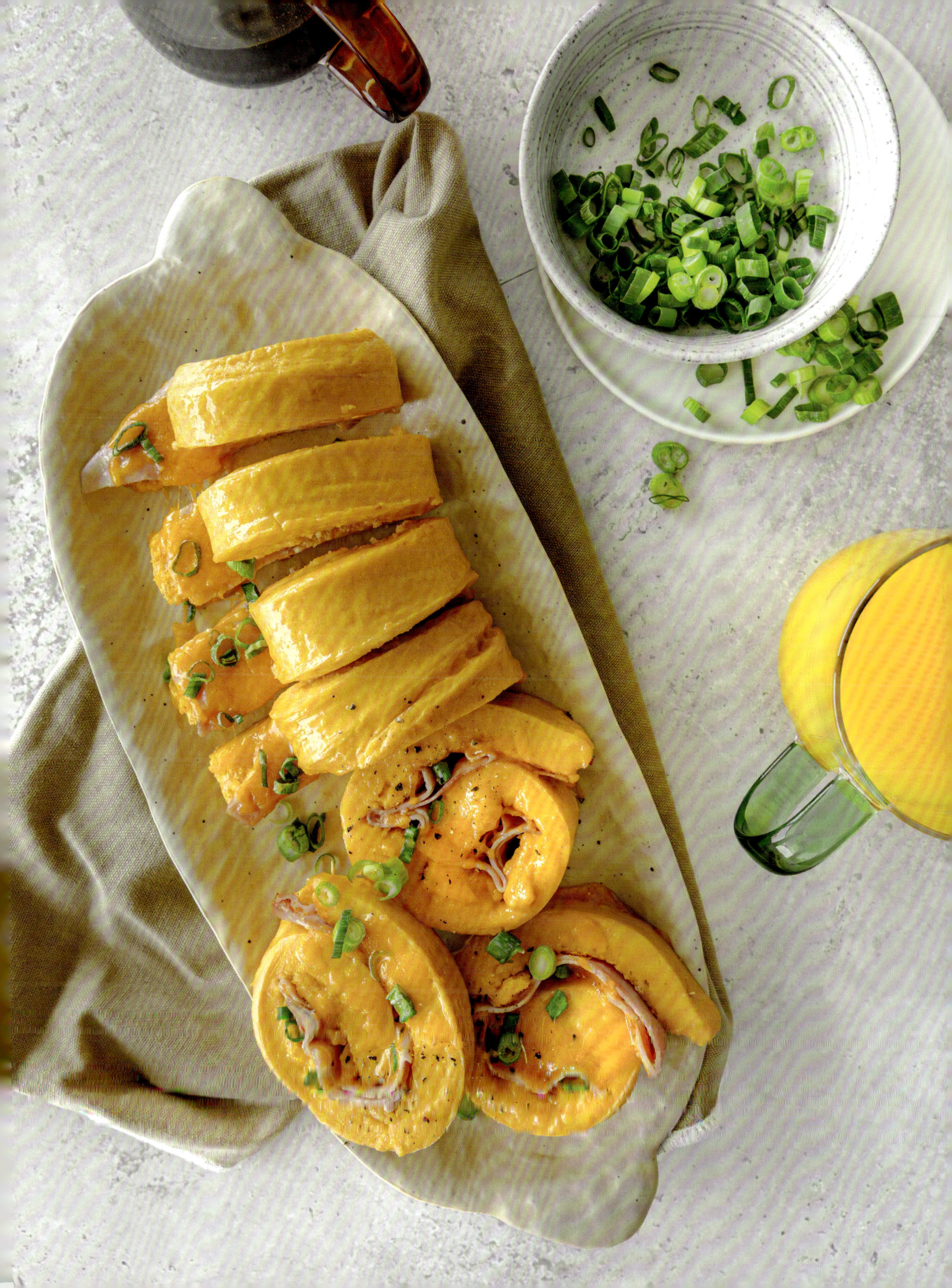

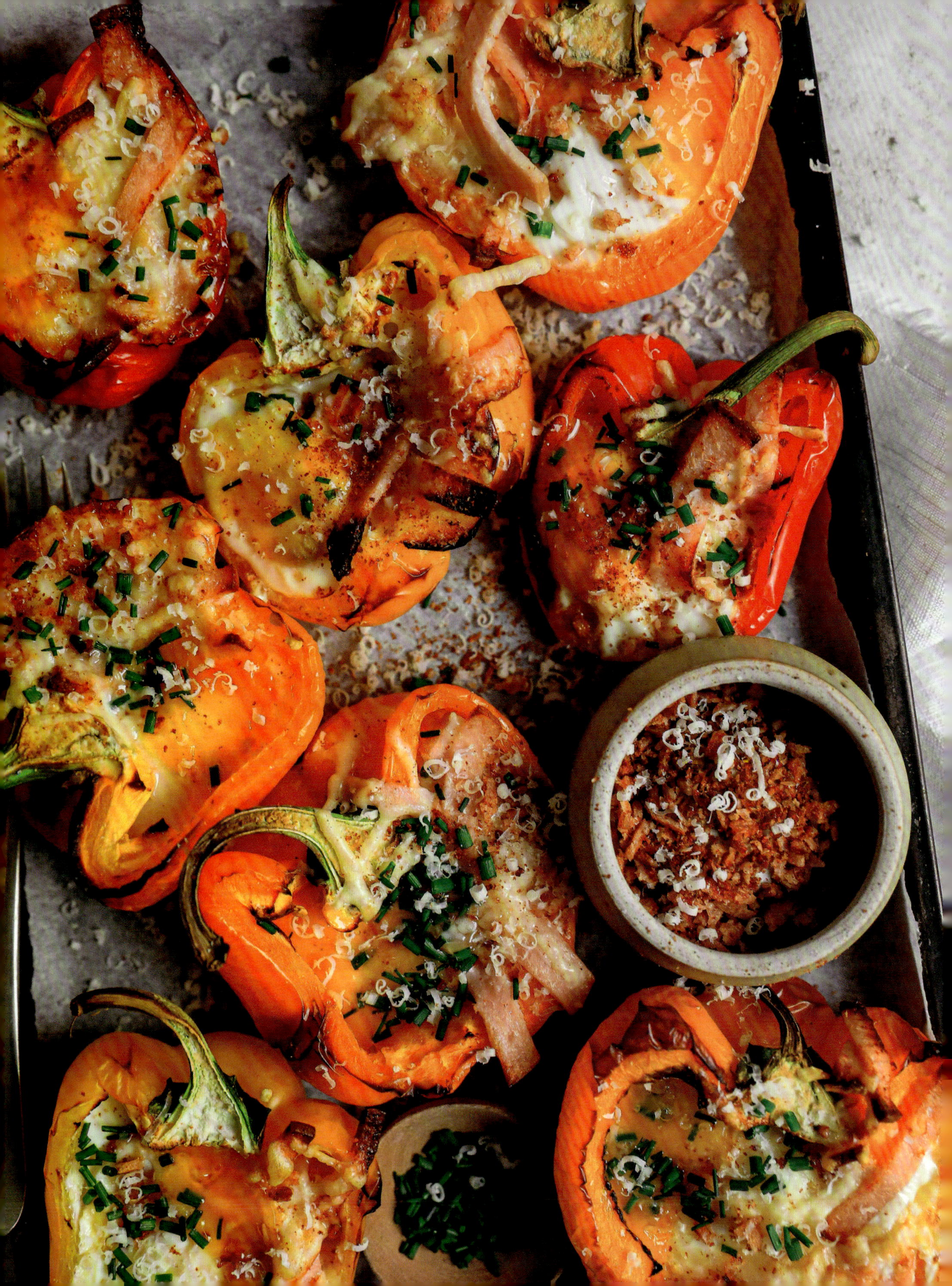

BREAKFAST STUFFED PEPPERS

2 large sweet bell peppers
Salt and pepper, to taste
¾ cup (90g) shredded low-fat cheddar cheese
2 tbsp (6g) diced chives
4 eggs
4 strips (104g) turkey bacon, diced

Make your mornings double-stuffed with one of my favorite second-breakfast options. I meal prep these on the regular, and they're just as good the next day. The yolk will firm up when reheated, so if you like your yolks runny, just make a fresh batch. However, if you're like me and don't discriminate between hard and soft yolks, reheat these bad boys by popping them in the oven at 350°F (180°C) for 7 to 9 minutes, and you'll start the day off satisfied. But please only keep these for 2 days—after that, they're as disappointing as that one-night stand you thought was a good idea at the time.

1. Preheat the oven to 350°F (180°C). Line a baking sheet with parchment paper.
2. Cut the bell peppers in half lengthwise, and remove the seeds and ribs. Season with salt and pepper.
3. On the prepared baking sheet, place the bell peppers flesh-side up and bake for 15 minutes to soften.
4. Keeping the oven on, remove the softened peppers from the oven and pour out any water that has pooled in the center of each pepper.
5. Sprinkle about ⅔ (60g) of the cheddar cheese and 1 tablespoon (3g) chives evenly over the four softened bell peppers.
6. One at a time, crack an egg and place it in the center of each bell pepper. Season with more salt and pepper.
7. Sprinkle the diced turkey bacon evenly on top of the bell peppers.
8. Sprinkle the remaining ⅓ (30g) of the cheddar cheese and 1 tablespoon (3g) chives on the peppers.
9. Bake for an additional 15 to 18 minutes, until the edges of the peppers darken and the cheese bubbles. Feel free to turn on the broiler for the last few minutes if you want a crispy top and less runny egg.

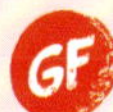

makes 2 stuffed peppers / 2 servings

NUTRITION (PER SERVING)

381 calories | **22g** fat
33.4g protein | **9.1g** net carbs

SAVORY OATS
WITH TEMPEH "BACON"

1 (8oz / 225g) block tempeh
1 tsp (3g) onion powder
1 tsp (3g) garlic powder
1 tsp (3g) paprika
½ tsp (1.5g) chili powder
½ tsp (2g) lemon pepper
⅛ tsp (250mg) cayenne pepper
⅜ tsp (2.25g) salt
½ cup (40g) quick oats
½ cup (120ml) Silk unsweetened almond milk
2 tbsp (18g) nutritional yeast
1½ cups (30g) kale, roughly chopped
½ cup (120g) button mushrooms, sliced
1 tbsp (15ml) coconut yogurt

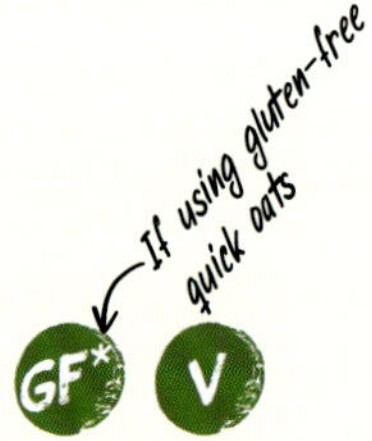

makes 1 serving

NUTRITION (PER SERVING)	
557 calories	**17g** fat
45g protein	**61g** net carbs

Bodybuilders love to confuse the muscles, but they never try to confuse the stomach, so I decided to take their diet staple and get a little weird with it (guaranteed gains for both you and the 'gram). This is a very rich dish, so don't skip the coconut yogurt. It really adds an element of freshness that balances the meal perfectly. When it comes to the tempeh bacon, you can eat it crumbled or keep it in strips. Looking to eat less meat? Use tempeh to replace the protein in other meatier recipes in this book. It even works wonders as an anabolic pizza topping. Trust me.

1. Preheat the oven to 425°F (220°C). Line a baking sheet with parchment paper.
2. Cut the tempeh into thin "baconlike" slices and place on the prepared baking sheet. Spray the top side with nonstick cooking spray.
3. In a small bowl, mix together the onion powder, garlic powder, paprika, chili powder, lemon pepper, cayenne pepper, and ⅛ teaspoon (750mg) salt.
4. Over the top of the tempeh, pour the spice mixture evenly. (Note: Seasoning both sides is not necessary.)
5. Bake the tempeh for 20 minutes, until golden brown and crispy. Set aside.
6. To a medium saucepan over medium-high heat, add the oats, almond milk, nutritional yeast, remaining ¼ teaspoon (1.5g) salt, and 1 cup (240ml) water. Stir the ingredients together and bring to a boil. Reduce the heat to low and let simmer until the oats are cooked all the way through and the mixture resembles a creamy porridge, 3 to 5 minutes. Set aside.
7. Spray a medium frying pan with nonstick cooking spray and place it over medium-high heat. Add the kale and mushrooms and sauté until the mushrooms are brown and the kale is wilted, 4 to 6 minutes.
8. Into a bowl, pour the savory oats and top with the tempeh "bacon," kale and mushrooms, and coconut yogurt.

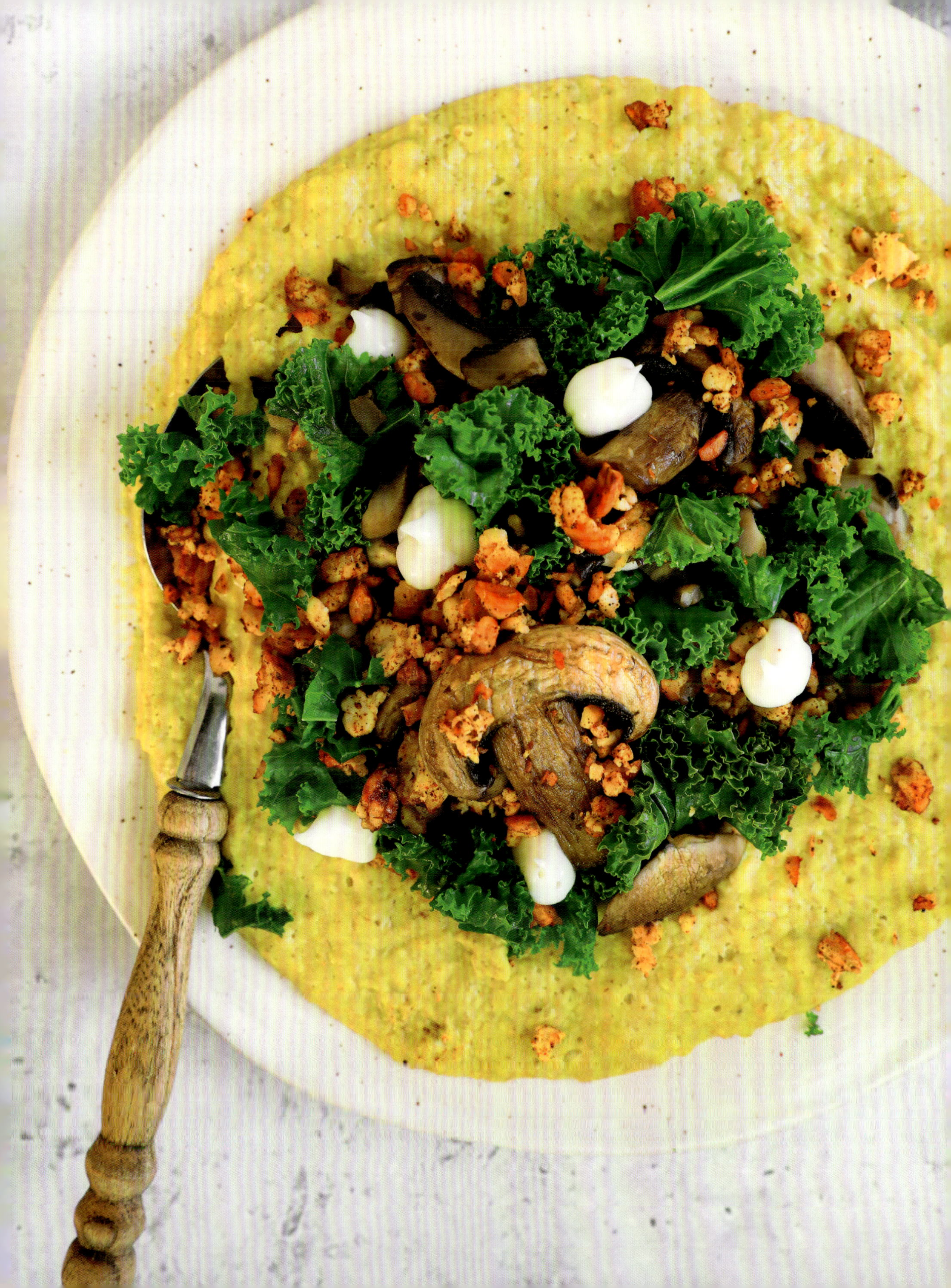

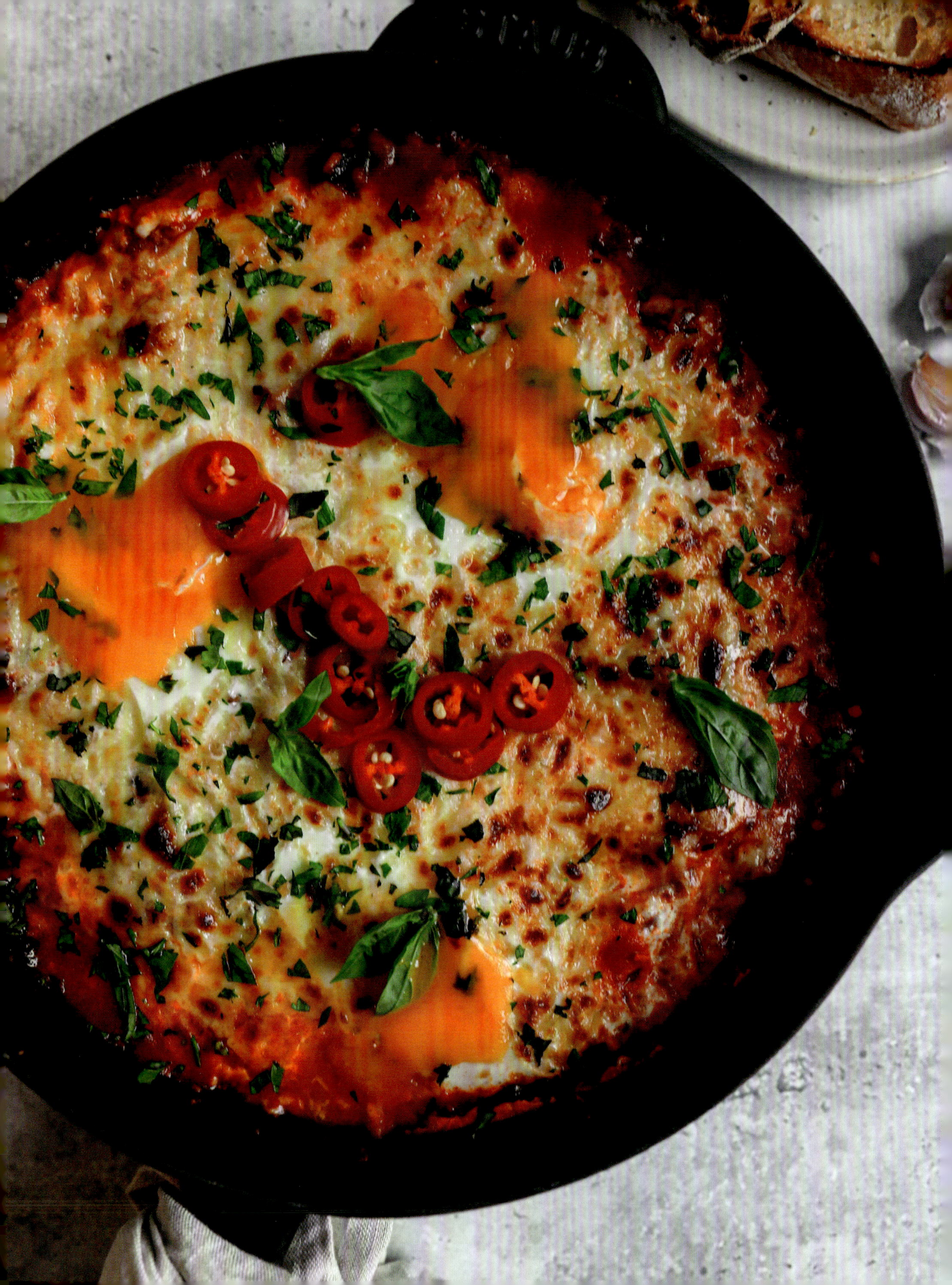

ITALIAN BAKED EGGS

1 garlic clove, finely diced
½ medium chile pepper, finely diced
1½ cups (45g) baby spinach
1 (14.5oz / 411g) can whole San Marzano tomatoes
Salt and pepper, to taste
4 tbsp (25g) Parmesan-and-herb seasoning
¼ cup (15g) fresh parsley, finely diced
¼ cup (15g) fresh basil, finely diced
3 eggs
⅓ cup (30g) shredded part-skim mozzarella cheese

Inspired by my summer escape at Maurizio's winery in Tuscany, this breakfast always got me out of bed in the morning, even though my legs were often weak. This is my take on the classic North African breakfast dish shakshuka, but I'm one-eighth Italian, so I'm drawing on what I know. To that end, I can't stress enough how important it is to get some good-quality canned tomatoes for this dish. The tomato sauce is the star of the show here, and we want it to taste like it was made with love by Nonna herself.

1. Preheat the oven to 350°F (180°C).
2. Heat a medium oven-safe frying pan over medium-high heat and spray it with nonstick cooking spray. Once the pan is hot, add the garlic, chile pepper, and spinach. Stir occasionally for 1 to 2 minutes, or until the spinach wilts.
3. To the pan, add the canned tomatoes. Using a spatula or wooden spoon, poke the tomatoes to break them apart into smaller chunks.
4. Reduce the heat to low and season with salt and pepper, along with the Parmesan-and-herb seasoning.
5. Add half the parsley and basil (7.5g each) to the sauce and stir to combine.
6. On top of the tomato-sauce mixture, crack the eggs, leaving space between each. Sprinkle the mozzarella on top of the eggs.
7. Bake for 10 to 15 minutes, or until the egg whites are set and the yolks are still runny. Keep an eye on them if you want a super runny yolk.
8. Remove from the oven and top with the remaining parsley and basil.

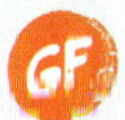

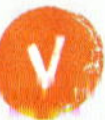

makes 1 serving

NUTRITION (PER SERVING)

460 calories | **25g** fat
31g protein | **28g** net carbs

HEALTHY FRIED CHICKEN AND WAFFLES WITH MUSTARD SYRUP

for the chicken:

2 chicken breasts, about 6oz (175g) each, cut in half horizontally
2 cups (490g) 1% buttermilk
1 cup (32g) cornflakes cereal
1 cup (115g) bread crumbs
½ tsp (1.5g) cumin
½ tsp (1.5g) chili powder
½ tsp (1.5g) garlic powder
Salt and pepper, to taste

for the sweet potato waffle:

2 cups (200g) shredded sweet potato
1 egg
4½ tbsp (67g) egg whites
1½ tbsp (12g) coconut flour
Salt and pepper, to taste

for the mustard syrup:

¼ cup (60ml) sugar-free maple syrup
¼ cup (60ml) chicken stock
1 tbsp (15ml) apple cider vinegar
1 tbsp (15ml) grainy mustard
1 tsp (6g) dried thyme
¼ tsp (1g) garlic powder

makes 2 servings

NUTRITION (PER SERVING)	
493 calories	**7.5g** fat
62g protein	**45g** net carbs

While I don't think the Colonel would approve of my healthy fried chicken, your gut and your self-respect certainly will. Be prepared to experience flavors you didn't think were possible to find in a healthy meal. This recipe might seem daunting, but it's actually pretty easy to make. The worst part will be cleaning the dishes when it's all done—because you'll wish you had more waffles. If you don't have a waffle maker and are in the market for one, check out my Kitchen Equipment Essentials on page 18 for my go-to recommendation.

1. **To make the chicken:** In a medium mixing bowl, place the chicken and buttermilk, making sure to submerge the chicken entirely. Let the chicken marinate in the fridge for at least 1 hour, but preferably 4 to 6 hours.
2. Once the chicken has marinated, in a blender or food processor, add the cornflakes, bread crumbs, cumin, chili powder, and garlic powder and season with salt and pepper. Blend until only a few chunks of cornflakes remain and pour the mixture into a large casserole dish. If you do not have a blender or food processor, pour the ingredients into a resealable plastic bag and crush with a rolling pin or heavy-bottom saucepan.
3. One piece at a time, remove the chicken breast from the buttermilk, and roll both sides in the cornflakes mixture until evenly coated. Spray both sides of the chicken with nonstick cooking spray.
4. Place the chicken in an air fryer at 425°F (220°C) for 13 to 15 minutes, flipping halfway. If you do not have an air fryer, bake in a conventional oven at 450°F (230°C) for 15 to 18 minutes, flipping halfway, or until the chicken reaches an internal temperature of 165°F (74°C).
5. **To make the sweet-potato waffle:** In a large mixing bowl, add the shredded sweet potato, egg, egg whites, and coconut flour and season with salt and pepper. Mix until the sweet potato is evenly coated.
6. On a heated and greased waffle iron, spread half the batter evenly and wait until cooked through. Repeat to make a second waffle.
7. **To make the mustard syrup:** In a small frying pan over medium-low heat, add the maple syrup, chicken stock, apple cider vinegar, mustard, thyme, and garlic powder. Simmer until the mustard syrup is heated, stirring often.
8. Top the waffles with the fried chicken and mustard syrup.

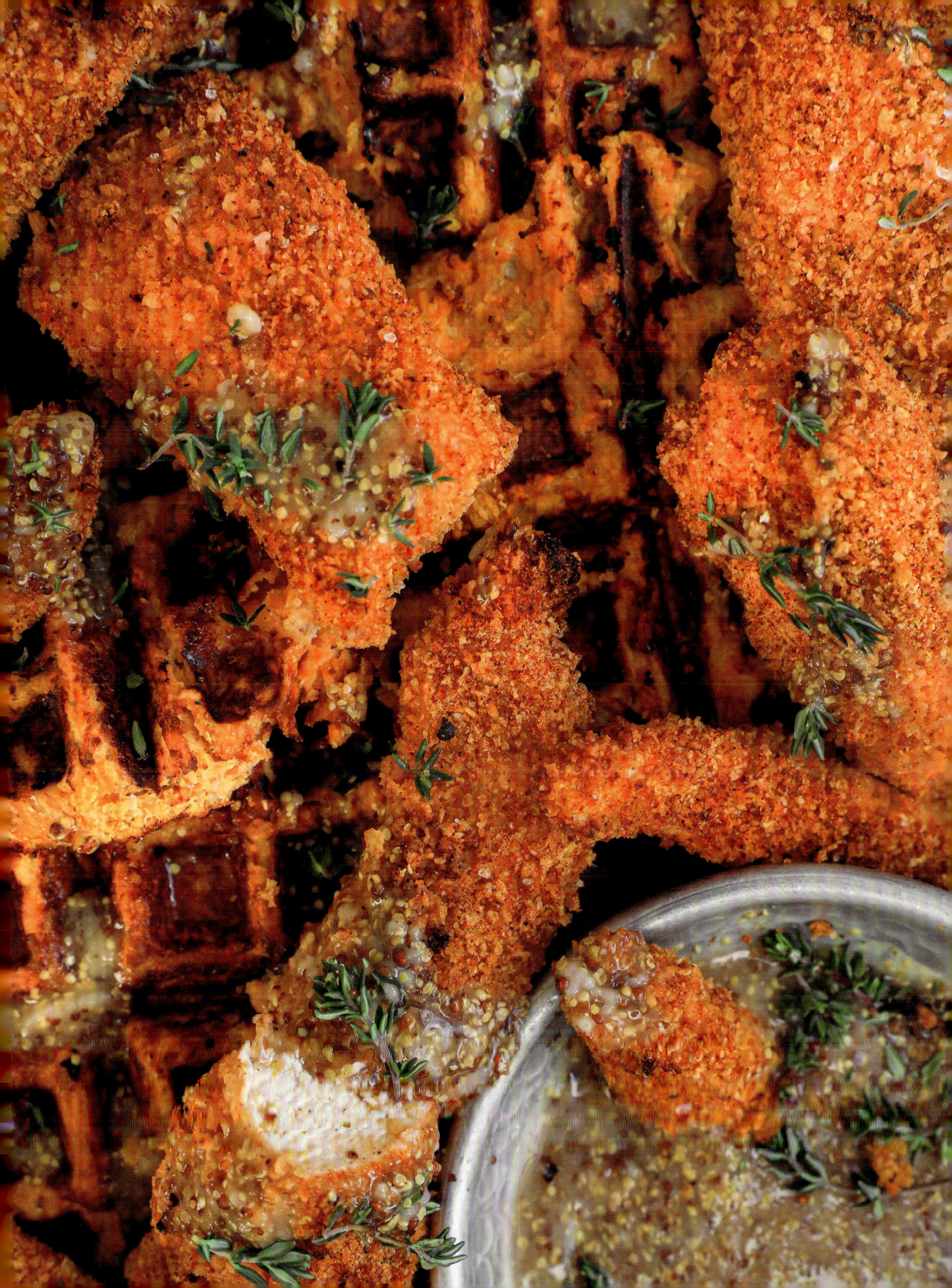

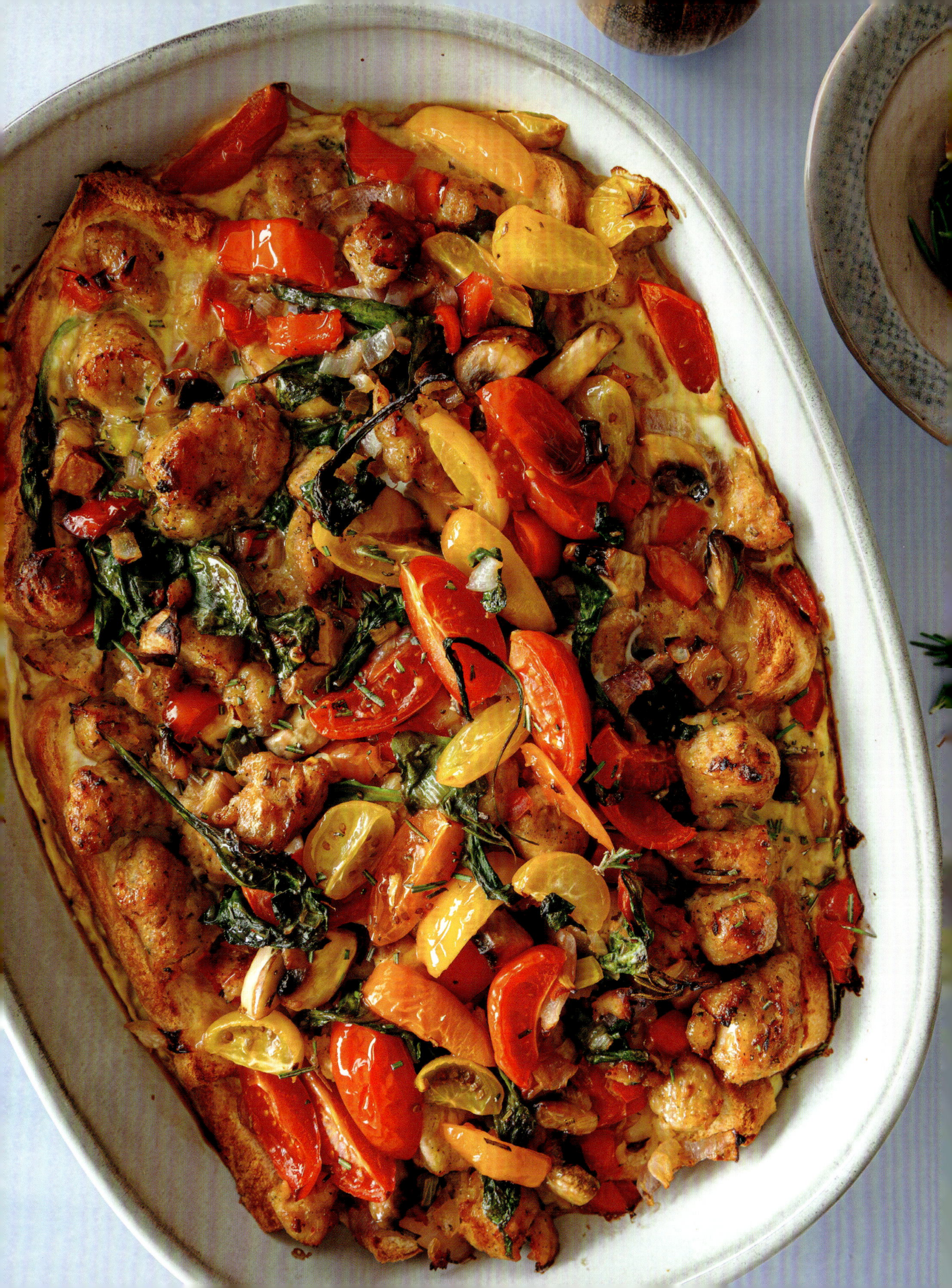

TURKEY-SAUSAGE BREAKFAST CASSEROLE

- 4 turkey sausages, about 11oz (375g) in total, casings removed
- 1 tbsp (1.5g) fresh rosemary, minced
- ¾ cup (180g) mushrooms, chopped
- 1 medium bell pepper, diced
- 1⅓ cup (150g) yellow or red onion, diced
- 1 garlic clove, minced
- Salt and pepper, to taste
- 2 cups (60g) spinach
- 5 eggs
- ¼ cup (60ml) milk of choice
- ¼ cup (22.5g) shredded part-skim mozzarella cheese
- 4–6 slices of bread
- ¼ cup (60g) cherry tomatoes, diced

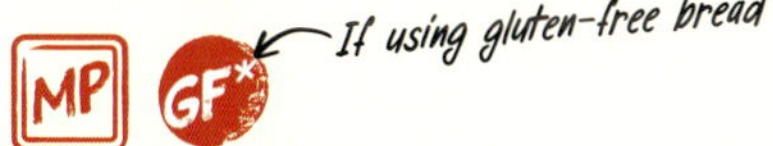

makes 5 servings

NUTRITION (PER SERVING)

[illegible] calories	**11g** fat
31g protein	**24g** net carbs

Perfect for meal prep, this casserole can feed you from Monday to Friday while fueling you for every workout in between. You can store the casserole in the fridge for up to 5 days by preportioning it and sealing each serving in airtight containers, or you can take the lazy way that I'm so fond of and just tightly cover the whole casserole dish with plastic wrap. To reheat, throw it in the microwave for 1 to 2 minutes, and you're good as gold. If you want to meal prep further in advance, cut the casserole into individual servings, and place in the freezer in an airtight container for up to 6 months. When you want to reheat it, stick it on a baking sheet in the oven at 375°F (190°C) for 9 to 12 minutes, and it'll taste as good as the day you made it.

1. Preheat the oven to 375°F (190°C).
2. Heat a large frying pan over medium-high heat and spray with nonstick cooking spray. Add the turkey sausages, breaking them apart with a spatula, and sauté until they are slightly brown and no longer pink.
3. Add the rosemary, mushrooms, bell pepper, onion, and garlic and season with salt and pepper. Sauté for 3 to 5 minutes, until the veggies soften. Add the spinach and sauté for an additional 1 to 2 minutes, until the spinach is wilted.
4. To a medium mixing bowl, add the eggs, milk, and cheese and stir to combine. Season with salt and pepper.
5. Spray an oven-safe 8 x 8-inch (20 x 20cm) casserole dish with cooking spray and place an even layer of sliced bread along the bottom.
6. To begin assembling the casserole, add half the egg mixture on top of the bread, followed by half the sausage-and-veggie mixture. Repeat this process with the remaining egg mixture, followed by the remaining sausage-and-veggie mixture. Top the casserole with a sprinkle of diced cherry tomatoes.
7. Bake for 30 to 35 minutes. If you like it extra crispy, leave the casserole in for an extra 5 minutes.
8. Let the casserole cool for 10 minutes and enjoy!

BREAKFAST PIZZA

for the pizza dough:

½ cup (115g) plain nonfat Greek yogurt
4½ tbsp (70g) egg whites
⅓ cup (40g) all-purpose flour
4 tsp (10g) coconut flour
¼ tbsp (4g) baking powder
1 tsp (3g) Italian seasoning
1 tsp (3g) garlic powder
½ tsp (1.5g) salt

for the toppings:

½ small onion, sliced
¼ bell pepper, sliced
¼ cup (60g) button mushrooms, chopped
2 eggs
Salt and pepper, to taste
⅓ cup (30g) shredded part-skim mozzarella cheese
2 turkey bacon strips, chopped
2 tbsp (30g) green onions, diced
2 tbsp (30ml) salsa (optional)

GF* V

*If using gluten-free all-purpose flour

makes 1 pizza / 1 serving

NUTRITION (PER SERVING)

620 calories	**15g** fat
58g protein	**63g** net carbs

As great as waking up to leftover pizza is, your mornings should start with a little more dignity—assuming you somehow didn't finish the whole pie the previous night. Here's a breakfast version that'll offer more protein and require less restraint. It's an easy win-win to start the day. Fair warning: This pizza dough will not resemble traditional pizza dough. It will be runny and difficult to shape. Don't freak out. Once you spread it on the baking sheet and let it do its thing in the oven, it'll reveal its gorgeous self.

1. Preheat the oven to 500°F (260°C). Line a baking sheet with parchment paper.
2. **To make the pizza dough:** To a medium mixing bowl, add the Greek yogurt and egg whites. Stir to create a soupy mixture.
3. In a separate medium bowl, combine the all-purpose flour, coconut flour, baking powder, Italian seasoning, garlic powder, and salt. Add the flour mixture to the Greek yogurt mixture and stir together into a liquidy pizza dough.
4. On the prepared baking sheet, spread the pizza dough into your desired shape. It is useful to have a cup of water beside you to rinse your fingers as you spread the dough, as it will easily stick to your fingers.
5. Bake for 8 to 10 minutes, until the dough is puffed up and golden.
6. **To prepare the toppings:** While the dough is in the oven, heat a medium skillet over medium-high heat and spray it with nonstick cooking spray. Add the onion, bell pepper, and mushrooms and sauté until softened, 5 to 7 minutes. Remove the veggies from the skillet and set aside.
7. In the same skillet, scramble the eggs and season with salt and pepper.
8. **To construct the pizza:** Over the crust, scatter the sautéed vegetables, followed by the scrambled eggs. Top with the cheese and turkey bacon, and place back in the oven for 3 to 4 minutes, until the cheese is melted and the turkey bacon is crisp.
9. Garnish with the green onion and salsa (if using).

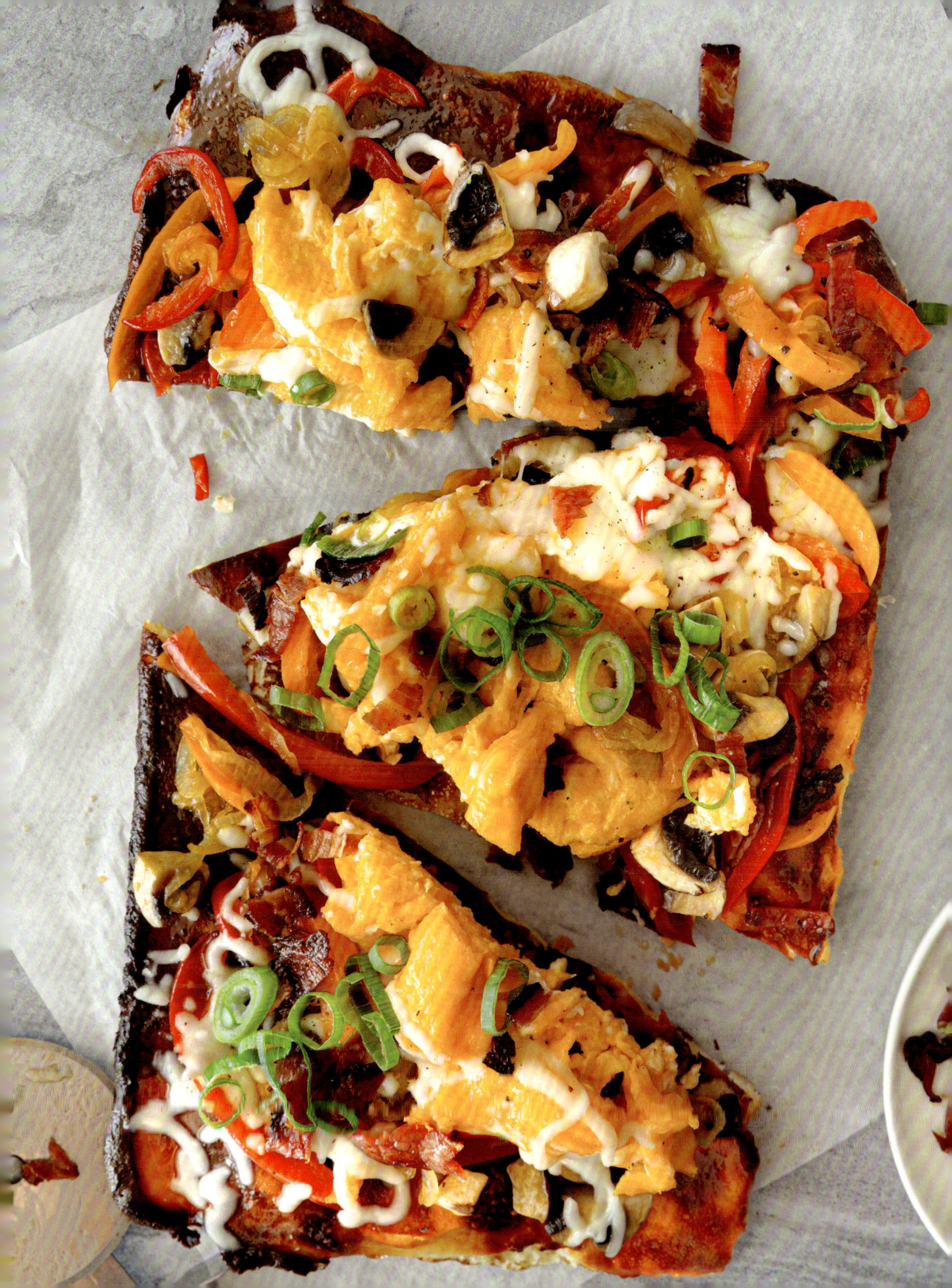

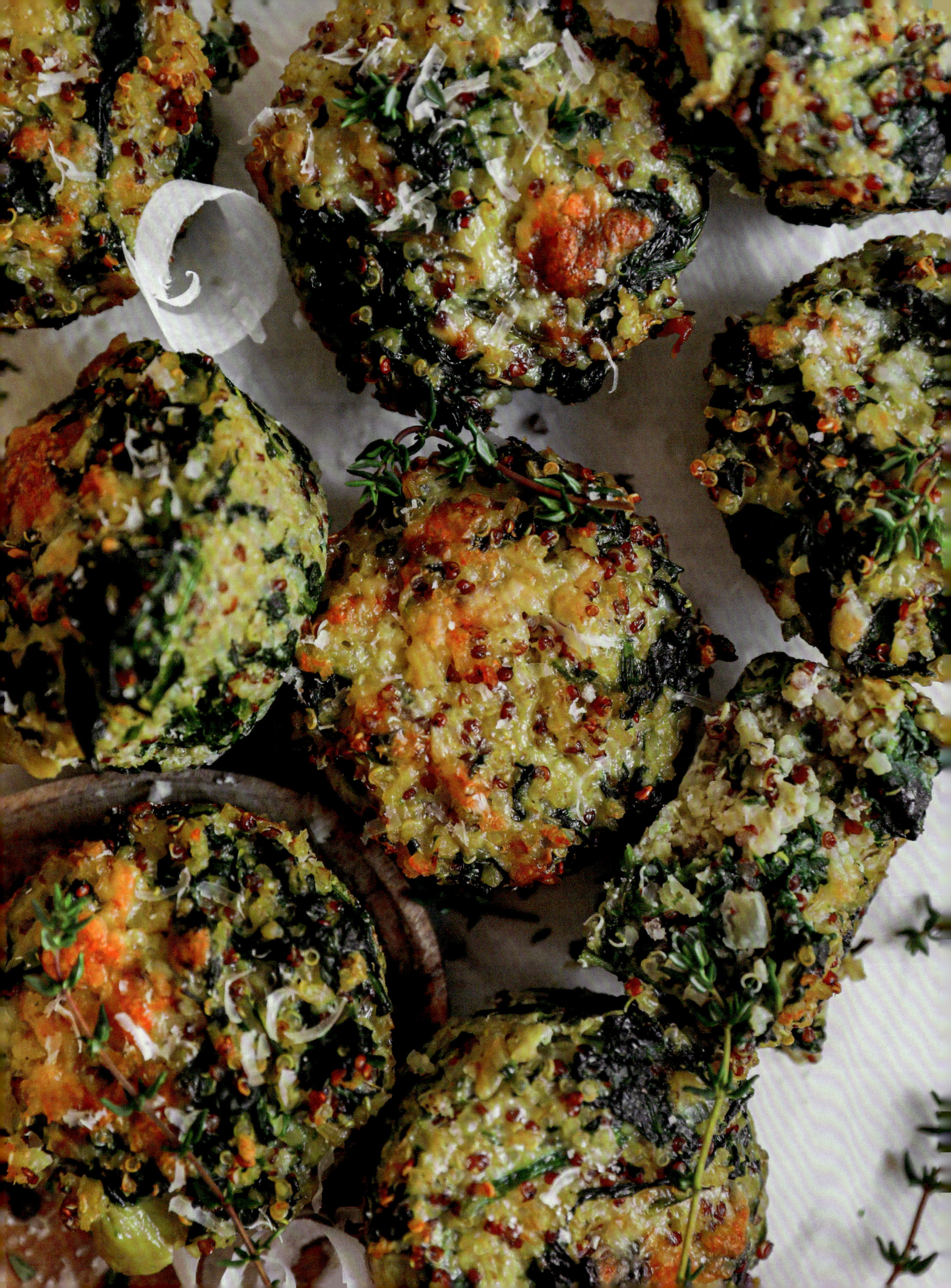

SAVORY QUINOA EGG BREAKFAST MUFFINS

1 cup (170g) dry quinoa, rinsed
1¼ cup (300g) frozen spinach
½ medium white onion, diced
2 eggs
¼ cup (30g) shredded low-fat cheddar cheese
1 tsp (3g) garlic powder
1 tsp (3g) dried oregano
Salt and pepper, to taste

Who said muffins had to be sweet? These savory quinoa muffins are loaded with fiber and protein, which will leave you feeling full and energetic while wiping away the memories of the chalky protein bars haunting your taste buds. A great meal-prep option, the muffins can be stored in the freezer in a plastic freezer bag or an airtight container for up to 6 months. When you want to grab a quick bite, microwave on high for 45 to 60 seconds, then let it sit for a minute so you don't burn your face off.

1. Preheat the oven to 350°F (180°C). Line a 12-cup muffin tray with liners.
2. To a medium saucepan over high heat, add the quinoa and 1¾ cups (420ml) water. Bring to a boil, then reduce the heat to medium-low and simmer for 10 to 15 minutes, until all the water has been absorbed by the quinoa. Fluff with a fork, then transfer to a large mixing bowl. Set aside to cool. (Note: This can be done up to 3 days in advance and stored in the fridge in an airtight container.)
3. Heat a large frying pan over medium-high heat and spray with nonstick cooking spray. To the pan, add the spinach and onions and sauté for 4 to 5 minutes, until the onions are soft and the spinach is thawed. Set aside.
4. To the mixing bowl with the cooled quinoa, add the eggs, cheese, garlic powder, and oregano and season with salt and pepper. Stir to combine.
5. To the quinoa mixture, add the cooked spinach and onions and stir to combine.
6. Scoop the quinoa mixture evenly into the prepared muffin tin.
7. Bake the muffins for 15 to 20 minutes, until the tops begin to brown. Let cool before serving.

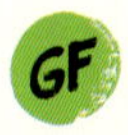

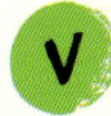

makes 12 muffins / 12 servings

NUTRITION (PER SERVING)

90 calories
2.5g fat
4.5g protein
12.5g net carbs

EGG TURKEY-BACON MUFFINS

6 turkey bacon strips, about 5½oz (156g) in total
6 eggs
Salt and pepper, to taste

If you've got an empty fridge but you're full of laziness, here's a recipe that'll make cooking so easy I almost didn't bother putting it in this cookbook. These muffins are peak simplicity in the kitchen, and if you prepare them ahead of time, you can make your morning even simpler. They keep well in the fridge for up to 4 days and heat up in the microwave in 60 to 90 seconds flat. Cook smart, not hard.

1. Preheat the oven to 350°F (180°C).
2. Around the inside perimeters of a 6-cup muffin or cupcake tray, place the turkey bacon strips in a circle. Spray the bottom of each muffin mold with nonstick cooking spray.
3. In the center of each turkey bacon-lined muffin cup, crack an egg. Season with salt and pepper.
4. Bake for 15 to 16 minutes. Remove from the oven and let sit for 10 minutes before serving.

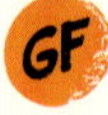

makes 6 muffins / 6 servings

NUTRITION (PER SERVING)

105 calories	**8g** fat
8g protein	**0.5g** net carbs

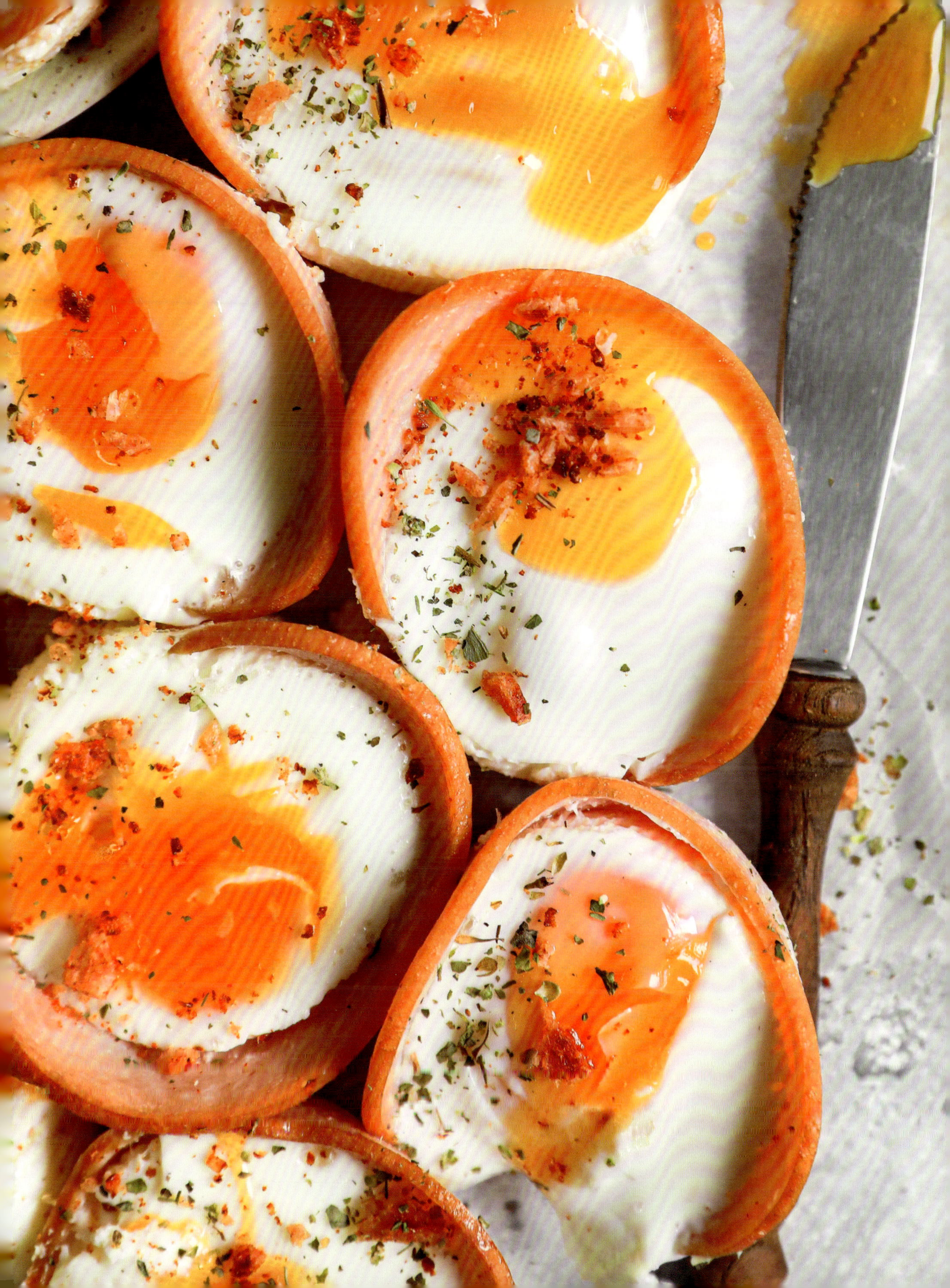

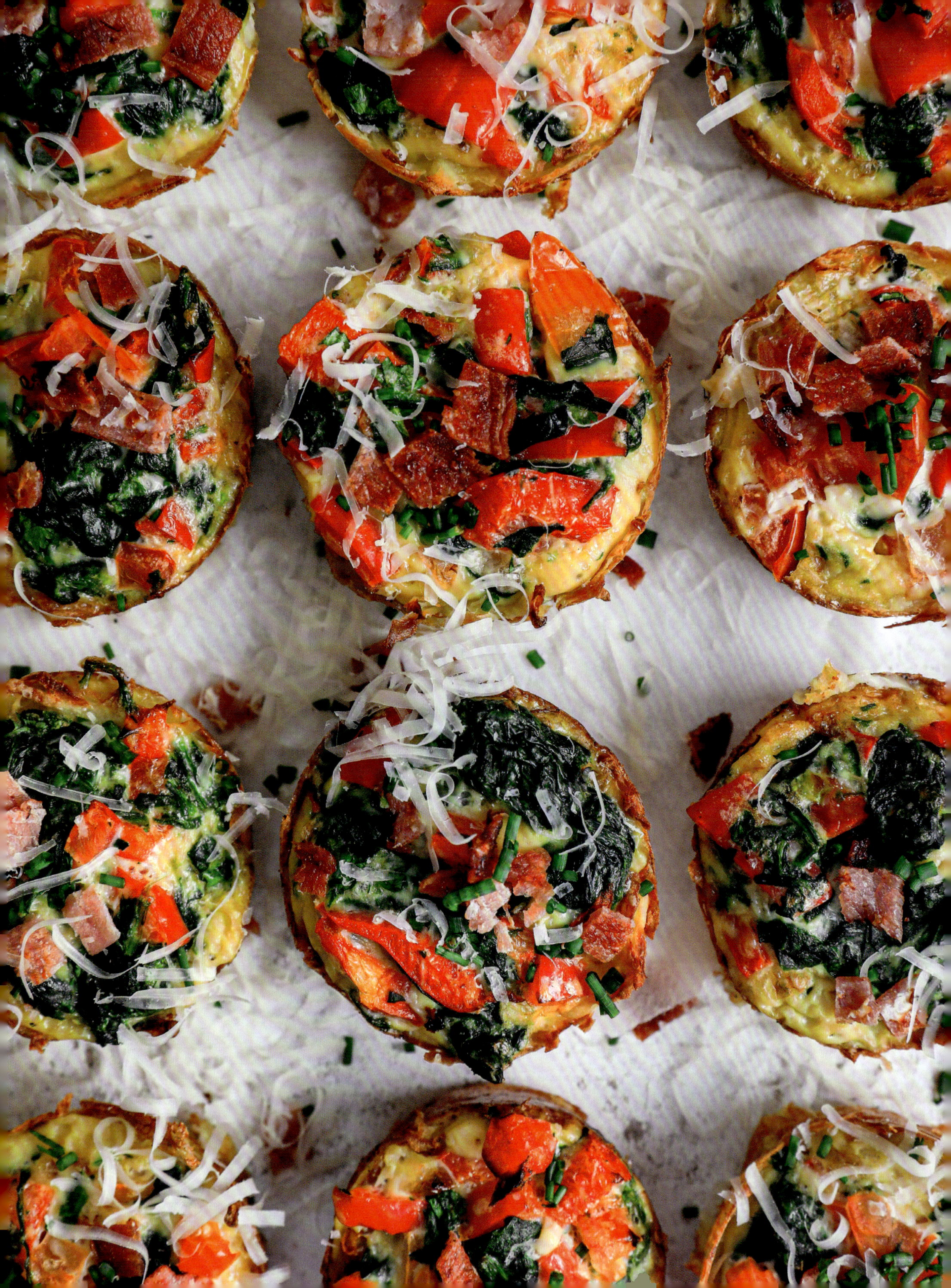

SHREDDED POTATO-WRAPPED QUICHES

4 eggs
½ cup (50g) shredded part-skim asiago cheese
Salt and pepper, to taste
2 heaping cups (about 300g) shredded russet potato, excess moisture squeezed out
¾ cup (80g) frozen spinach, thawed and drained
1 jalapeño, diced
¼ red bell pepper, diced
2 tbsp (17g) store-bought bruschetta mix
1 turkey bacon strip, diced

They say you are what you eat, and these shredded potato-wrapped quiches will definitely help you get those washboard abs you've always dreamed of. And they taste good too. This recipe is super easy to change around to fit your goals. You can skip the yolks and go all egg whites if you're trying to cut back on the fats, add whatever veggies you like to your filling, or even skip the filling entirely and just carb load on potato cups.

1. Preheat the oven to 425°F (220°C).
2. To a medium bowl, add 1 of the eggs and about 3 tablespoons (20g) of the cheese. Season with salt and pepper and stir to combine.
3. To the same bowl, add the shredded potato. Fold until evenly coated.
4. Spray 8 molds of a muffin tray with nonstick cooking spray. Coat each mold with the potato mixture, pressing down in the center to create cups.
5. Bake for 15 minutes, or until crispy.
6. While the potato cups are baking, to a medium bowl, add the remaining 3 eggs, the remaining cheese, the spinach, jalapeño, bell pepper, and bruschetta mix. Season with more salt and pepper and stir to combine.
7. When the potato cups are golden and crisp, remove them from the oven. Fill each mold with the egg mixture, and top with the turkey bacon.
8. Bake for another 7 to 10 minutes, until the egg is cooked through.
9. Remove from the oven, let cool, and enjoy!

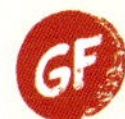

makes 8 quiches / 8 servings

NUTRITION (PER SERVING)

90 calories	**4g** fat
6g protein	**7.5g** net carbs

EGG-WHITE VEGETABLE FRITTATA

2 cups (170g) frozen broccoli florets, thawed
2 cups (500g) egg whites
½ tsp (1.5g) garlic powder
½ tsp (1.5g) onion powder
½ tsp (1.5g) Italian seasoning
Salt and pepper, to taste
⅓ cup (30g) shredded part-skim mozzarella cheese
1 tbsp (15ml) yellow mustard (optional)
Hot sauce (optional)
1 tbsp (15ml) salsa (optional)

This is the first dish I ever made on my channel, and for good reason. I ate this frittata every single morning for years, and never got sick of it. With the perfect combination of being low calorie, high protein, and full of volume, this is an all-time winning staple of mine. A little tip if you're a fan of extra crisp: When your frittata is puffed up and cooked, switch your oven to broil for 1 minute and keep an eye on it. Let the top get browned and the cheese bubble, and then take it out before you end up with a charred kitchen fail.

1. Preheat the oven to 425°F (220°C).
2. Spray a medium oven-safe skillet with nonstick cooking spray, and scatter the broccoli florets along the bottom.
3. Pour the egg whites over the broccoli and add the garlic powder, onion powder, and Italian seasoning. Season with salt and pepper.
4. Place the skillet on the middle rack of the oven and bake for 10 to 15 minutes, until the egg whites are cooked through.
5. Remove the skillet from the oven, sprinkle with the shredded mozzarella, and bake for an additional 5 minutes, until the frittata is golden and puffed.
6. Let the frittata cool. Then, if using, garnish with the mustard, hot sauce, and salsa for extra flavor.

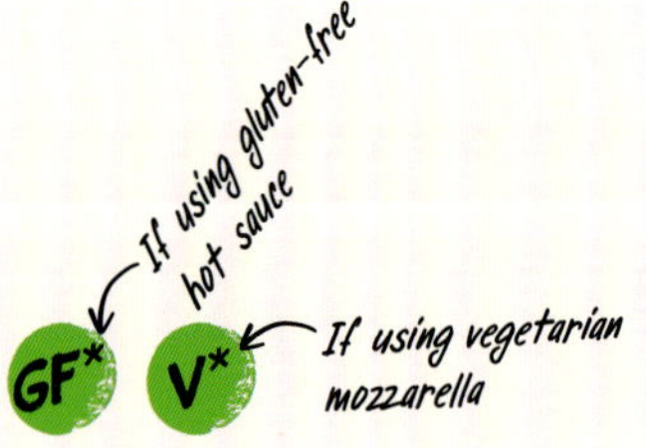

makes 1 frittata / 1 serving

NUTRITION (PER SERVING)	
290 calories	**6g** fat
61g protein	**19g** net carbs

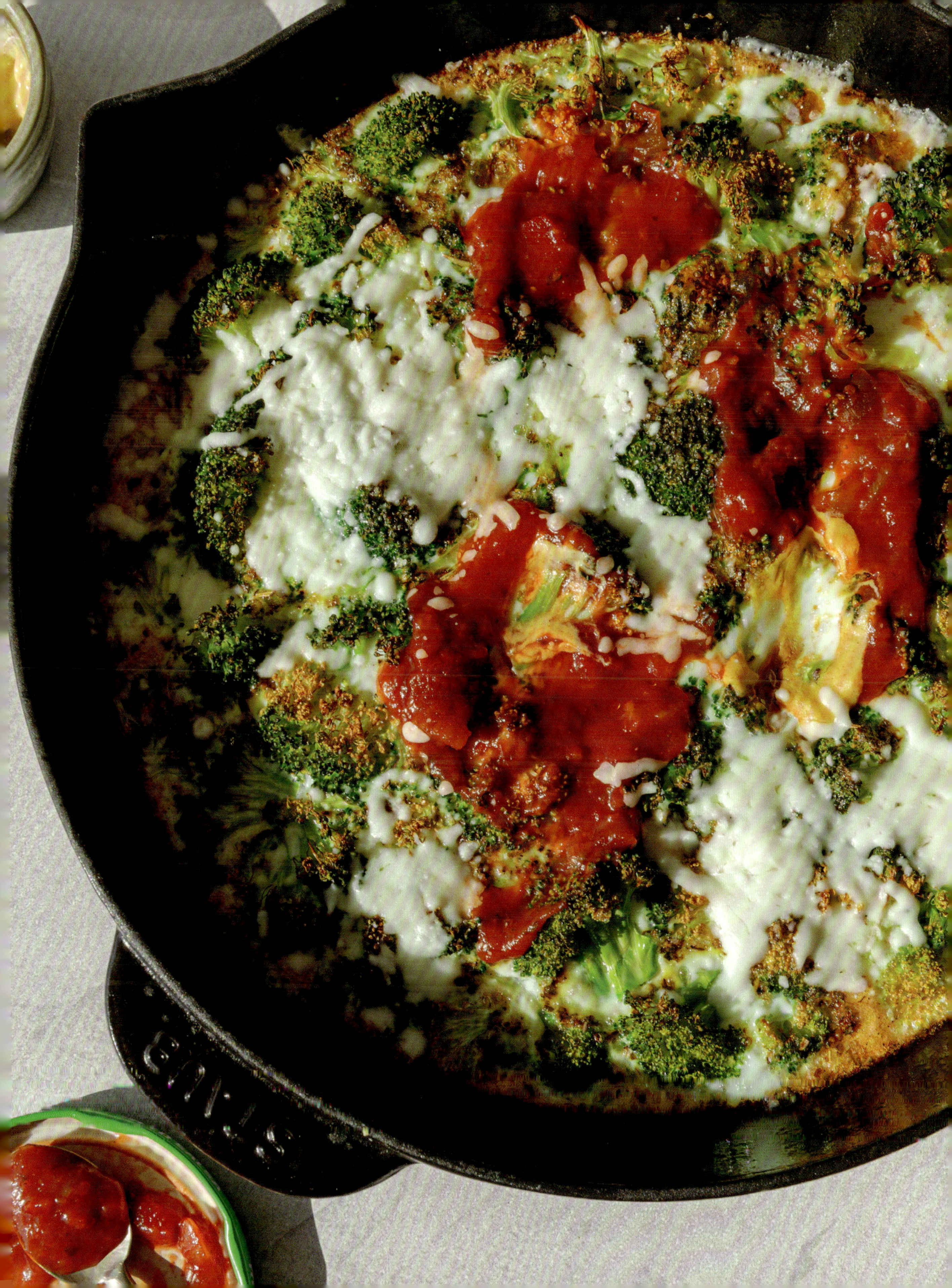
STAUB

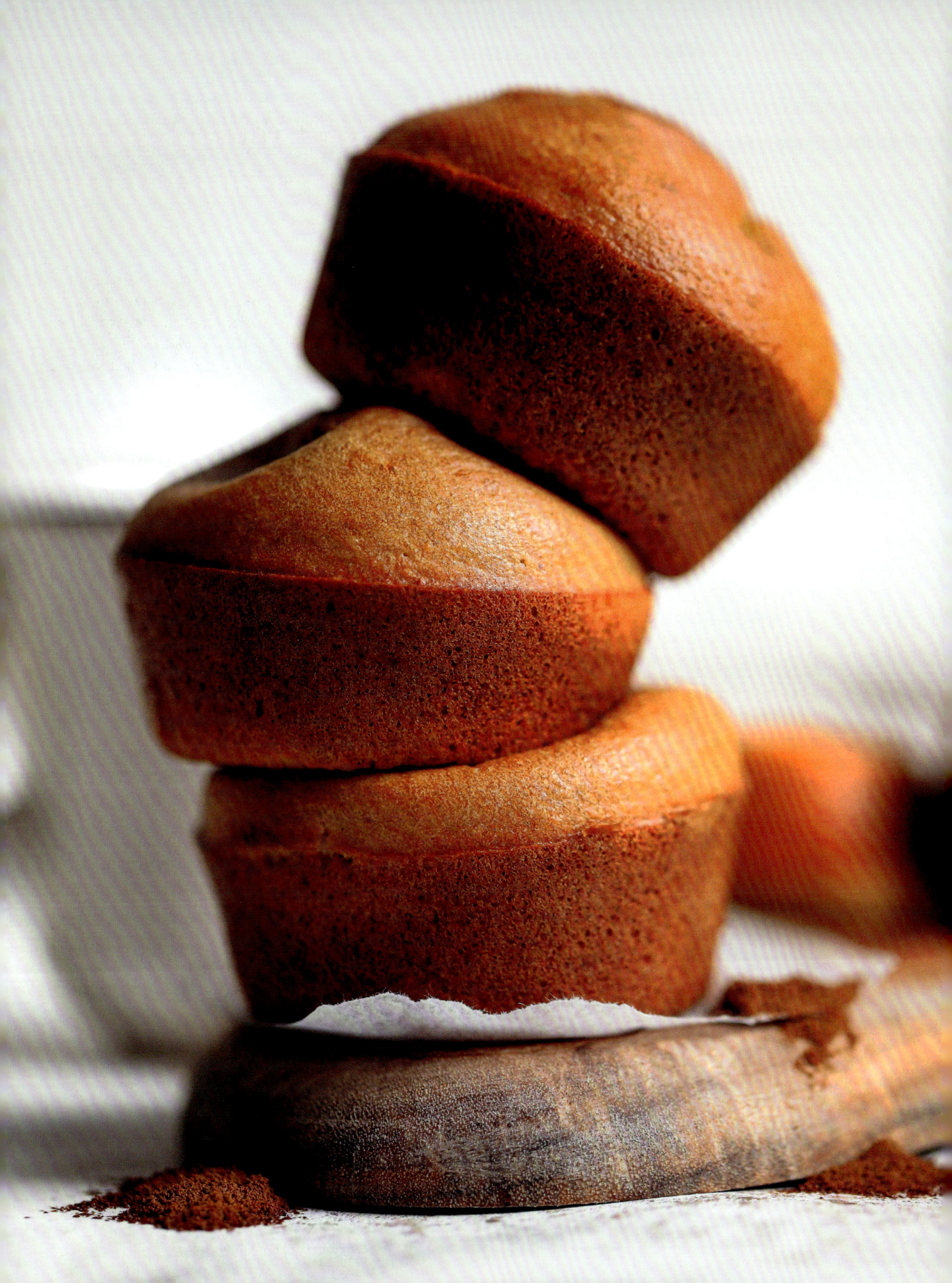

PROTEIN COFFEE MUFFINS

¾ cup (100g) almond flour
1 scoop (31g) protein powder
1 tsp (5g) baking powder
¼ cup (60g) plain nonfat Greek yogurt
¼ cup (60ml) Silk unsweetened cashew milk
1¼ tbsp (18g) egg whites
2 tsp (10ml) vanilla extract
1 oz (30ml) brewed espresso
¼ cup (60ml) sugar-free maple syrup

While I'll never add anything to my coffee, it doesn't mean I won't add coffee to the other things I enjoy. Prepare these muffins ahead of time, and keep them on hand to stay sane for those rush-hour traffic jams on your way to work. They stay fresh on your counter for 2 to 3 days, or in your fridge covered in plastic wrap for 5 to 7 days. The muffins do get a little dense in the fridge, so a little 20-second zap in the microwave will do wonders if you want that straight-out-the-oven mouth experience.

1. Preheat the oven to 350°F (180°C). Line 8 molds of a muffin tray with liners.
2. To a large mixing bowl, add the almond flour, protein powder, and baking powder. Stir to combine.
3. To the same bowl, add the Greek yogurt, cashew milk, egg whites, vanilla extract, espresso, and maple syrup and mix until smooth.
4. Into the prepared muffin tray, pour the mixture so the molds are just over halfway full.
5. Bake for 15 minutes, until the muffins are brown and slightly puffed, or a toothpick inserted into the center of a muffin comes out clean.
6. Remove from the oven and let sit for 5 to 10 minutes before serving.

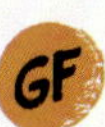

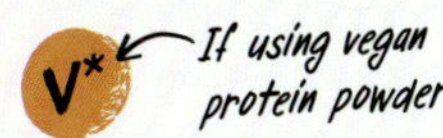

makes 8 muffins / 8 servings

NUTRITION (PER SERVING)

90 calories
4.5g fat
9g protein
4g net carbs

CHOCOLATE-CHIP PROTEIN MUFFINS

½ cup (52g) PB2 Powdered Peanut Butter
1 cup (240ml) unsweetened apple sauce
½ cup (60g) almond flour
1 tsp (5g) baking powder
2 scoops (62g) vanilla protein powder
½ cup (80g) semisweet chocolate chips

Who doesn't like waking up to a warm muffin? Refer to Johnny Sins for tips on how to butter it. If you don't have any PB2 Powdered Peanut Butter on hand, this recipe works just as well with any nut butter that tickles your fancy. Just make sure it's smooth—we don't want to steal the chocolate chips' thunder. These muffs keep fresh at room temperature for 2 to 3 days, or in your fridge covered in plastic wrap for 5 to 7 days. Grab and go, or reheat in the microwave for 20 to 30 seconds, and start your day strong.

1. Preheat the oven to 350°F (180°C). Spray 8 molds of a muffin tray with nonstick cooking spray or use paper liners.
2. In a large bowl, mix the PB2 Powdered Peanut Butter with a small amount of water. Stir and continue adding water until it resembles a thin peanut butter.
3. To the PB2 mixture, add the apple sauce, almond flour, baking powder, and protein powder. Stir into a smooth batter. Add the chocolate chips and stir to combine.
4. Into the prepared muffin tray, pour the batter, filling the molds three-fourths of the way to the top.
5. Bake on the middle rack for 15 to 18 minutes, until the muffin tops are puffed up and golden, or a toothpick inserted into the center of a muffin comes out relatively clean (not goopy!).
6. Let cool for at least 10 minutes before serving.

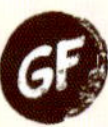

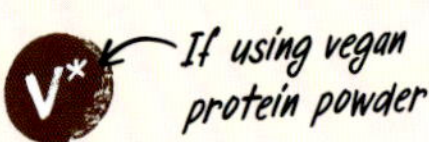

makes 8 muffins / 8 servings

NUTRITION (PER SERVING)	
135 calories	**4.5g** fat
13g protein	**10g** net carbs

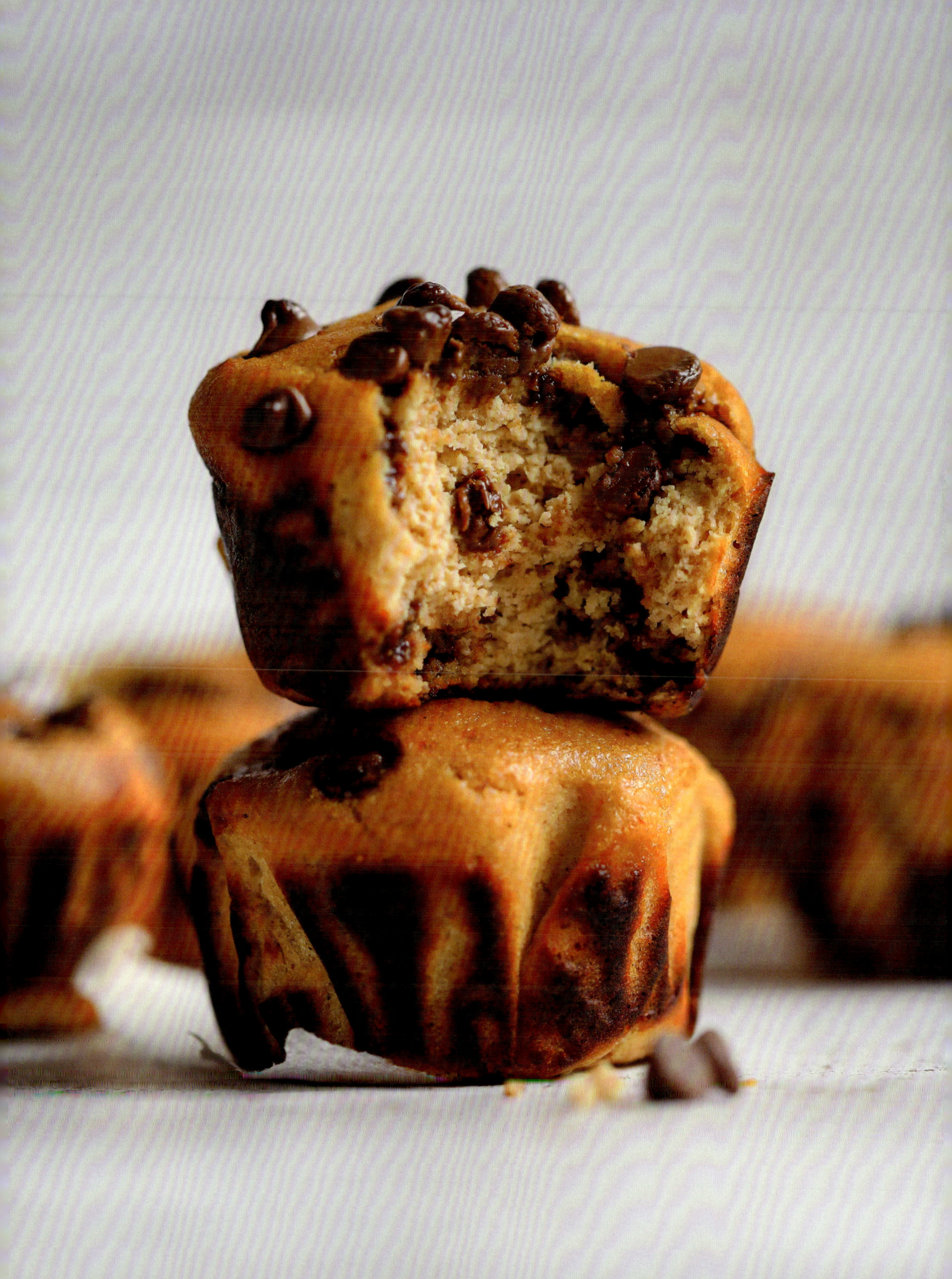

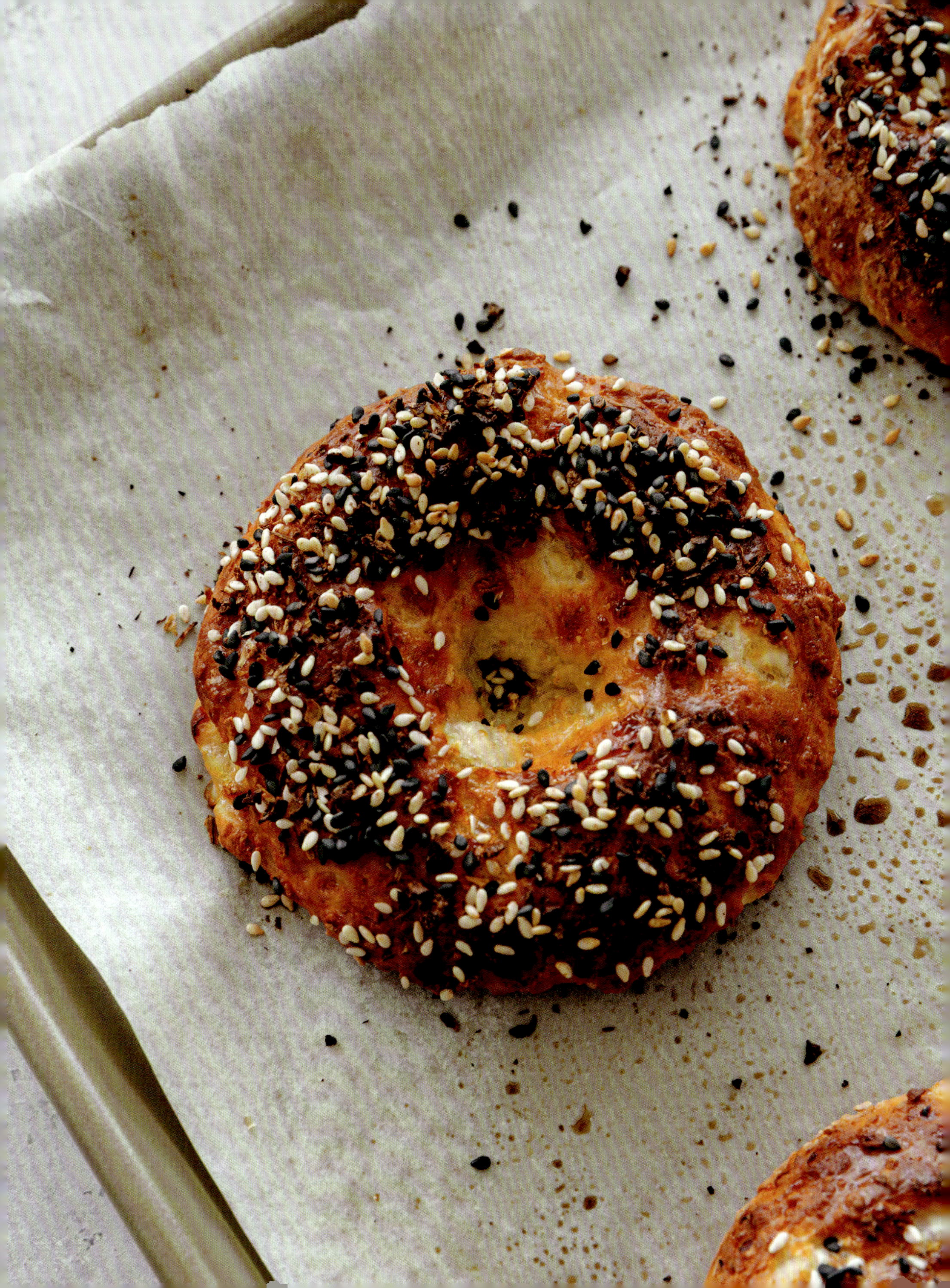

COTTAGE-CHEESE PROTEIN BAGELS

¾ cup (90g) all-purpose flour
¾ cup (150g) unflavored whey protein powder
1 tbsp (15g) baking powder
1 tsp (3g) salt
2 tsp (6g) garlic powder
1½ cups (340g) 2% cottage cheese, strained, or 1½ cups (345g) 2% plain Greek yogurt, strained
4¼ tbsp (67g) egg whites, beaten
Everything bagel seasoning (optional)

After making these protein bagels, I'm convinced that the Black Eyed Peas were talking about cottage cheese when they sang about those "lovely lady lumps." This recipe calls for you to strain your cottage cheese, and I find the easiest way is to line a strainer with a cheesecloth or coffee filter, add the cottage cheese, let it drain over a bowl for at least 30 minutes, and press gently if needed. This will leave the cottage cheese denser, drier, and easier to mold. On another note, I know that unflavored protein powder isn't a staple in everyone's pantry, so if you don't have any, you can use more all-purpose flour instead. Just note that your macros will change. You can top your bagels with your favorite seasoning, herb, or seed—or mix and match if you feel like really shaking things up.

1. Preheat the oven to 375°F (190°C). Line a baking sheet with parchment paper. If using an air fryer, spray the basket with nonstick cooking spray and forgo preheating the oven.
2. In a large mixing bowl, whisk together the flour, protein powder, baking powder, salt, and garlic powder until combined.
3. Add the cottage cheese and mix for 1 to 2 minutes, until the mixture starts to separate into small lumps.
4. Using your hands, knead the dough in the bowl for 2 to 3 minutes, until it is smooth and no longer sticks to your hands.
5. Cut the dough into 6 equal pieces and roll each piece into a ball. With your finger, poke a hole in the center of each ball, then stretch the hole to at least 2 inches in width, as it will shrink when baked.
6. On the lined baking sheet or in the prepared air fryer basket, place the shaped bagels. Brush the tops with the egg whites and sprinkle with a modest amount of everything bagel seasoning (if using).
7. If using the oven, bake on the top rack for 25 to 30 minutes, or until puffed up and golden. If using an air fryer, air fry at 300°F (150°C) for 20 to 22 minutes, until the bagels are puffed up and golden.
8. Let the bagels cool on the baking sheet for at least 20 minutes before slicing.
9. Serve as is or sliced and topped with your favorite spread.

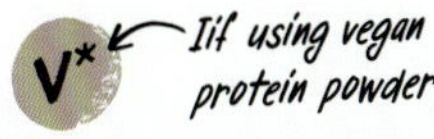

makes 6 bagels / 6 servings

NUTRITION (PER SERVING)

143 calories
1.3g fat
17.3g protein
14.5g net carbs

FRENCH TOAST PROTEIN BAGELS

- 1 cup (230g) vegan nonfat Greek yogurt
- ½ cup (60g) self-rising flour
- ½ cup (80g) casein-whey blend vanilla protein powder
- 4 tsp (20g) cinnamon
- 1½ tbsp (15g) raisins
- 3 tbsp (45ml) melted coconut oil
- 1 tbsp (12g) Swerve brown sugar
- 1 tsp (5ml) vanilla extract

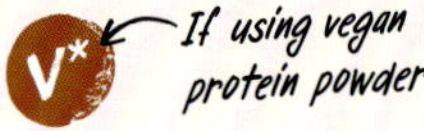

makes 4 bagels / 4 servings

NUTRITION (PER SERVING)

222 calories	**10.7g** fat
11g protein	**18.5g** net carbs

Instead of giving you guys another simple anabolic French toast recipe, I figured I'd give you something far better, so I added a hole. Now you have a breakfast with a fun, interactive component. A couple of things I should point out to make sure your bagels live up to their full potential: 1) Go out and get that self-rising flour. All-purpose flour will leave these bagels flat, and we want some bounce. 2) Using a protein powder with a casein-whey blend really is the key to a moist, fluffy texture, which is why it's always been my preferred powder (for baking).

1. Preheat the oven to 375°F (190°C). Line a rimmed baking sheet with parchment paper.
2. In a medium mixing bowl, combine the Greek yogurt, flour, protein powder, 3 teaspoons (15g) of the cinnamon, and the raisins. Mix with a fork or spatula until the ingredients are well incorporated and a dough begins to form. Dust your hands lightly with flour if the dough feels sticky.
3. Shape the dough into a smooth ball and divide it into 4 equal portions. Using the palms of your hands, roll each portion into a ball. Place the balls on the prepared baking sheet and gently press the tops with the palm of your hand to slightly flatten them.
4. Using your finger or a shot glass, create a 1-inch (2.5cm) hole in the center of each dough ball to form the bagel shape. Set aside.
5. In a small bowl, combine the coconut oil, brown sugar, vanilla extract, and the remaining 1 teaspoon (5g) cinnamon. With a spoon, stir the mixture until it forms a smooth, thin sauce.
6. Drizzle the sauce evenly over the tops of the bagels using the spoon to create a streaky appearance.
7. Bake on the center rack of the oven for 15 to 20 minutes, or until the bagels are golden brown and have expanded to nearly double their original size. Let them cool on the baking sheet for at least 10 minutes before slicing.

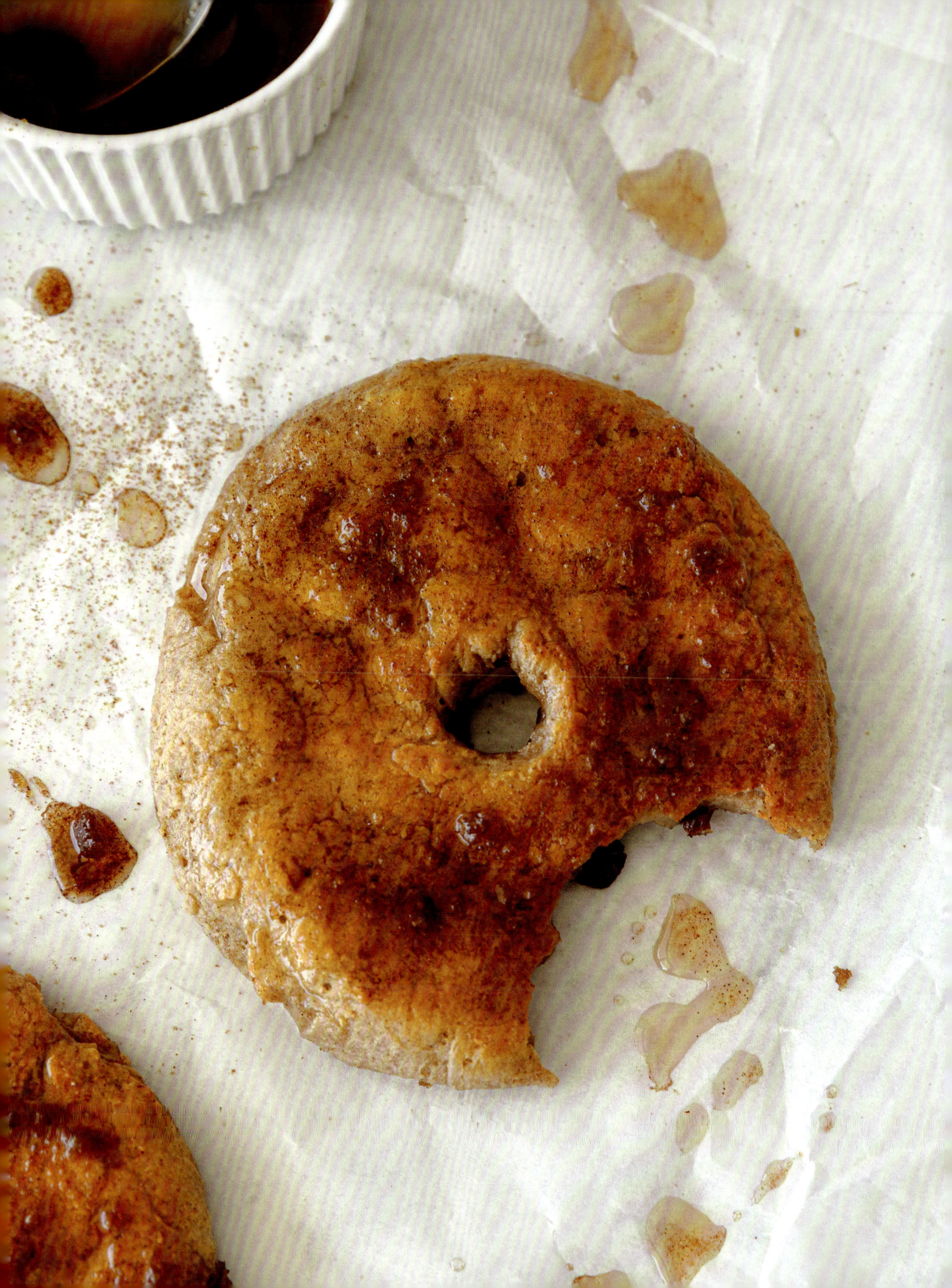

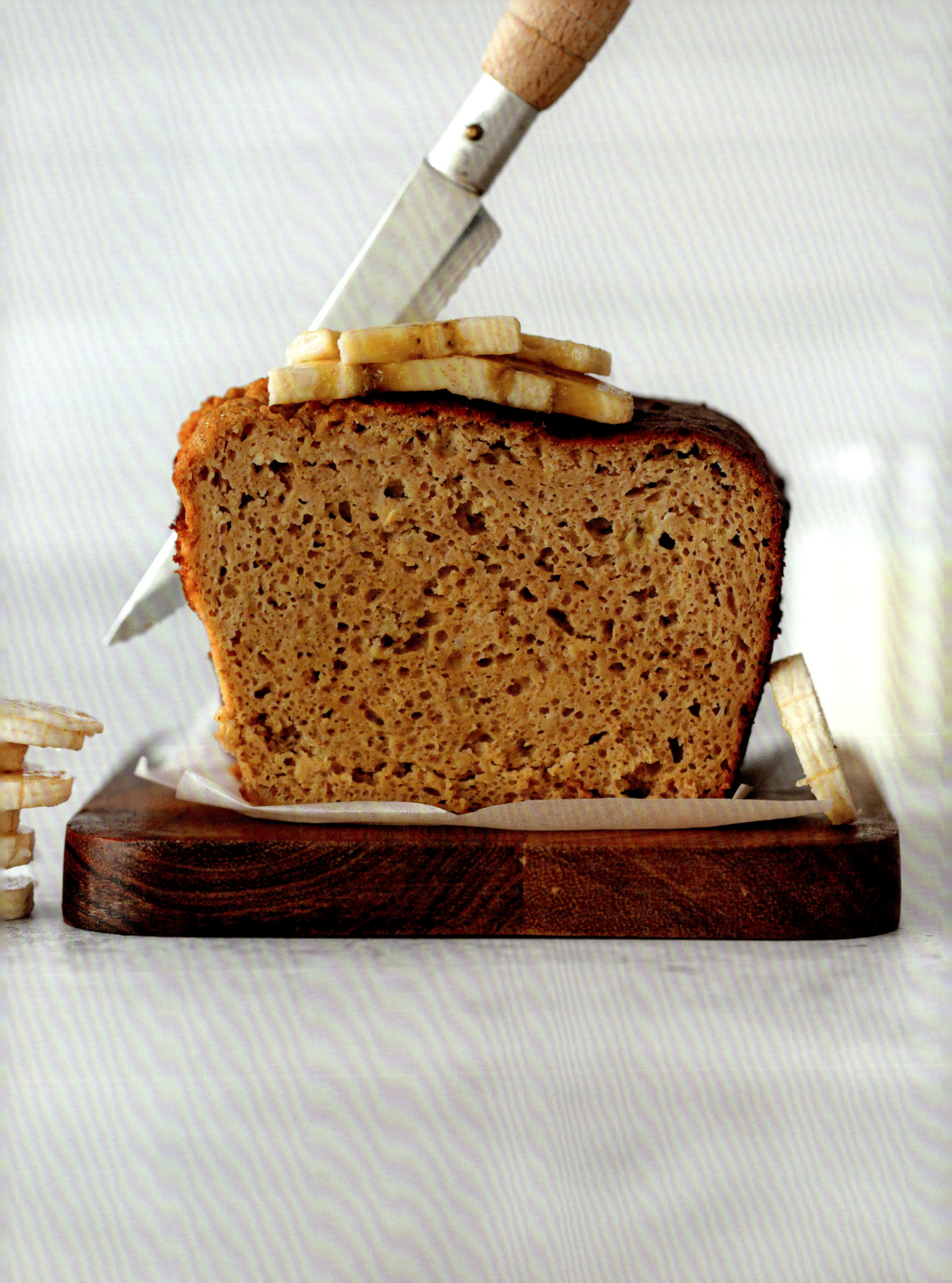

PROTEIN BANANA BREAD

2 large ripe bananas
1 egg
½ cup (120ml) Silk unsweetened cashew milk
½ cup (115g) nonfat Greek yogurt
1 tsp (5ml) vanilla extract
½ cup (80g) vanilla protein powder
½ cup (60g) all-purpose flour
½ cup (96g) Swerve brown sugar
2 tsp (10g) baking powder
Pinch of salt
1 tsp (3g) cinnamon

Does anyone ever actually plan on making banana bread? Because to me, banana bread is just a socially acceptable way of admitting we ignored our bananas for a week and now have no choice but to turn them into a cake. With my banana bread, you can at least boast protein gains at the same time. If you manage to use enough self-restraint to have leftover loaf for the next few days, store it in the fridge in a sealed container. If it seems a little dense, microwave on high for 20 seconds, and it will get its second wind.

1. Preheat the oven to 350°F (180°C). Line the bottom and sides of an 8½ x 4½-inch (21.5 x 11cm) loaf pan with parchment paper.
2. In a large mixing bowl, using a large fork or wooden spoon, mash the bananas until they reach a chunky liquid consistency.
3. Add the egg, cashew milk, Greek yogurt, and vanilla extract and stir until the mixture is well combined.
4. In a separate mixing bowl, whisk together the protein powder, flour, brown sugar, baking powder, salt, and cinnamon. Add the dry ingredients to the bowl with the wet ingredients and gently fold together until a thick, pale batter forms.
5. Into the prepared loaf pan, pour the batter and smooth the top with a spatula.
6. Bake on the middle rack for 40 minutes, or until the top rises and turns golden brown.
7. Remove from the oven and let the banana bread cool in the pan for 15 minutes. Carefully transfer the loaf to a wire rack to finish cooling before slicing into 10 even pieces.
8. Serve and enjoy!

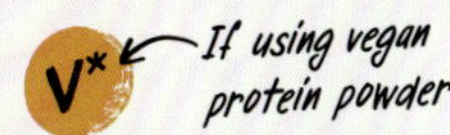

makes 1 loaf / 10 servings

NUTRITION (PER SERVING)

134 calories	**1g** fat
10g protein	**21g** net carbs

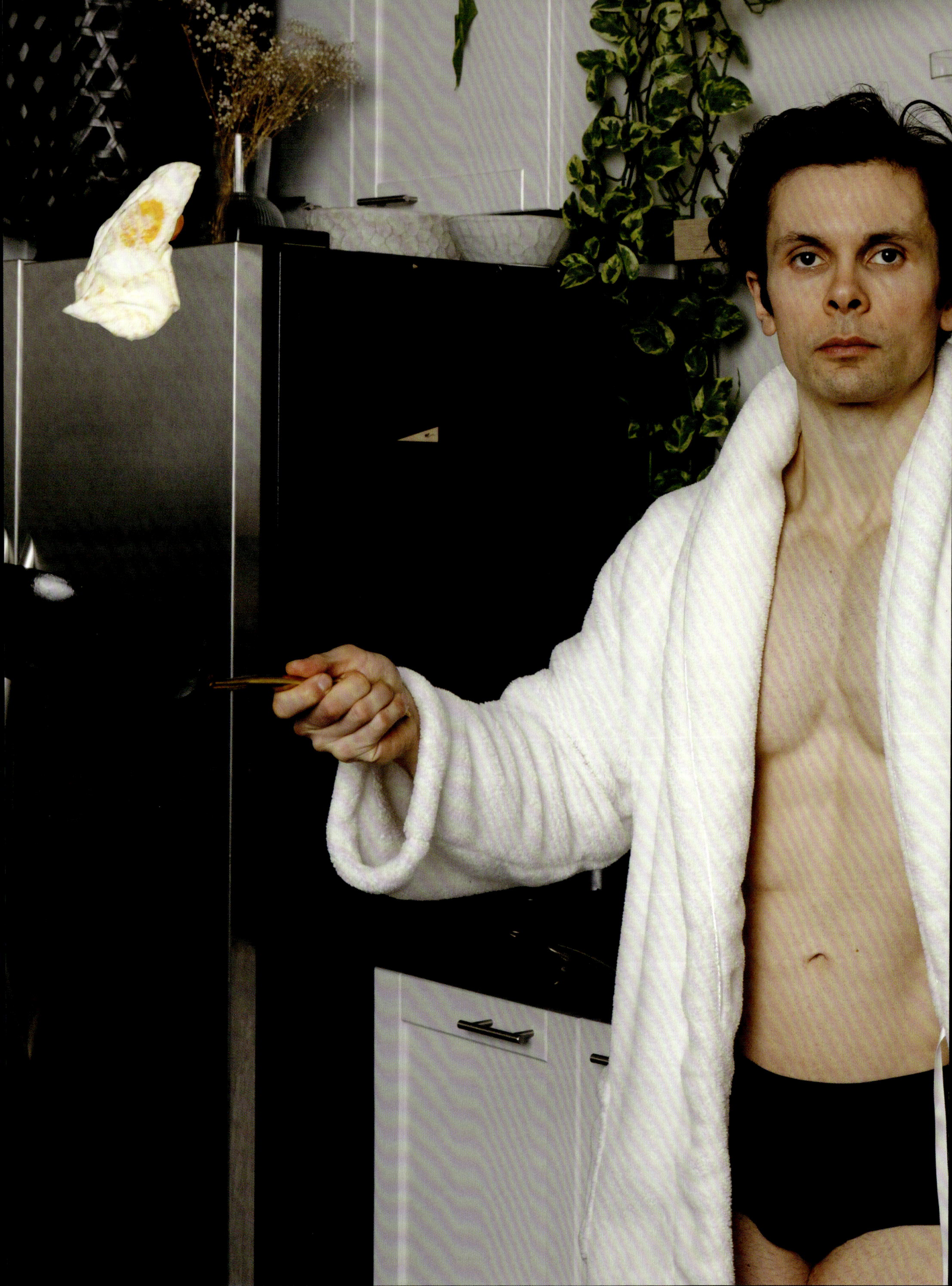

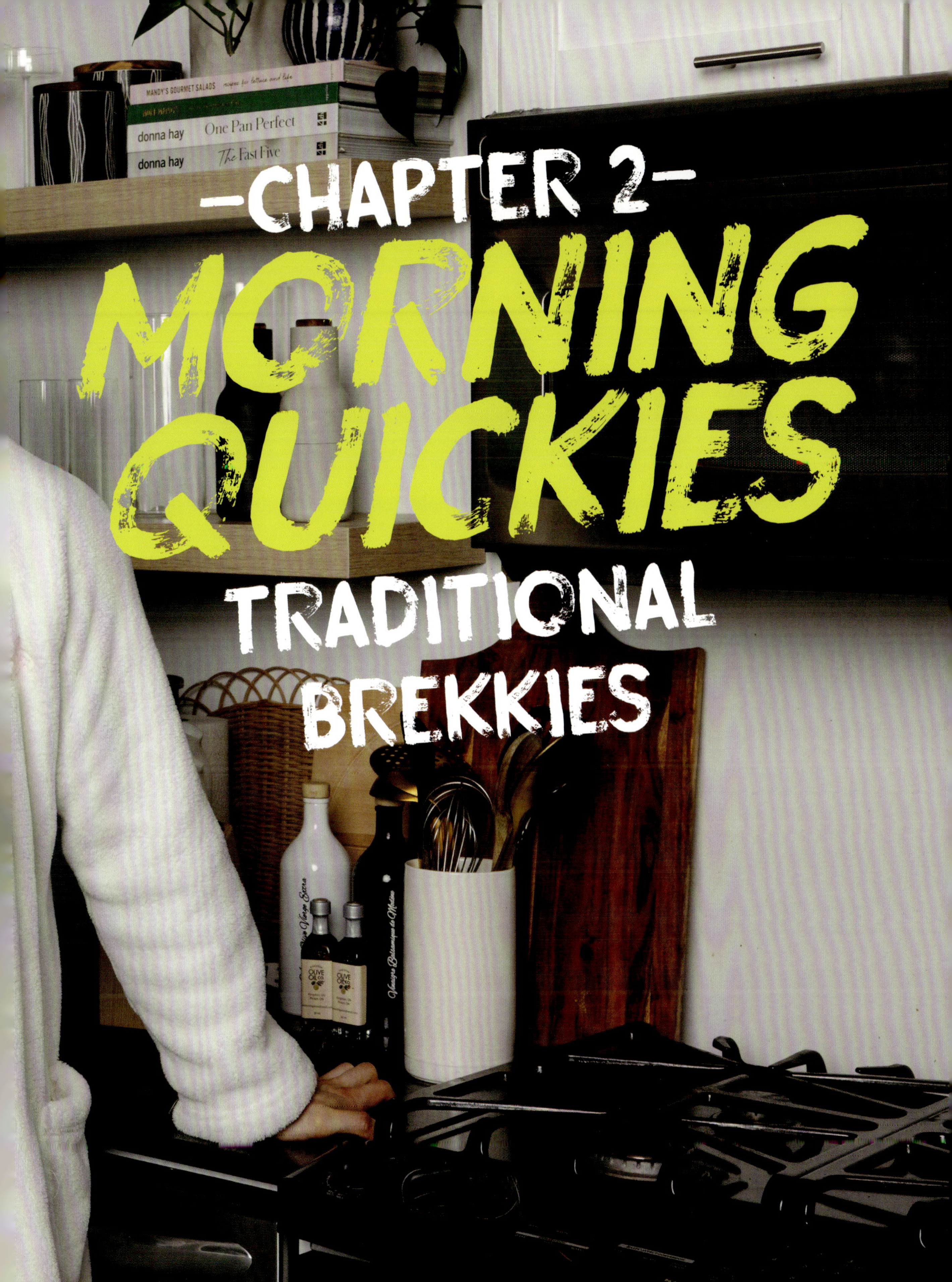

–CHAPTER 2–
MORNING QUICKIES
TRADITIONAL BREKKIES

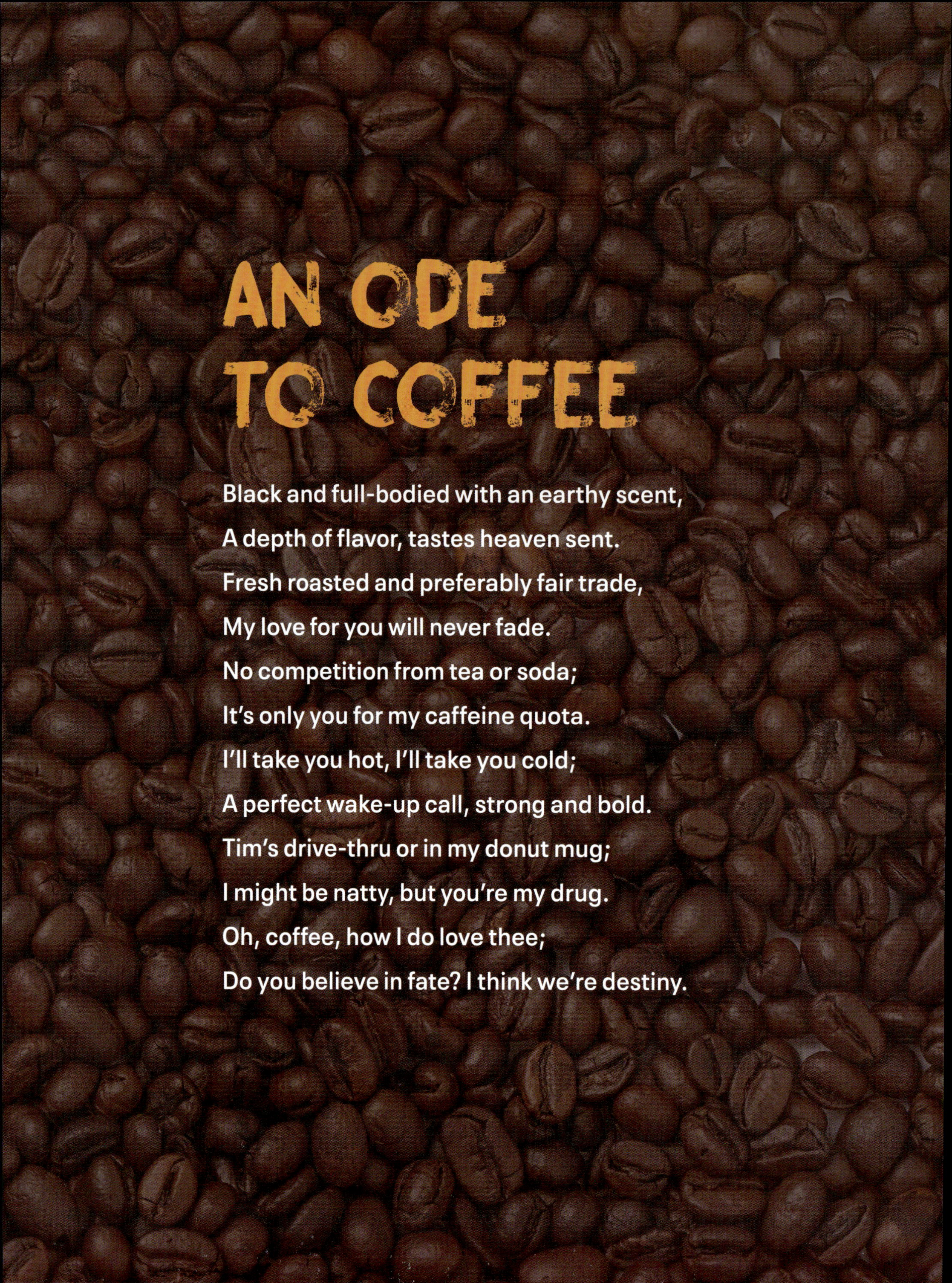

AN ODE TO COFFEE

Black and full-bodied with an earthy scent,
A depth of flavor, tastes heaven sent.
Fresh roasted and preferably fair trade,
My love for you will never fade.
No competition from tea or soda;
It's only you for my caffeine quota.
I'll take you hot, I'll take you cold;
A perfect wake-up call, strong and bold.
Tim's drive-thru or in my donut mug;
I might be natty, but you're my drug.
Oh, coffee, how I do love thee;
Do you believe in fate? I think we're destiny.

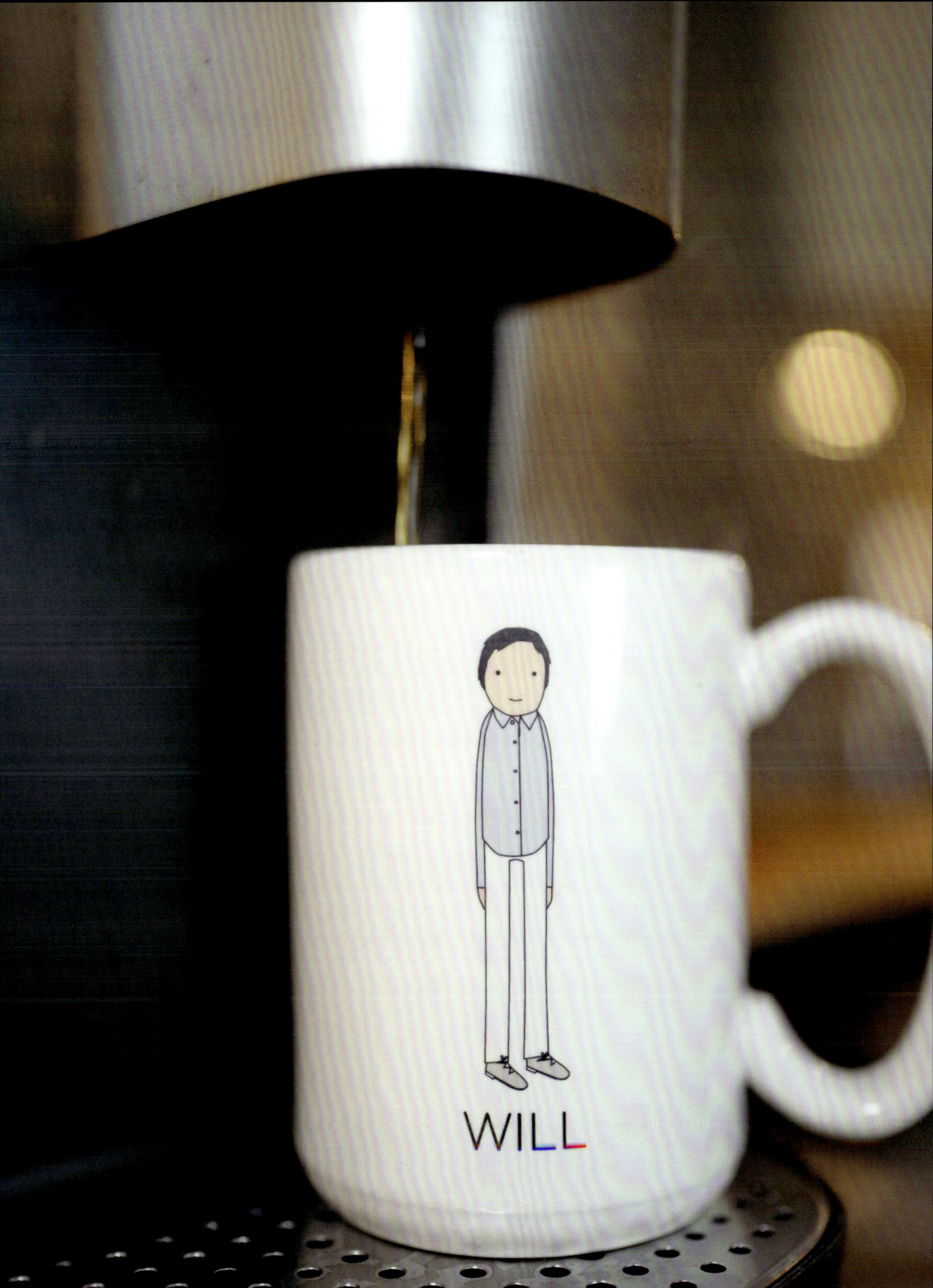
WILL

BREAKFAST QUESADILLA

for the quesadilla:

¼ small red onion, finely sliced
¼ small green bell pepper, finely sliced
1 garlic clove, diced
Salt and pepper, to taste
2 eggs
2 low-calorie tortillas
⅓ cup (40g) shredded low-fat cheddar cheese
1–2 tbsp (3.75–7.5g) cilantro, roughly chopped

for the delicious creamy dip:

2 tbsp (30g) nonfat Greek yogurt
2 tbsp (30ml) salsa

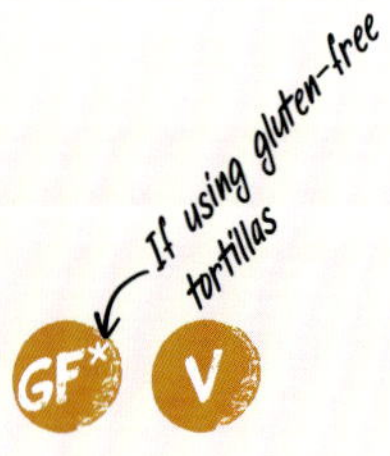

makes 1 quesadilla / 1 serving

NUTRITION (PER SERVING)

409 calories
13g fat
27g protein
42g net carbs

As a child, only visits from Santa or the Tooth Fairy could turn me into a morning person. As a grown-up, I've enjoyed being able to add this breakfast quesadilla to the list. If an early-morning feed isn't your bag, this recipe can be modified to make a more substantial lunch or dinner by swapping the egg out for some shredded rotisserie chicken, ground meat, or pan-fried tofu. Heck, keep the egg in too. If cilantro tastes like soap to you, use some diced green onions instead. We have no hard-and-fast rules in our kitchen.

1. **To make the quesadilla:** Heat a large frying pan over medium-high heat and spray it with nonstick cooking spray. Add the red onion, bell pepper, and garlic and season with salt and pepper. Sauté for 6 to 7 minutes, until softened. Set aside.
2. Spray the frying pan once again with nonstick cooking spray. Into the pan, crack the eggs. Let them cook sunny side up. Once the whites begin to set, burst the egg yolk with a spatula, then flip them and cook for an additional 30 seconds. Remove the eggs from the pan and set aside.
3. **To assemble the quesadilla:** To the heated frying pan, add one tortilla and sprinkle with half (15g) of the cheddar cheese. Add half of the cilantro, followed by the sautéed vegetables, then the cooked eggs.
4. Over the eggs, add the remaining cheddar and the remaining cilantro. Top with the second tortilla and grill on each side for 3 to 4 minutes, until the cheese is melted and the tortilla is golden brown and crisp.
5. **To make the delicious creamy dip:** To a small bowl, add the Greek yogurt and salsa and mix. Top the quesadilla with the dip, or dip your sliced quesadilla into the sauce as you enjoy.

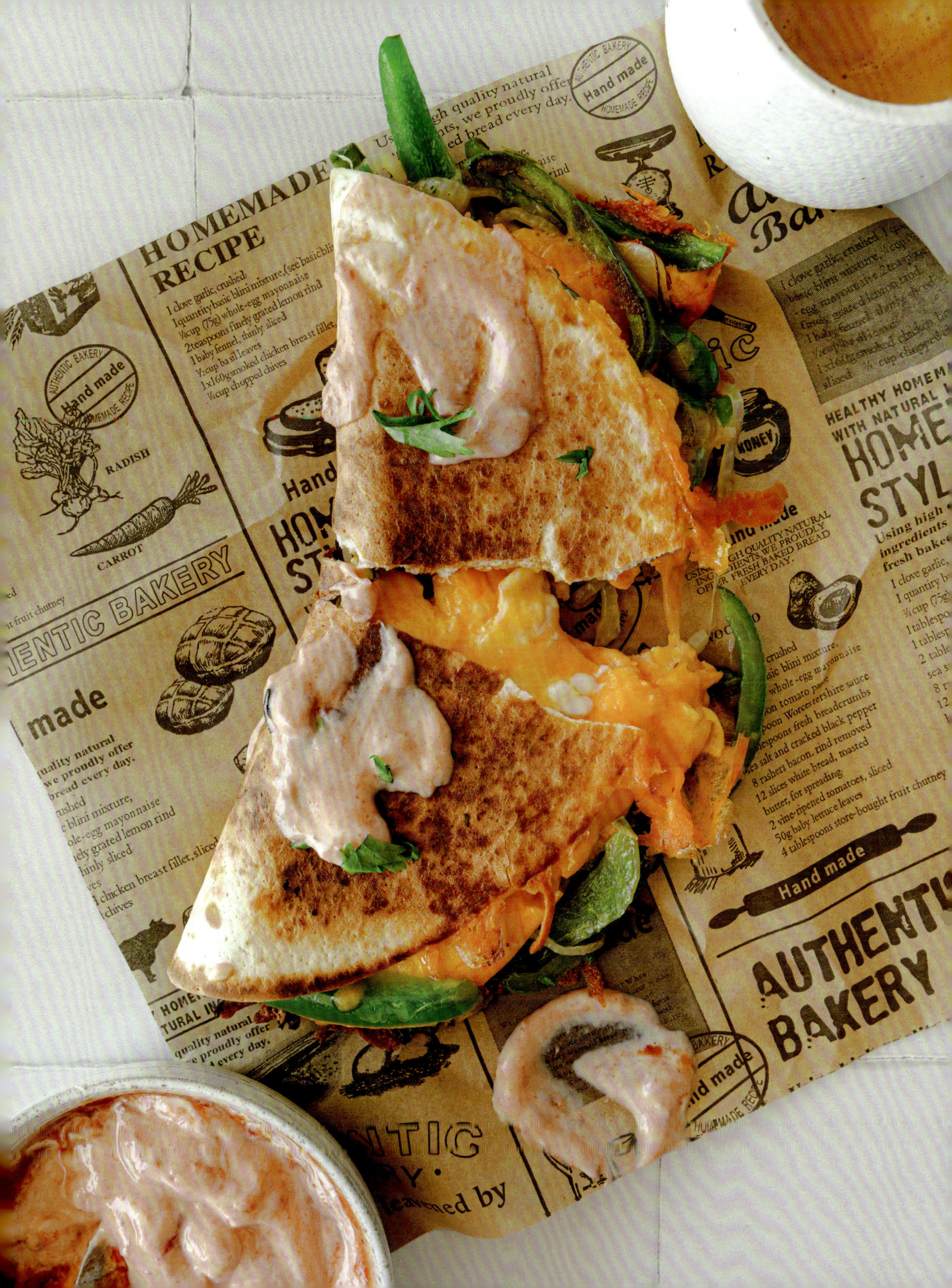
HOMEMADE
RECIPE
1 clove garlic, crushed
Hand made
RADISH
CARROT
HONEY
HEALTHY HOMEM
WITH NATURAL
HOME
STYL
Hand made
AUTHENTI
BAKERY

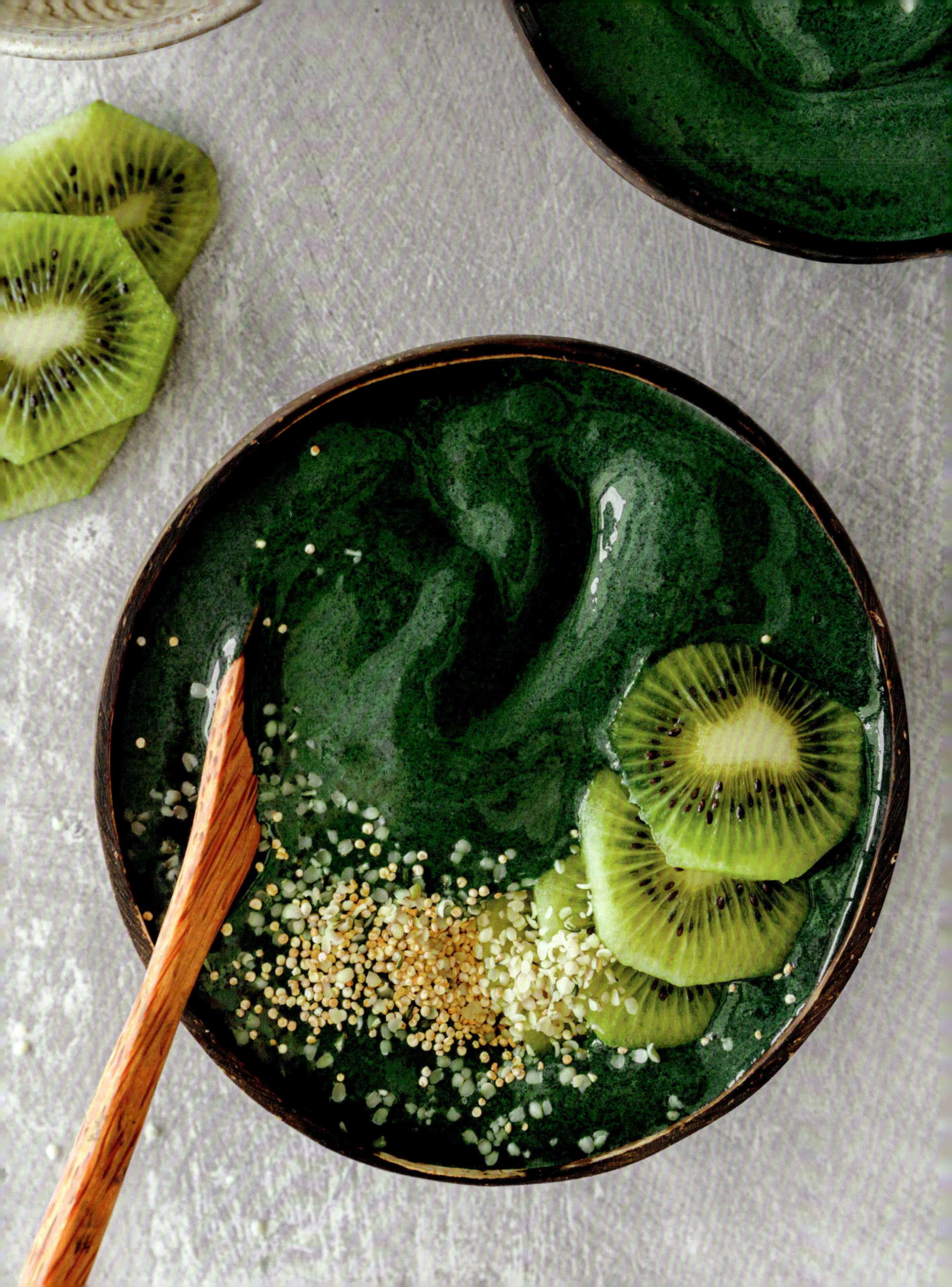

VEGAN MACA BOWL

2 tbsp (10g) dry quinoa
¾ cup (100g) frozen blueberries
¾ cup (100g) frozen strawberries
2½ tbsp (15g) spirulina powder
2 cups (240ml) Silk unsweetened cashew milk
¼ cup (50g) vegan protein powder
1 tsp (5g) maca powder
1 large handful of ice
2½ tbsp (20g) hemp hearts
1 medium kiwi, sliced

Packed with so much health, this is the only bowl you'll need to hit for a full post-Vegas bender recovery. Maca is a root also known as Peruvian ginseng, and is rich in calcium, amino acids, and iron. More importantly, it is a well-known aphrodisiac, so keep this recipe in your arsenal if you have a guest to impress. Working in tandem with spirulina, which can help with muscle recovery and endurance, this smoothie bowl has it all. To change up your toppings, another go-to combo of mine is chia seeds, blackberries, and thinly sliced pear. Now run along, and enjoy all the benefits this dish has to offer.

1. Heat a small saucepan over medium-high heat. Once hot, add the quinoa. The quinoa will begin to make popping sounds immediately. Shake the saucepan frequently to keep the quinoa from burning. Cook for 1 to 2 minutes, until puffed up. Set aside.
2. To a blender, add the blueberries, strawberries, spirulina powder, cashew milk, protein powder, maca powder, and ice. Blend until smooth. The texture should be far thicker than a smoothie. Add more ice if the consistency is too thin or more cashew milk if it's too thick.
3. Into a bowl, pour the blended mixture. Top with the puffed quinoa, hemp hearts, and kiwi slices. Feel free to explore and add other fruits and toppings that you desire.

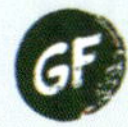

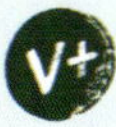

makes 1 serving

NUTRITION (PER SERVING)

550 calories | **17g** fat
47g protein | **52g** net carbs

PB&J PROTEIN PANCAKE

for the pancake:

1 medium banana, peeled
2 eggs
1 scoop (31g) peanut-butter protein powder
1 tsp (4g) Stevia sweetener (optional)
2 tbsp (13g) PB2 Powdered Peanut Butter, mixed with water to desired consistency

for the strawberry compote:

1 cup (140g) frozen strawberries
1 tbsp (15ml) lemon juice

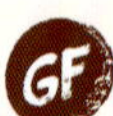

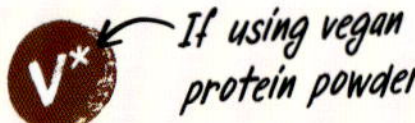

makes 1 large pancake / 1 serving

NUTRITION (PER SERVING)

428 calories	**12g** fat
39g protein	**39g** net carbs

A taste of childhood that's truly free of trauma, this pancake will take you back in time while helping your gains make a leap forward. If your gym partner gets tired of their unseasoned egg whites and oats, this recipe is easy to double or triple, so you can share the love. You can also pour the batter in smaller rounds if you prefer your breakfasts tall and stacked. We're inclusive here. If you like your pancakes on the sweeter side, the Stevia sweetener will be your best friend. Add some sugar-free maple syrup if you really want to turn up the flavor, you sweet-freak.

1. **To make the pancake:** To a large bowl, add the banana. Using a fork, mash the banana until it resembles a clumpy paste.
2. Add the eggs, protein powder, and Stevia (if using) and mix until evenly combined into a thick batter.
3. Preheat a large frying pan over medium-high heat and spray it with nonstick cooking spray.
4. Into the heated pan, pour the pancake batter and cook for about 5 minutes on each side, flipping when bubbles form on the top and the edges begin to set.
5. **To make the strawberry compote:** While the pancake is cooking, to a small pot over medium-high heat, add the strawberries and lemon juice. As the strawberries begin to thaw and cook, use a mixing spoon to break up the fruit and stir together. Remove the compote from the heat after 5 to 7 minutes, once the strawberries soften and are heated through.
6. Pour the hot strawberry compote over the protein pancake, top with the PB2 mixture, and enjoy!

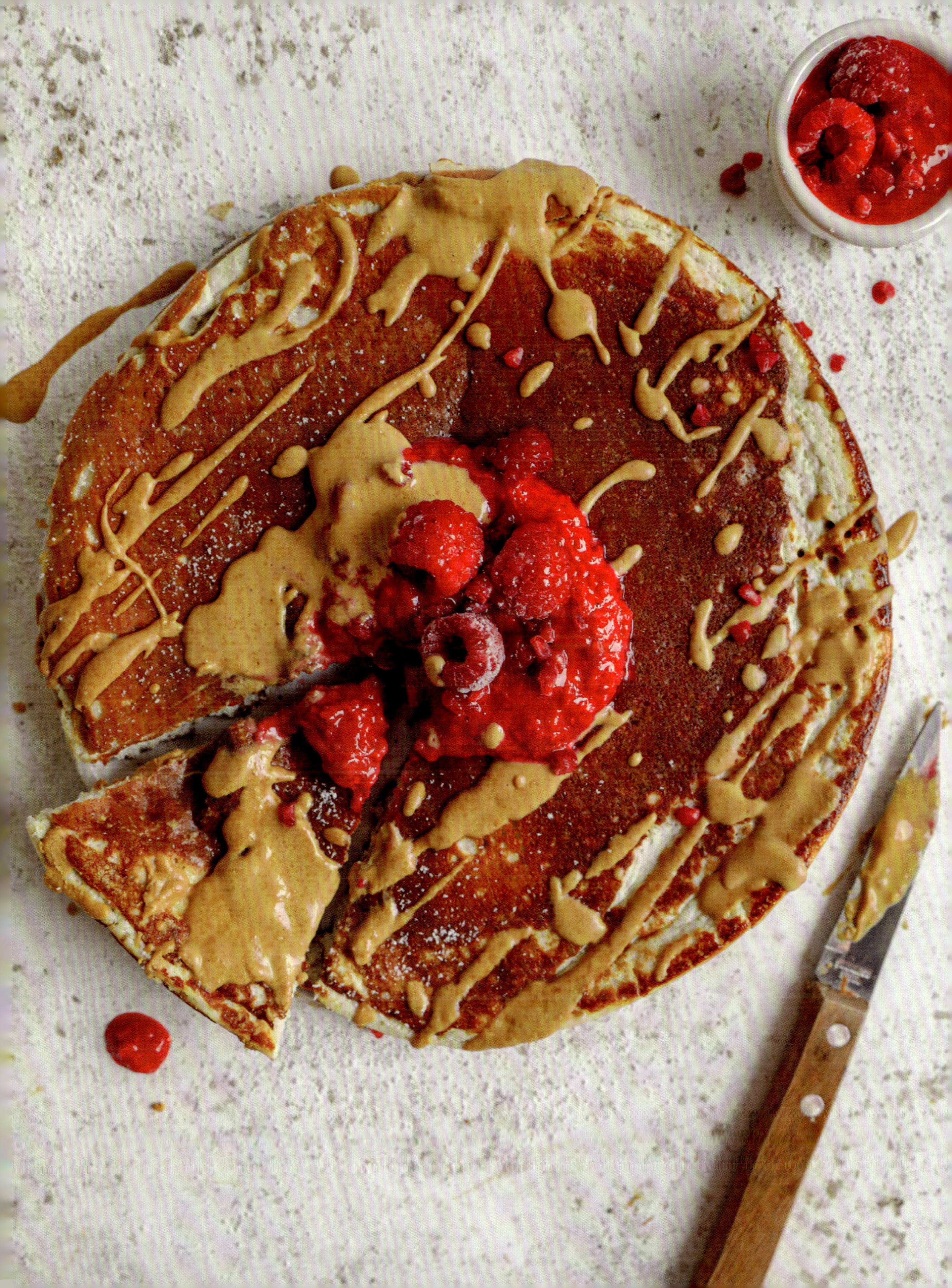

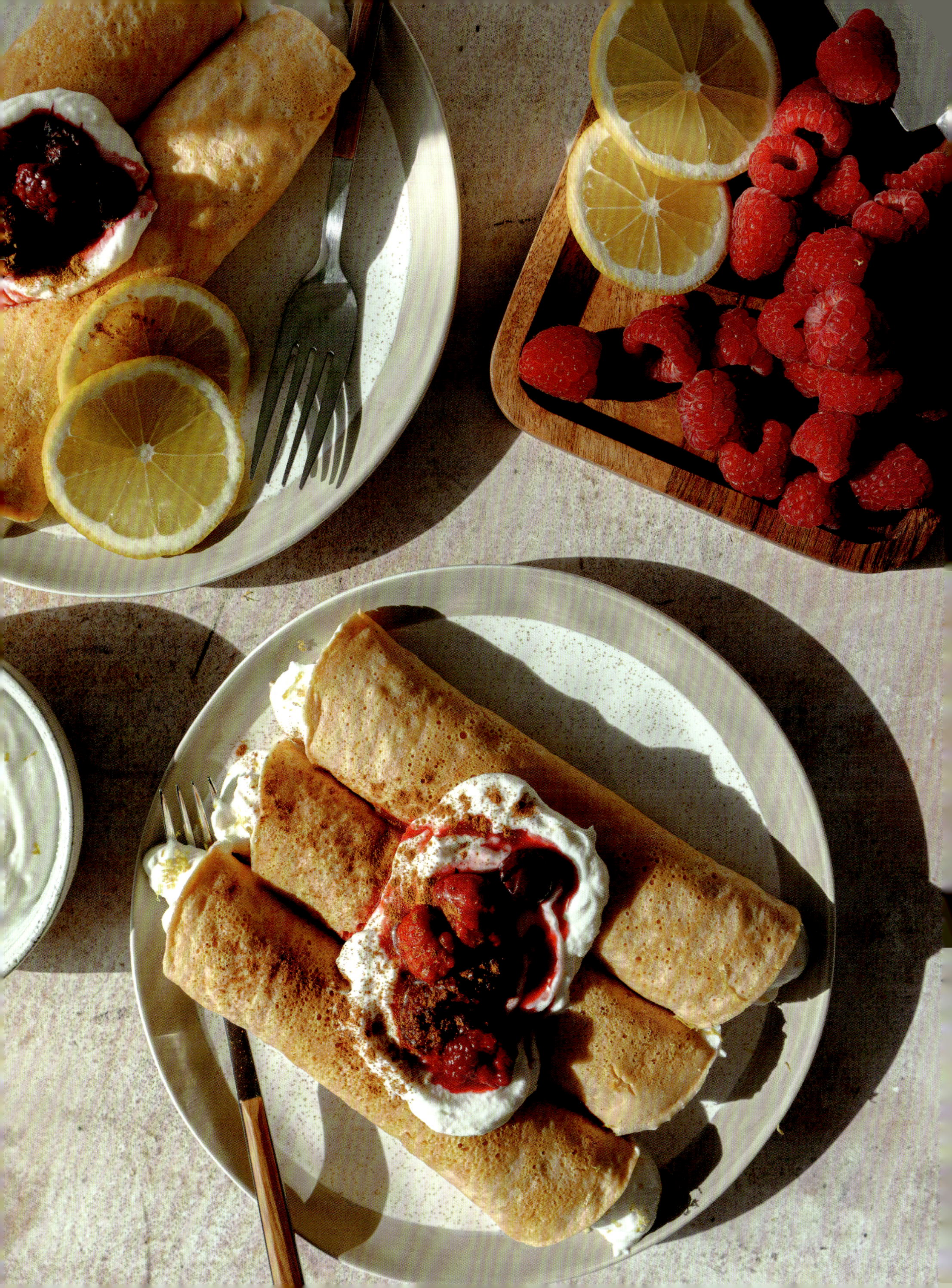

LEMON-RICOTTA PROTEIN CREPES

for the lemon-ricotta filling:
8oz (226g) low-fat ricotta cheese
1 tsp (5ml) vanilla extract
2 tsp (8g) Stevia sweetener
Zest of 1 lemon
4 tbsp (60ml) Silk unsweetened cashew milk

for the crepes:
2 eggs
1 scoop (31g) vanilla protein powder
2 tbsp (30ml) Silk unsweetened cashew milk
½ tsp (1.5g) cinnamon, to garnish

for the berry topping:
½ cup (40g) frozen berries
1 tsp (4g) Stevia sweetener

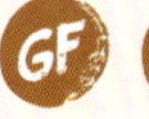

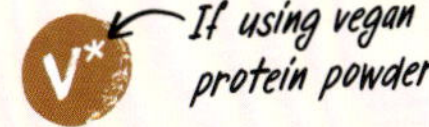

makes 2 servings

NUTRITION (PER SERVING)

269 calories	**11g** fat
26g protein	**12g** net carbs

One of my kitchen's most versatile cheeses, ricotta can go both ways by contributing a thick, creamy goodness in any dish, whether it's sweet or savory. The lemon zest will perk you up, as the light and fluffy crepes show you what it means to be properly filled. If you happen to be one of the few people on Earth who owns a crepe maker, this will be the easiest way to ensure your crepes turn out thin and crispy. For the rest of the world, a frying pan will work just fine—just be sure to add way less batter than you think to the center of your pan, and tilt and swirl the pan to coat the entire bottom. You want the batter to be so thin, it should almost be see through. Do this, and you'll have the perfect crepe every time.

1. **To make the lemon-ricotta filling:** To a blender, add the ricotta, vanilla extract, Stevia, lemon zest, and 2 tablespoons (30ml) of the cashew milk. Blend until smooth and fluffy, slowly adding in the remaining 2 tablespoons (30ml) cashew milk as needed. Set aside.
2. **To make the crepes:** Preheat a medium frying pan over medium-high heat and spray it with nonstick cooking spray.
3. To a large bowl, add the eggs and whisk. Add the protein powder and cashew milk and mix well until there are no clumps, creating a crepe batter.
4. Into the heated pan, pour a very thin, almost translucent layer of batter. Tilt and swirl the pan to coat the entire bottom, and let cook for 1 minute per side, until the batter bubbles and the edges set. Remove the crepe from the pan and repeat until all the batter has been used.
5. In the center of each crepe, place 2 heaping tablespoons of the lemon-ricotta filling and roll the crepe around the filling into a long tube shape.
6. **To make the berry topping:** In a microwave-safe bowl, place the berries and heat until the berries are thawed. Mix in the Stevia.
7. Pour the berries over the crepes, sprinkle with the cinnamon, and you're all set with this epic creation.

BREAKFAST BURRITOS WITH HOMEMADE SWEET-POTATO WRAPS

for the sweet-potato wraps:

2 large sweet potatoes (360g)
1 cup (120g) all-purpose flour

for the burritos:

½ white onion, chopped
⅓ cup (80g) button mushrooms, chopped
2 eggs
6½ tbsp (100g) egg whites
Salt and pepper, to taste
⅓ cup (20g) cilantro, roughly chopped
⅔ cup (60g) shredded part-skim mozzarella
2 tbsp (30ml) salsa

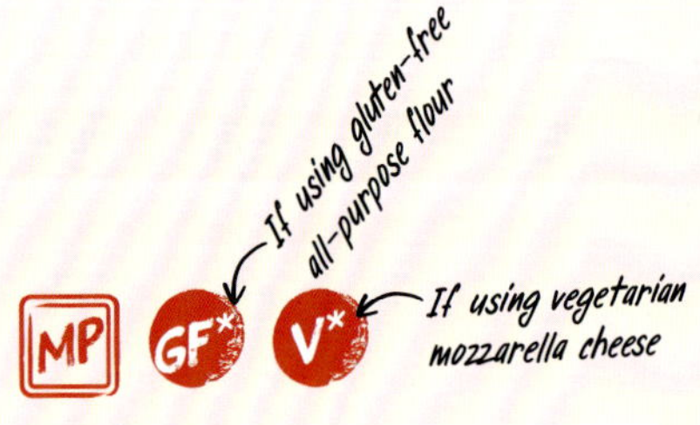

makes 2 burritos / 2 servings

NUTRITION (PER SERVING)	
310 calories	**8.5g** fat
19.5g protein	**39g** net carbs

Nobody likes overprocessed, store-bought wraps. So, if you're going to wrap it up, avoid the taste of latex with something homemade, and fill it with all your classic breakfast faves. These sweet potato wraps are perfect to meal prep alongside your protein and veg, and this recipe gifts you with three extra wraps that you can use for days. They keep fresh covered at room temperature for about a week, and while they're the perfect burrito vessel, they also work as a flatbread crust, a naan or roti substitute, or cut into pieces as chips (air fry or bake them for more crisp).

1. **To make the sweet-potato wraps:** Pierce each sweet potato 3 to 4 times with a fork, and microwave on high for 7 to 8 minutes, flipping them halfway through. The potatoes should be soft and cooked through. Let cool slightly, then remove the skin.
2. In a large mixing bowl, mash the potatoes. Add the flour and knead together with your hands until the mixture forms a dough ball.
3. Flour a clean, flat surface and roll the dough into a tube about 2 inches (5cm) thick. Cut the dough into 5 equal pieces and roll each into flat circles 8 to 9 inches (20 to 23cm) in diameter.
4. In a medium skillet over medium-high heat, place the wraps one at a time. Flip the wrap every 30 seconds until it starts to bubble and brown spots appear, 2 to 3 minutes. Set aside.
5. **To make the burritos:** Spray the same hot skillet with nonstick cooking spray and add the onion and mushrooms. Sauté for 5 to 6 minutes, or until the onions are translucent and the mushrooms are brown. Remove from the pan and set aside.
6. To a small bowl, add the eggs and egg whites and season with salt and pepper. Whisk to combine.
7. Reduce the heat under the skillet to medium and spray it again with nonstick cooking spray. When the pan is hot, add the egg mixture and stir often with a spatula until the eggs set and thicken into a scramble. Once no visible liquid remains in the pan, remove the eggs.
8. **To assemble:** To the center of each sweet-potato wrap, add the scrambled eggs, sautéed veggies, cilantro, cheese, and salsa. Wrap them up and chow down!

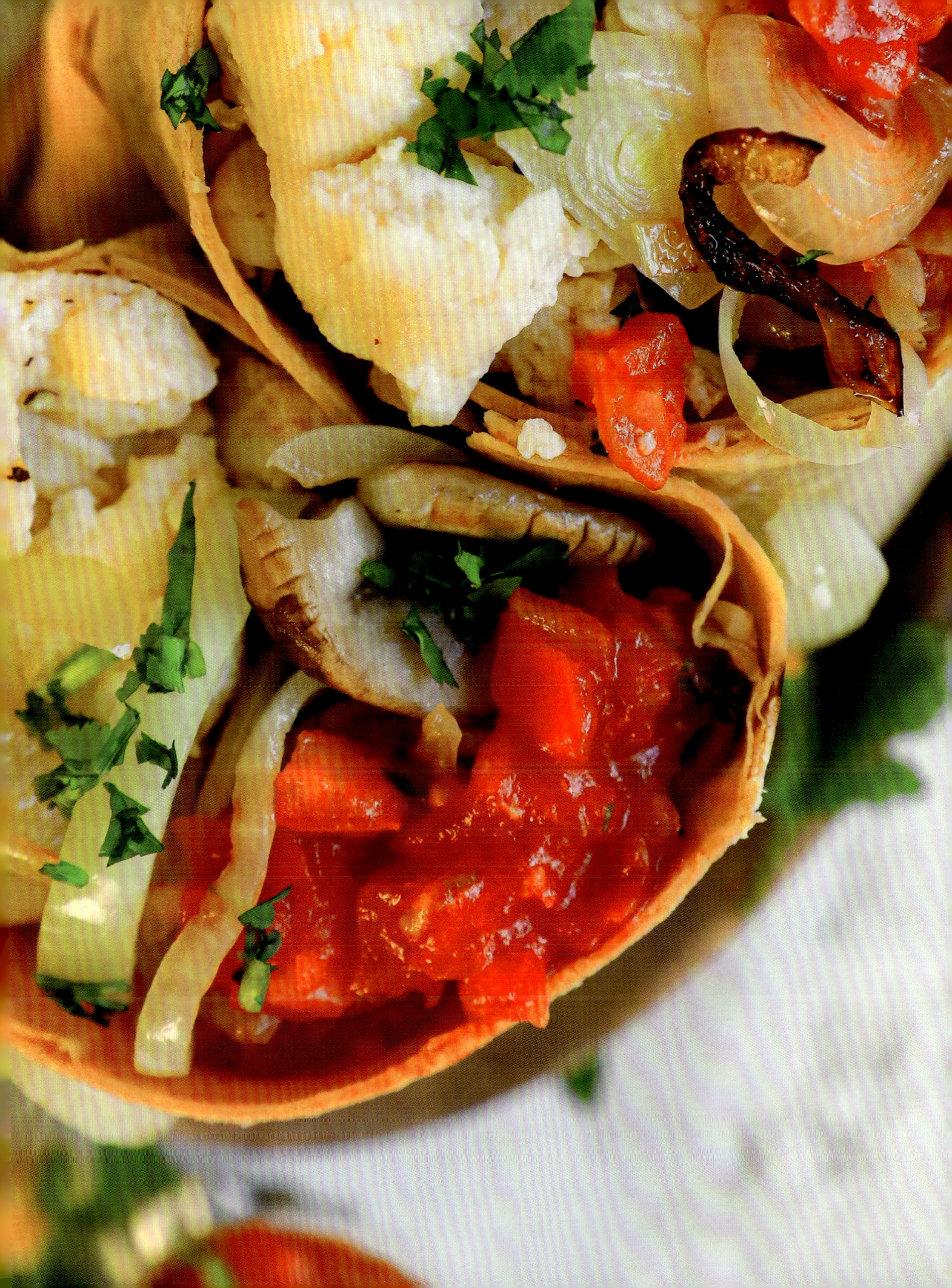

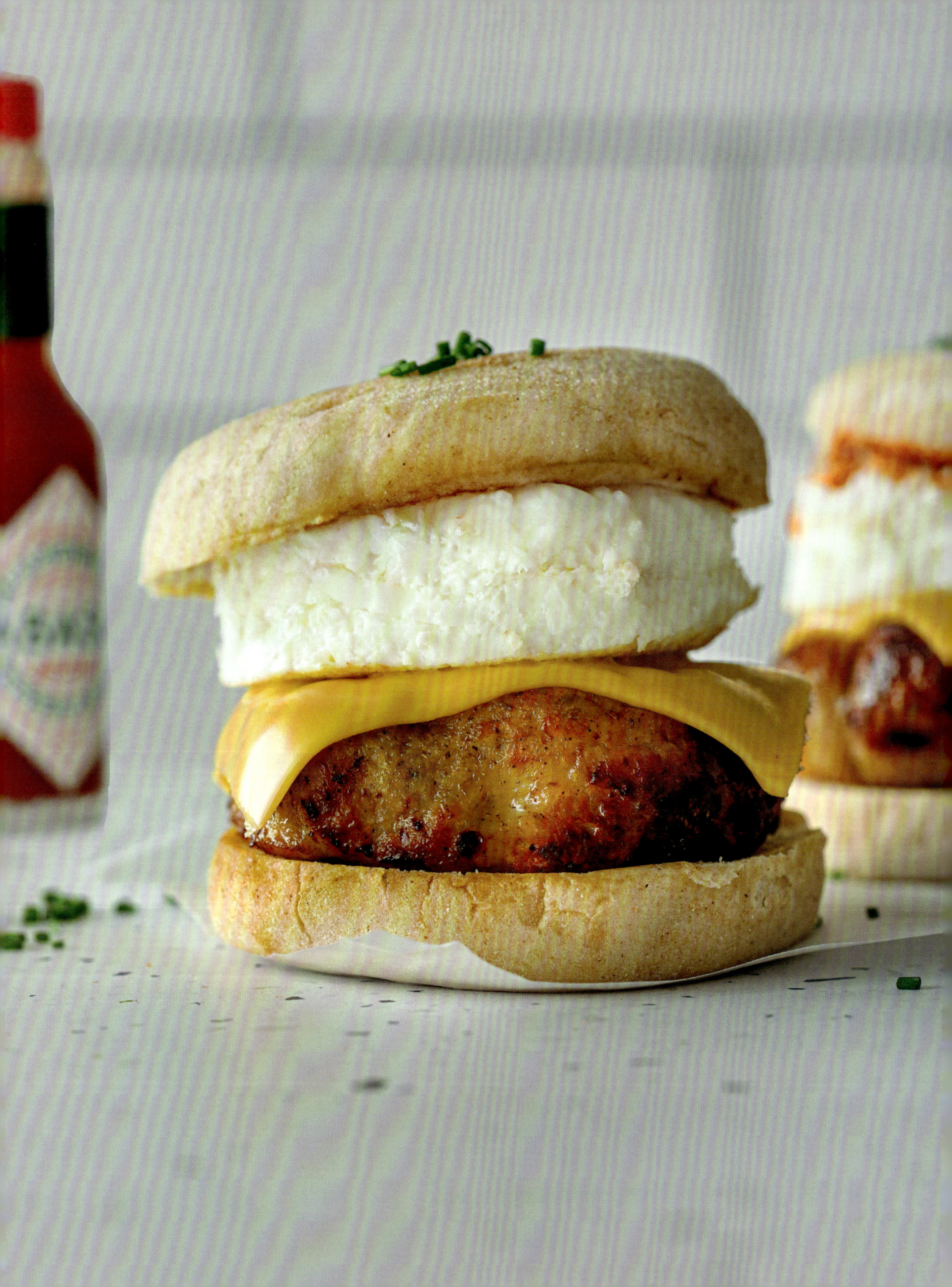

HEALTHY SAUSAGE AND EGG McWILLS

2 turkey sausages (about 188g), casings removed
2 English muffins, cut in half and toasted
6½ tbsp (100g) egg whites
Salt and pepper, to taste
2 slices low-fat cheddar cheese
Hot sauce (optional)

I am so confident that you'll love this healthier take on a Sausage McMuffin that I named it after myself. The only thing yolked in this recipe will be you at the gym if you eat the McWill on the regular. To make a big batch of sausage patties for the week, you can skip uncasing the sausages, and just mix 1 pound (450g) of ground turkey with salt, pepper, garlic powder, onion powder, and your favorite herb. Form the mixture into five patties, pan-fry them for 4 to 5 minutes, and store them in the fridge for up to 5 days or in the freezer for up to 6 months.

1. Heat a medium frying pan over medium-high heat and spray it with nonstick cooking spray.
2. Flatten and shape each sausage into a circular patty. In the hot pan, place the patties. Cook until brown and crispy on the outside and no longer pink in the center, 4 to 5 minutes per side. Remove the sausages from the pan.
3. Spray the same frying pan with nonstick cooking spray again, add the egg whites, and season with salt and pepper. Fry until firm and cooked through, about 1½ minutes.
4. Remove the egg whites from the pan and cut them in half. Fold each in half so it can fit on the English muffin.
5. On the bottom half of each English muffin, place a sausage patty, followed by the cheese slices, the egg whites, and the top of the English muffin. Top with the hot sauce (if using).

makes 2 sandwiches / 2 servings

NUTRITION (PER SERVING)

282 calories **6g** fat
32g protein **25g** net carbs

ZUCCHINI HASHBROWNS

2 large zucchinis
Salt, to taste
2 tbsp (6g) chives, minced
½ cup (55g) powdered Parmesan cheese
1 tsp (3g) dried oregano
2 garlic cloves, diced
1 egg
Pepper, to taste

If you want to spend the morning with a clown, that's your call, but with this recipe in your life, you'll always have a healthier choice than McDonald's. These hashbrowns are already deliciously special on their own, but if you want to crank it up a notch, top them with a thick tomato slice, a fried egg, and a crack of pepper, and you'll have a more complete meal. If you're looking to meal prep, you can freeze a batch of these in a sealed container, and to heat them up, bake them in the oven at 425°F (220°C) for 10 to 12 minutes, or in the air fryer at 400°F (200°C) for 5 to 6 minutes, and presto.

1. Preheat the oven to 400°F (200°C). Line a baking sheet with parchment paper.
2. Using the large side of a box grater, grate the zucchinis into a large bowl and sprinkle generously with salt. Mix and set aside for 20 minutes while the salt draws moisture from the zucchini.
3. Transfer the zucchini to a large cheese cloth or kitchen towel and squeeze out the excess liquid.
4. Return the zucchini to the large bowl and add the chives, Parmesan, oregano, garlic, and egg and season with salt and pepper. Mix until well combined.
5. Onto the prepared baking sheet, portion the zucchini mixture into 6 equal hash brown patties.
6. Bake for 20 minutes until golden brown and crispy.

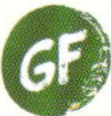

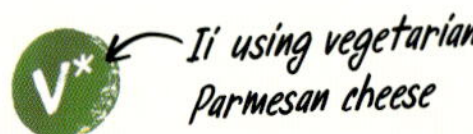

makes 6 hashbrowns / 6 servings

NUTRITION (PER SERVING)

110 calories	**7g** fat
9g protein	**3g** net carbs

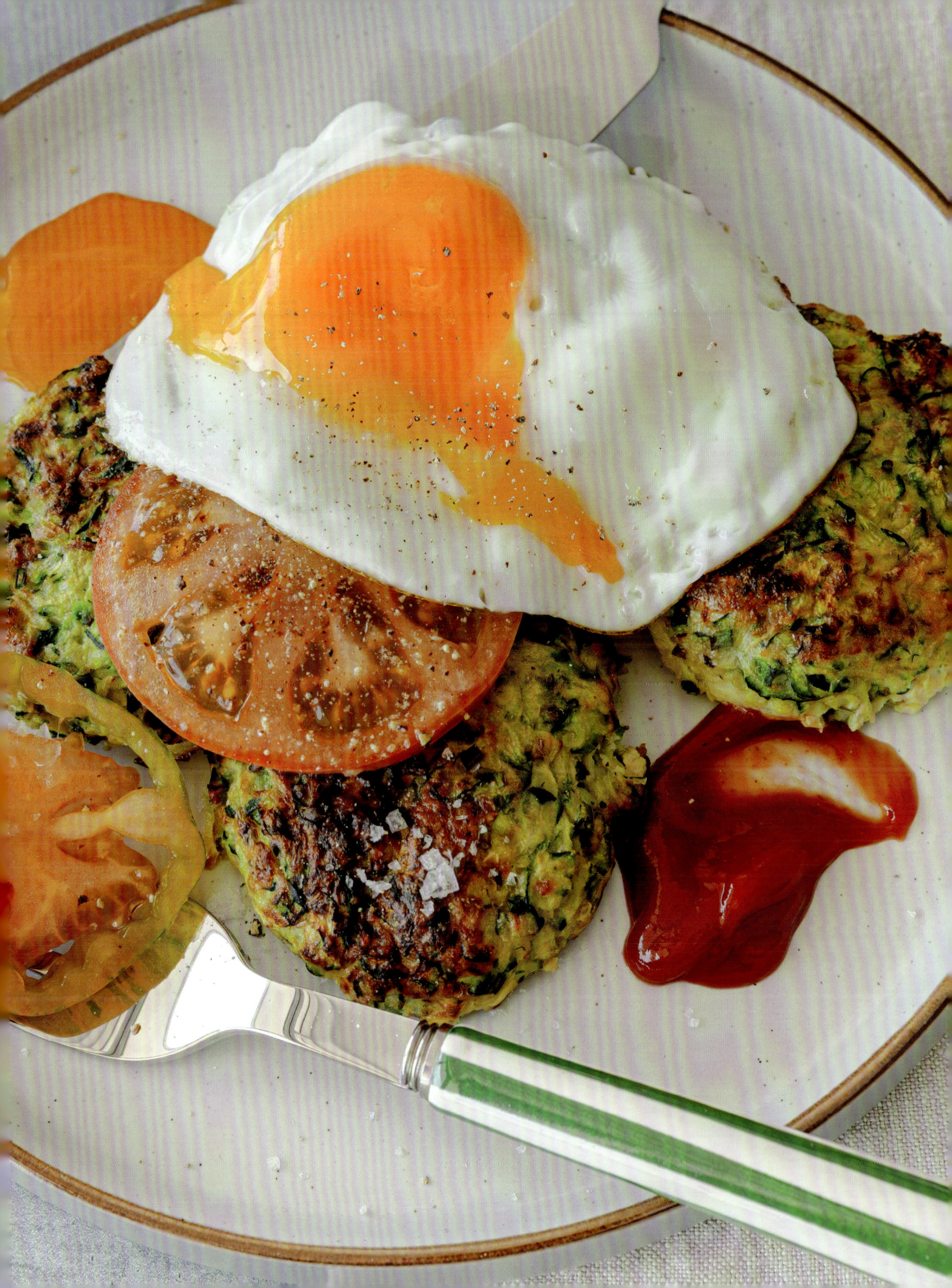

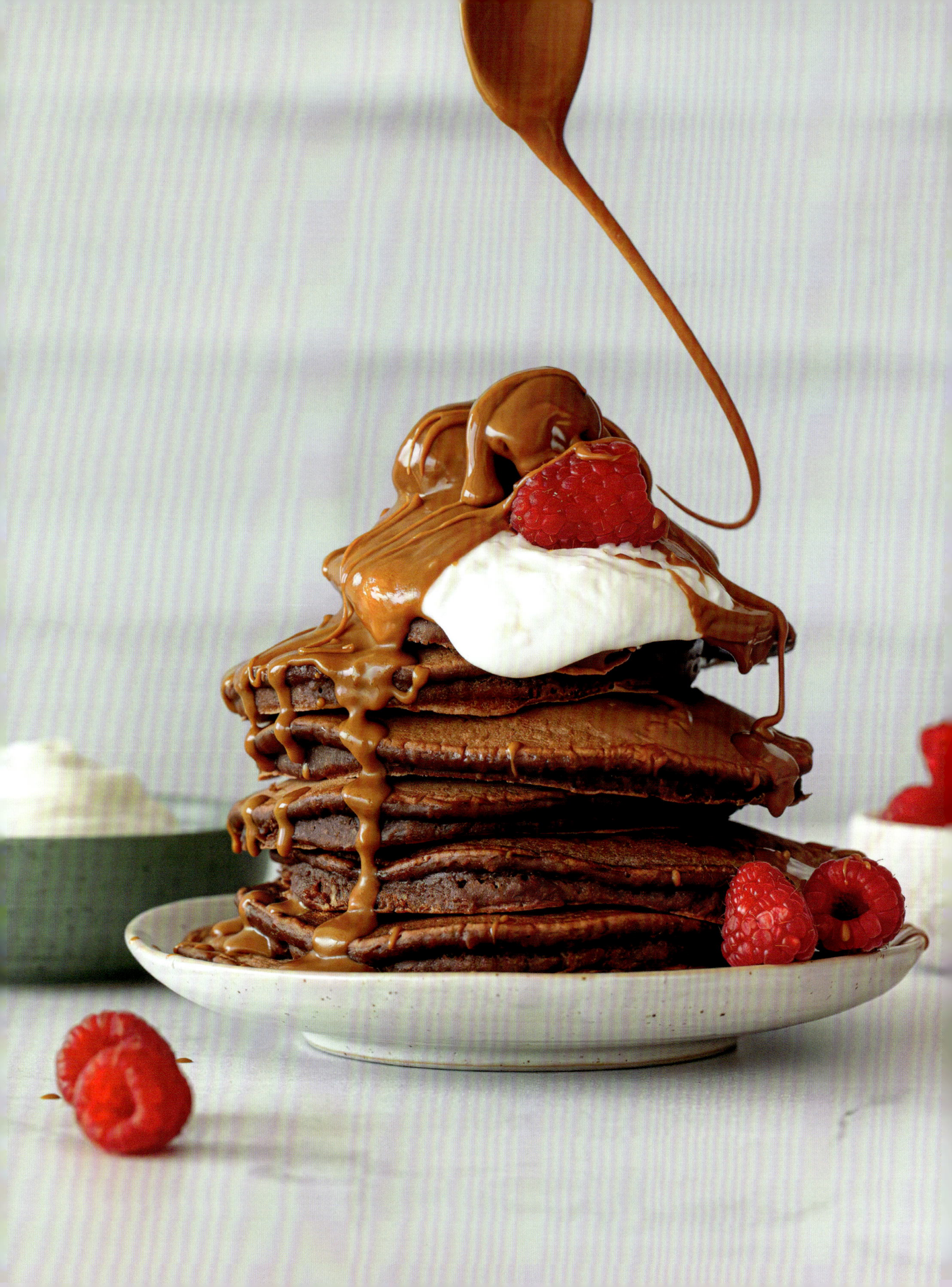

CHOCOLATE PROTEIN PANCAKE

1 egg
6½ tbsp (100g) egg whites
1 scoop (31g) protein powder of choice
2 tsp (4g) cocoa powder
3 tbsp (22.5g) coconut flour
½ tsp (2.5g) baking soda
2–4 tbsp (30–60ml) Silk unsweetened cashew milk
½ cup (115g) nonfat Greek yogurt
Fresh raspberries, to garnish
2 tbsp (13g) PB2 Powdered Peanut Butter, mixed with water to desired consistency

If a molten chocolate lava cake doesn't fit into your macros, try this chocolate protein pancake recipe instead. It's not going to taste the same, but if you close your eyes, your imagination can convince your tongue of anything. If you want to get as close as possible to tricking yourself into believing you're eating a dessert, use a casein-whey-blend protein powder. This will give the pancake an airier, cakier texture than traditional whey protein. While I prefer one supersize pancake, if you prefer a tower, you can divide your batter into three or four smaller pancakes and stack them like you're playing competitive Jenga. You can layer Greek yogurt between each pancake if you really wanna get fancy with it.

1. To a large bowl, add the egg and egg whites and whisk until thoroughly combined. Add the protein powder, cocoa powder, coconut flour, and baking soda and mix. While stirring the batter, slowly add the cashew milk until it reaches a thick, airy cake-batter consistency.
2. Heat a large skillet over medium-high heat and spray it with nonstick cooking spray.
3. Into the heated skillet, pour the pancake batter and cook for 2 to 3 minutes, or until the edges start to look dry. Flip the pancake and cook for an additional 1 to 2 minutes.
4. Plate the pancake and top with Greek yogurt and raspberries, and drizzle with the PB2 mixture. Eat up!

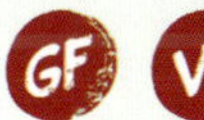

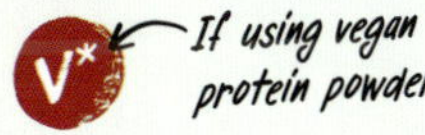

makes 1 pancake / 1 serving

NUTRITION (PER SERVING)

510 calories
11g fat
75g protein
28g net carbs

3-MINUTE BREAKFAST SANDWICH

1 English muffin, cut in half
2 eggs
1 tsp (1g) chives, finely chopped
⅓ cup (40g) shredded low-fat cheddar cheese
Salt and pepper, to taste
3 slices (55g) Black Forest ham

Don't worry about sleeping through your alarm; this morning quickie is guaranteed to finish before you even reach the final verse of your fave T Swift track. When I'm on the go, I'm not picky about the temperature of my meat, but if you want to heat up your ham before adding it to the middle of your sandwich, you can fry it in a separate pan while your eggs are cooking. You'll have an extra dish to clean, but we all have to make sacrifices for the things that truly matter to us.

1. Heat a large nonstick frying pan over medium heat and spray it with nonstick cooking spray.
2. On one side of the pan, place the English muffin halves facedown. On the other side of the pan, crack the eggs side by side and puncture the yolks with a spatula.
3. Once the eggs are mostly cooked through, sprinkle them with the chives and cheese and season with salt and pepper.
4. Place the toasted English muffins facedown over the eggs and let sit for 30 seconds.
5. Flip the whole sandwich over, egg-side up, and place the ham into the middle of the sandwich. Fold the sandwich closed and remove from the heat.

makes 1 sandwich / 1 serving

NUTRITION (PER SERVING)

425 calories	**21g** fat
36g protein	**23g** net carbs

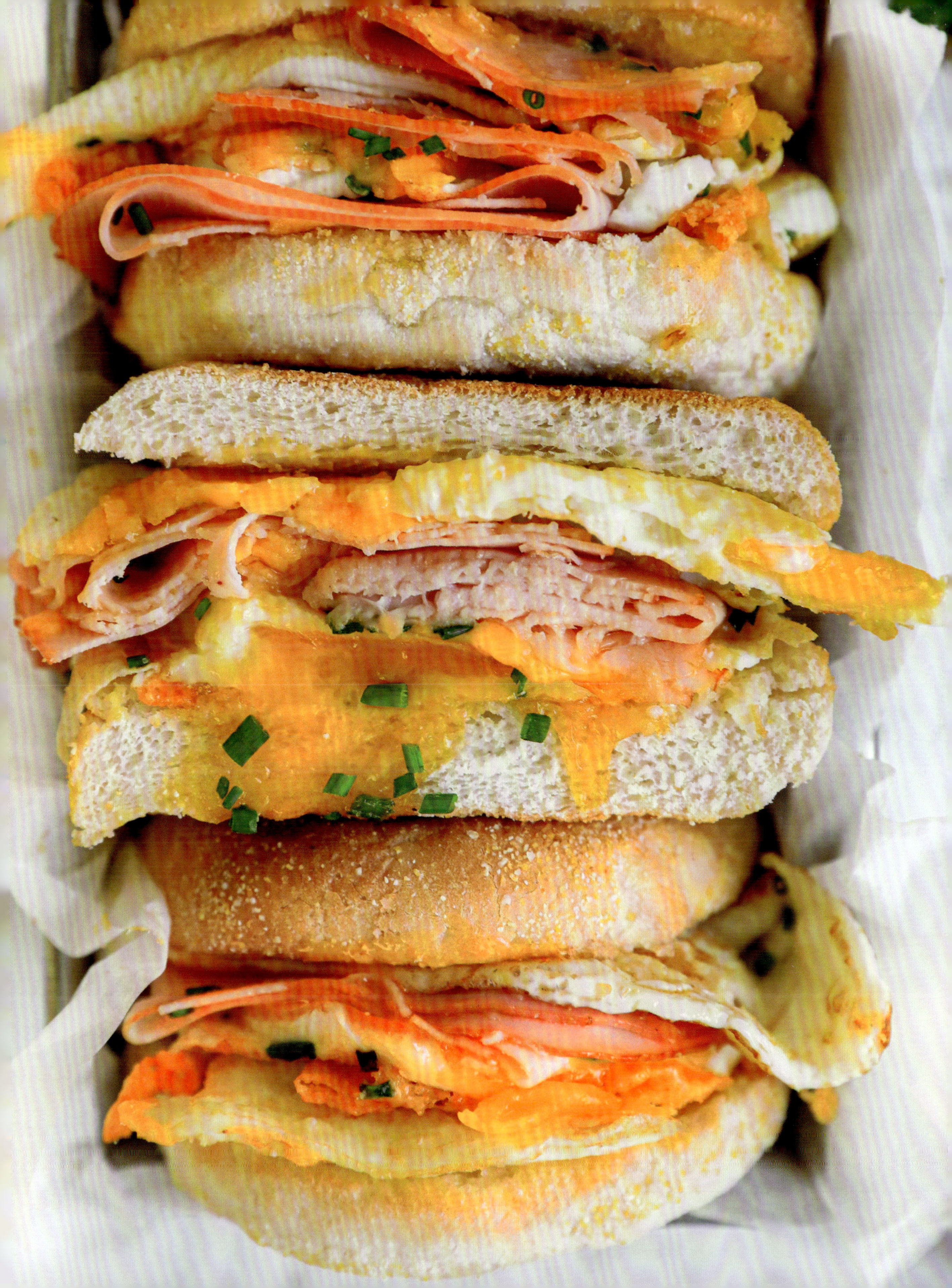

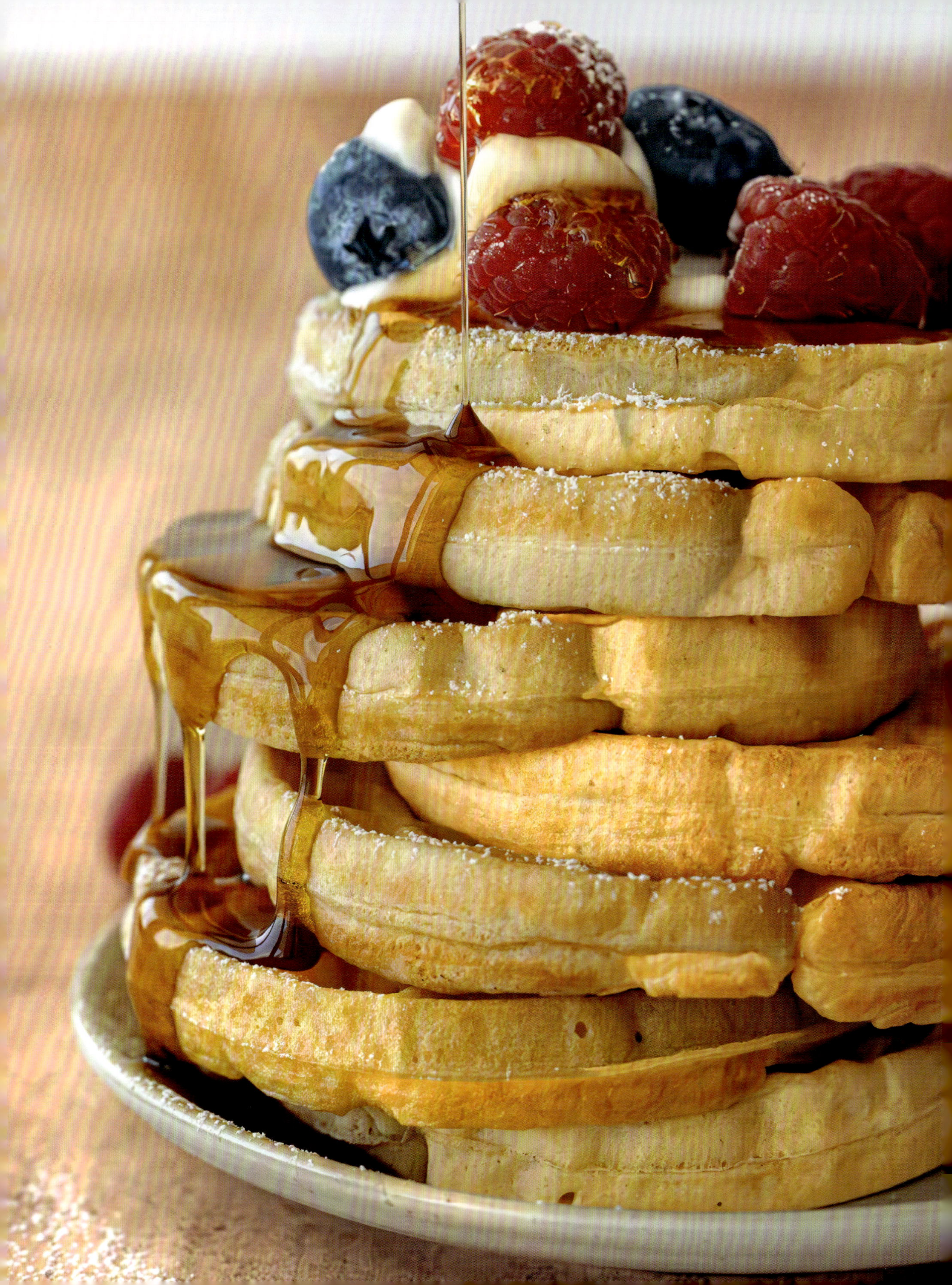

PROTEIN WAFFLES

8½ tbsp (130g) egg whites
⅔ cup (150g) cottage cheese
2 scoops (62g) protein powder of choice
8 tsp (20g) coconut flour
½ tsp (2.5g) baking powder
1 tsp (3g) cinnamon
1 tsp (4g) Stevia sweetener
2 tbsp (30ml) sugar-free maple syrup
1 tbsp (15g) nonfat Greek yogurt
Fresh fruit of choice (optional)

One of my all-time staple breakfasts, these waffles are a protein bomb that'll have you hitting PRs both your bros and your girl appreciate—as long as she accepts the increased risk of an accidental Dutch ovening. I use coconut flour for this recipe because I find that it makes a crispier waffle. If you prefer a fluffier, cakier waffle, all-purpose flour might be a good swap for you.

1. Preheat the waffle maker.
2. To a large mixing bowl, add the egg whites, cottage cheese, protein powder, coconut flour, baking powder, cinnamon, and Stevia. Stir together until the mixture resembles a chunky batter.
3. Spray both sides of the waffle iron with nonstick cooking spray. Scoop the batter into the center of the waffle maker, leaving space around the edges, and close the lid. Remove when the waffle maker indicates the waffle is cooked. Repeat until you have used all the batter.
4. Top the waffles with the maple syrup, Greek yogurt, and fresh fruit of choice (if using).

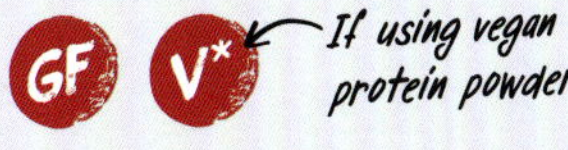

makes 1 serving

NUTRITION (PER SERVING)

538 calories	**5g** fat
97g protein	**24g** net carbs

MICROWAVE BREAKFAST BOWL

1 tbsp (14g) light margarine
1 egg
3 tbsp (45ml) Silk unsweetened cashew milk
Salt and pepper, to taste
¼ cup (37.5g) chopped red bell pepper
¼ cup (15g) chopped cilantro
¼ cup (60g) chopped grilled chicken breast
2 tbsp (14g) shredded low-fat cheddar cheese
1–2 slices low-calorie bread, broken into bite-size pieces
Hot sauce (optional)

This bowl is a great recipe when you want to make a meal out of something other than the takeout containers stacked in your fridge. Throw any veggies and protein into a bowl with cheese, and you'll be making microwave magic in no time. You can make a million different variations of this recipe, as long as you have the basics down pat. Switch the cheddar for feta and the cilantro for chopped spinach, throw in some fresh dill, and you have a Greek breakfast bowl. Meatless Monday? Scrap the chicken, and add tempeh bacon and mushrooms. What's your favorite combo?

1. To a microwave-safe bowl, add the margarine and microwave until melted.
2. Add the egg and cashew milk. Season with salt and pepper and whisk. Add the bell pepper, cilantro, chicken, and cheese and stir to combine.
3. Gently fold in the bread pieces until completely coated. Let the mixture sit for 1 to 2 minutes, allowing the bread to absorb the egg.
4. Microwave on high for 2 minutes, or until the mixture is firm and pulls away from the edges of the bowl. Top with the hot sauce for some spice (if using).

makes 1 serving

NUTRITION (PER SERVING)	
370 calories	**14g** fat
28g protein	**33g** net carbs

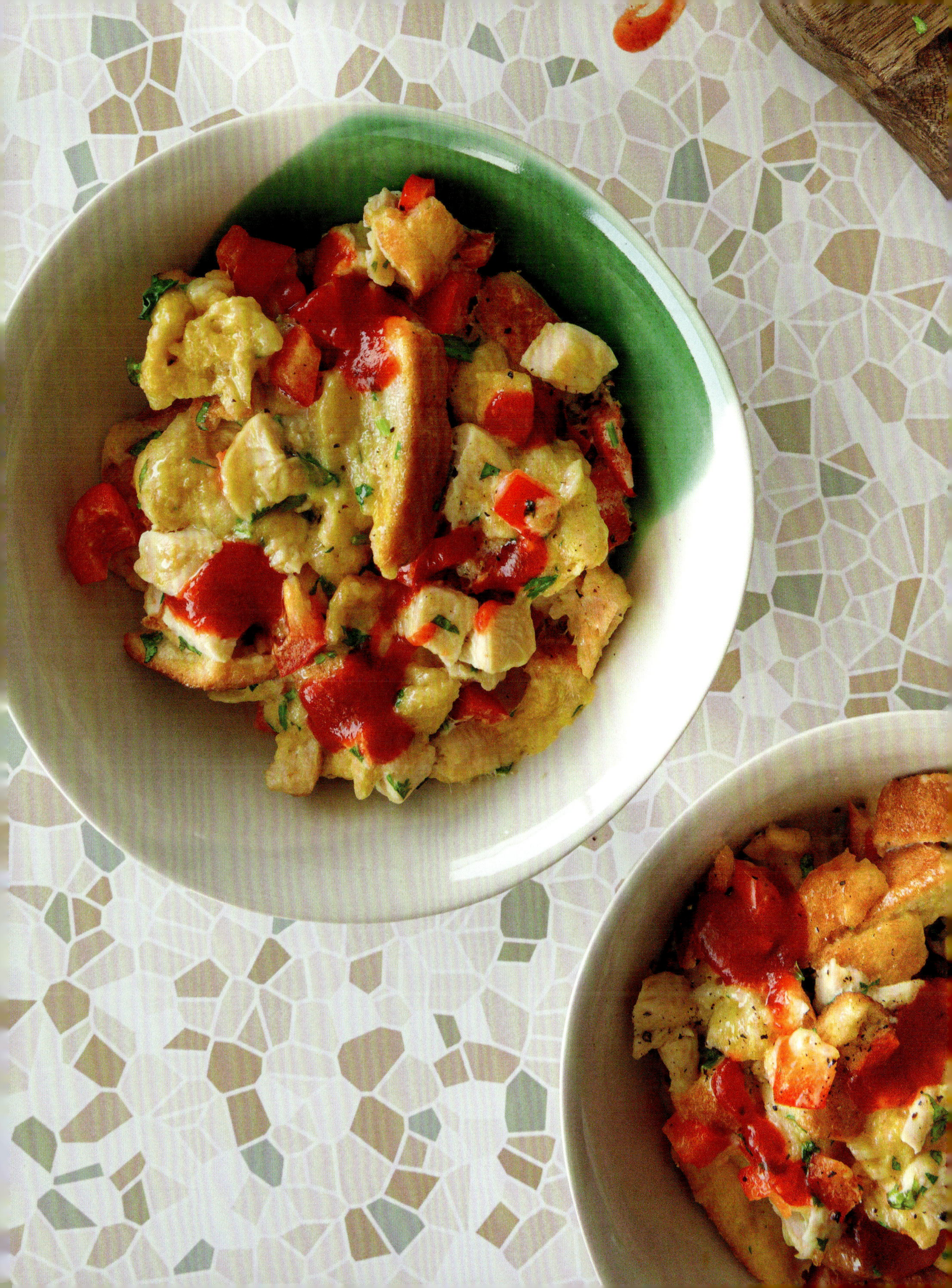

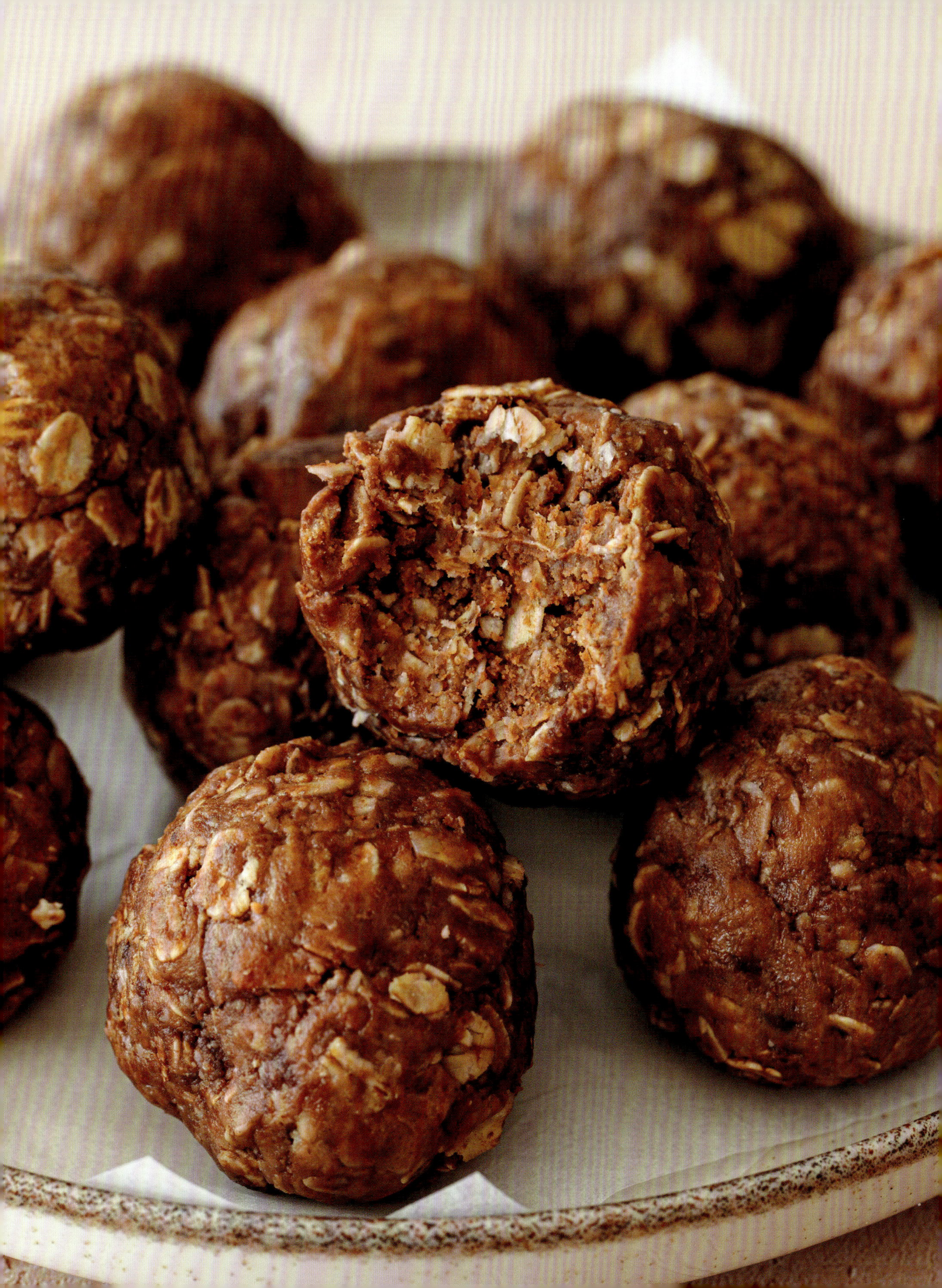

CHOCOLATE PEANUT BUTTER NO-BAKE ENERGY BALLS

- 1 cup (104g) PB2 Powdered Peanut Butter
- 2 scoops (62g) chocolate peanut-butter protein powder
- 1½ cups (120g) quick oats
- ¼ cup (60ml) sugar-free maple syrup
- 2 tbsp (20g) chocolate chips

By manipulating my nuts and using the powdered instead of the real thing, I've made this calorie-dense morning snack more diet friendly while retaining the full taste. Feel free to use peanut butter, almond butter, or any kind of smooth nut butter, instead of the powdered variety—just remember to adjust your macros accordingly. The protein powder flavor is also really up to you, because what *doesn't* taste good with peanut butter and chocolate chips?

1. To a large mixing bowl, add the PB2 Powdered Peanut Butter. Slowly add room temperature water and stir until it reaches the consistency of a creamy peanut butter (about ¾ cup [180ml] water in total).
2. Add the protein powder, oats, maple syrup, and chocolate chips. Mix until combined.
3. With your palms, roll the mixture into large, tightly packed golf-ball-size spheres. This can be done with gloves to avoid sticky hands.
4. Place the balls in the fridge to let them firm up or eat right away! If you're storing them in the fridge, place the balls in a single layer on a plate and cover.

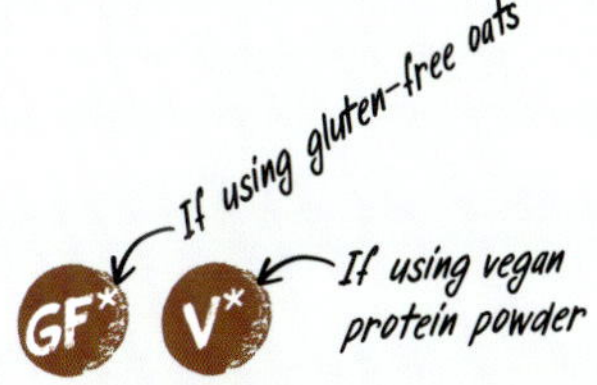

makes 6 balls / 6 servings

NUTRITION (PER SERVING)

155 calories	**3.5g** fat
15g protein	**33g** net carbs

PB&J PROTEIN ROLL UP

5 tbsp (40g) protein pancake mix
1 scoop (31g) protein powder
3¼ tbsp (50g) egg whites
½ cup (50g) Silk unsweetened cashew milk
Sprinkle of cinnamon
7½ tsp (15g) PB2 Powdered Peanut Butter
3 tsp (15g) creamy peanut butter
4 tbsp (80g) sugar-free strawberry jam

Everyone's favorite sandwich when they were kids has gone through puberty right alongside us. And bonus points for me, because this version comes without a crust you have to beg your mom to cut off. More protein, the same taste of childhood. If you're wondering what protein pancake mix would be best, I use Kodiak Power Cakes, but any "just add water" mix will work just as great. As for which protein powder flavor is superior? I'd go for vanilla, peanut butter, or even snickerdoodle.

1. To a medium mixing bowl, add the pancake mix, protein powder, egg whites, cashew milk, and cinnamon and lightly whisk together for 30 seconds to 1 minute, until a thick batter is formed.
2. Spray a large frying pan with nonstick cooking spray and heat over medium-high heat. Into the heated pan, pour the batter, tilting the pan and using a spatula to ensure the batter covers the entire bottom. Let cook for 3 to 4 minutes, until the top starts to bubble and the edges are set. Flip the pancake and cook for an additional 2 to 3 minutes. Remove from the heat and set aside.
3. While the pancake is cooking, in a small bowl, mix the PB2 Powdered Peanut Butter with 1½ tbsp (23ml) water and stir together until it is creamy and there is no dry powder remaining.
4. To the PB2 mixture, add the peanut butter and stir together.
5. Place the pancake on a large plate and spread the peanut-butter mixture and jam evenly over its surface.
6. Starting from one edge, roll the pancake into a long log. Cut in half and enjoy!

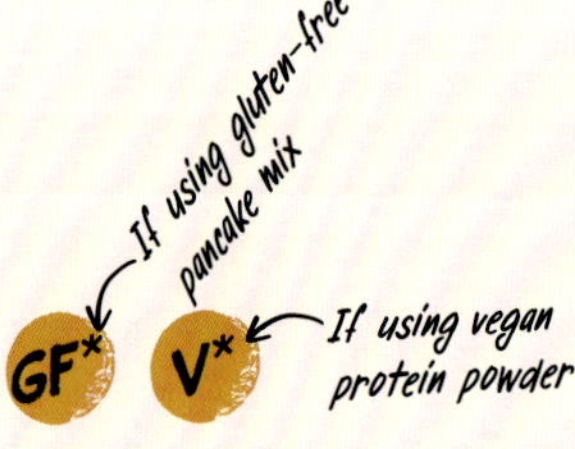

makes 1 serving

NUTRITION (PER SERVING)

486 calories	**10.5g** fat
45g protein	**32g** carbs

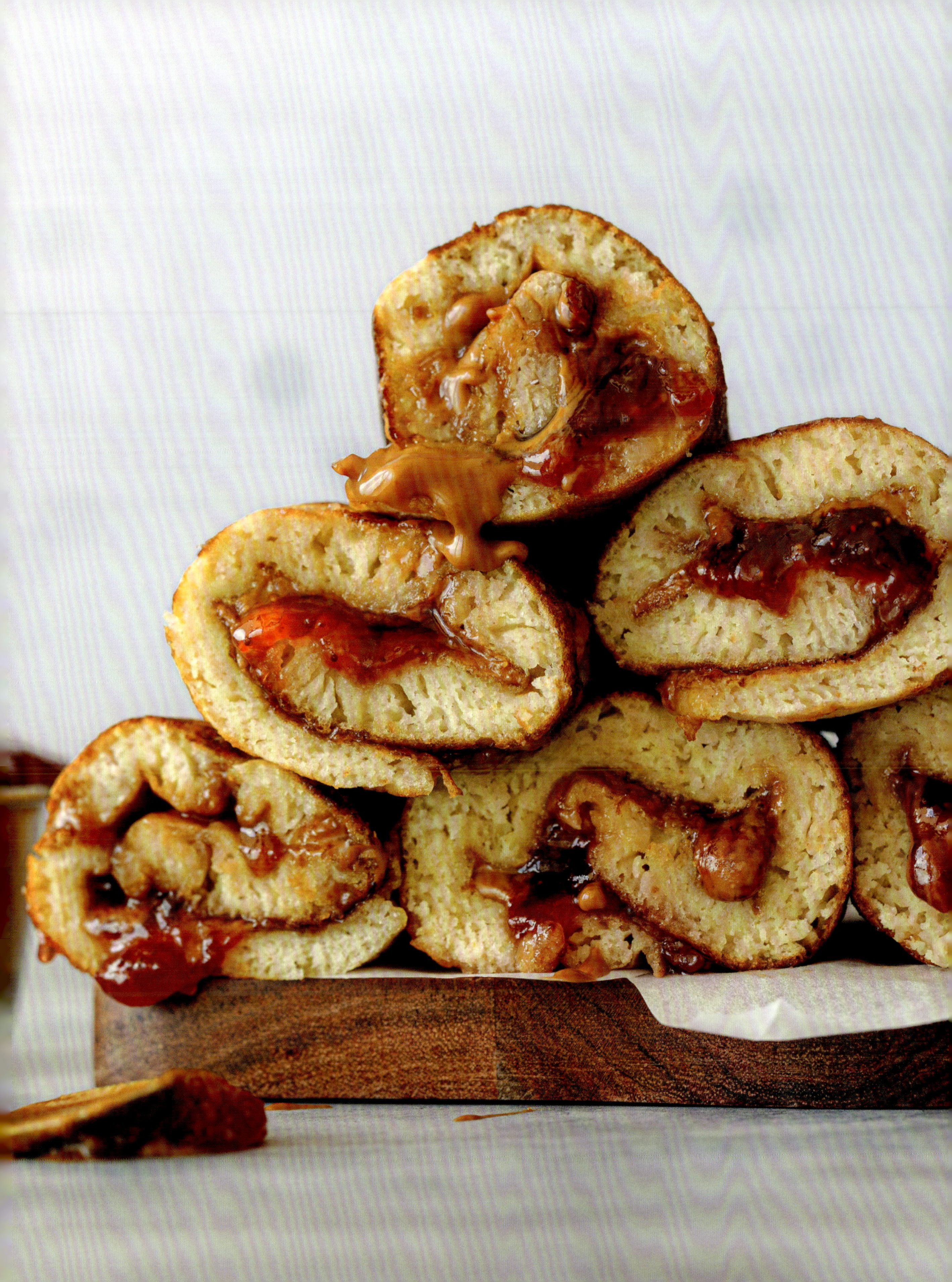

BREAKFAST TOAST 3 WAYS

Some people say breakfast is the most important meal of the day—I say it's just an excuse to eat fancy toast. Why settle for plain butter or jam when you can have Autumn on Toast, packed with cozy pumpkin goodness? Or maybe you're feeling a little extra and want Katie's Sweet Cottage-Cheese Toast? And then there's Ricotta Be Kiddin' Me Spread (because I had to), bringing creamy, herby, lemony heaven that can go sweet *or* savory. Whichever way you slice it, these toasts prove one thing: Even the most basic breakfast should never be boring.

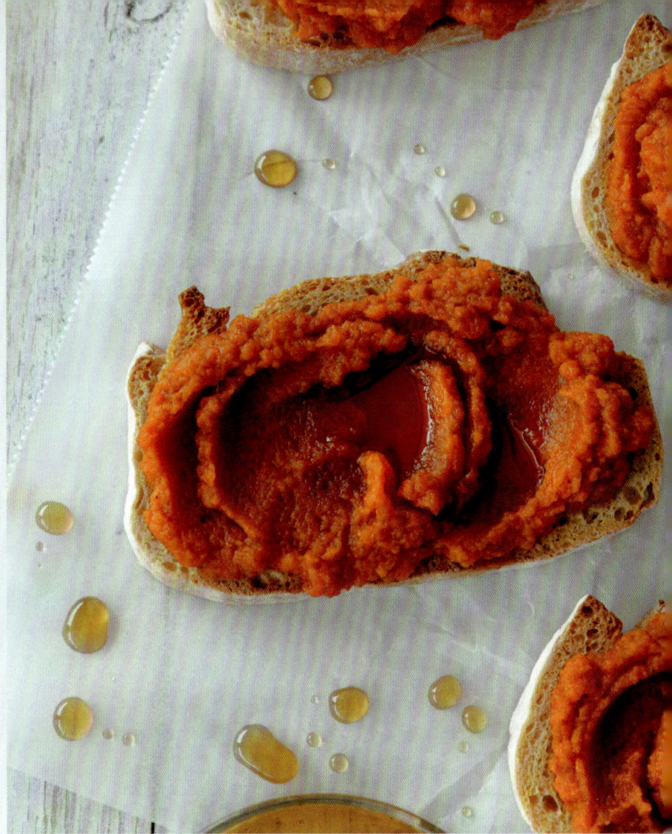

makes 4 pieces of toast each / 4 servings each

NUTRITION (PER SERVING)

Autumn on Toast

233 calories	**3.8g** fat
6.2g protein	**43g** net carbs

Katie's Sweet Cottage-Cheese Toast

265 calories	**1.8g** fat
20g protein	**32.5g** net carbs

Ricotta Be Kiddin' Me Spread

287.5 calories	**10.3g** fat
17g protein	**32g** net carbs

AUTUMN ON TOAST

- 1 (15oz / 425ml) can pumpkin purée
- 4½ tbsp (67.5ml) maple syrup
- 1 tbsp (12g) Swerve brown sugar
- ¼ cup (60ml) Silk unsweetened cashew milk
- ¾ tsp (2.25mg) ground cinnamon
- ¼ tsp (750mg) ground ginger
- ¼ tsp (750mg) ground clove
- ¼ tsp (750mg) ground nutmeg
- 4 slices of toasted sourdough bread

1. Place a medium saucepan over medium-high heat. Add the pumpkin purée, maple syrup, brown sugar, cashew milk, cinnamon, ginger, clove, and nutmeg. Stir until the ingredients are well combined.
2. Bring the mixture to a boil, then reduce the heat to low and simmer gently.
3. Cook the spread for 15 minutes, stirring occasionally, until it thickens and has a slightly sticky consistency.
4. Remove the saucepan from the heat and allow the spread to cool slightly. Serve warm or cold on the toasted sourdough.

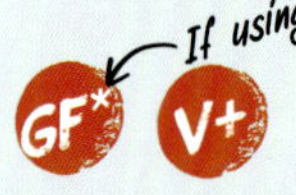

*If using gluten-free bread

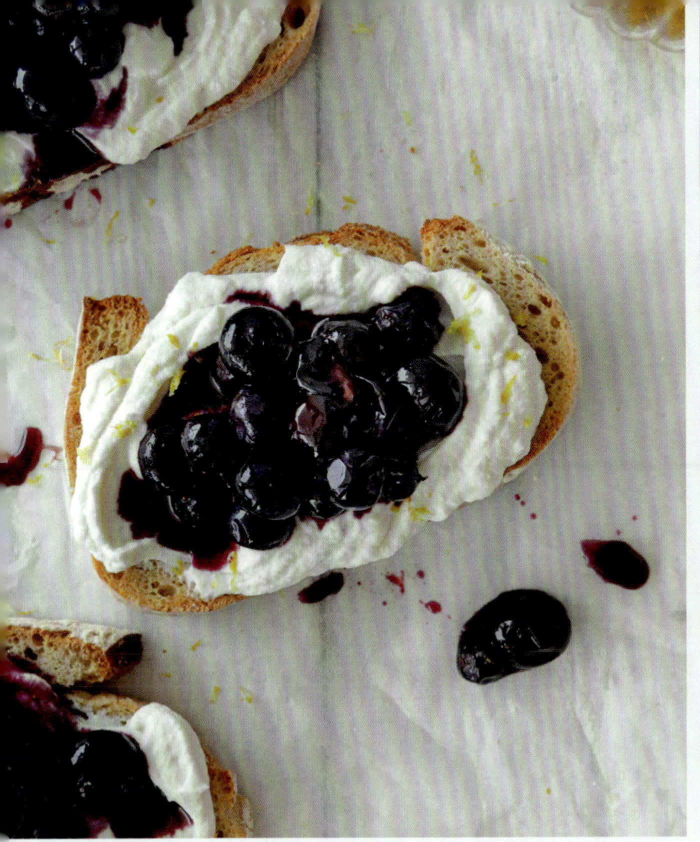

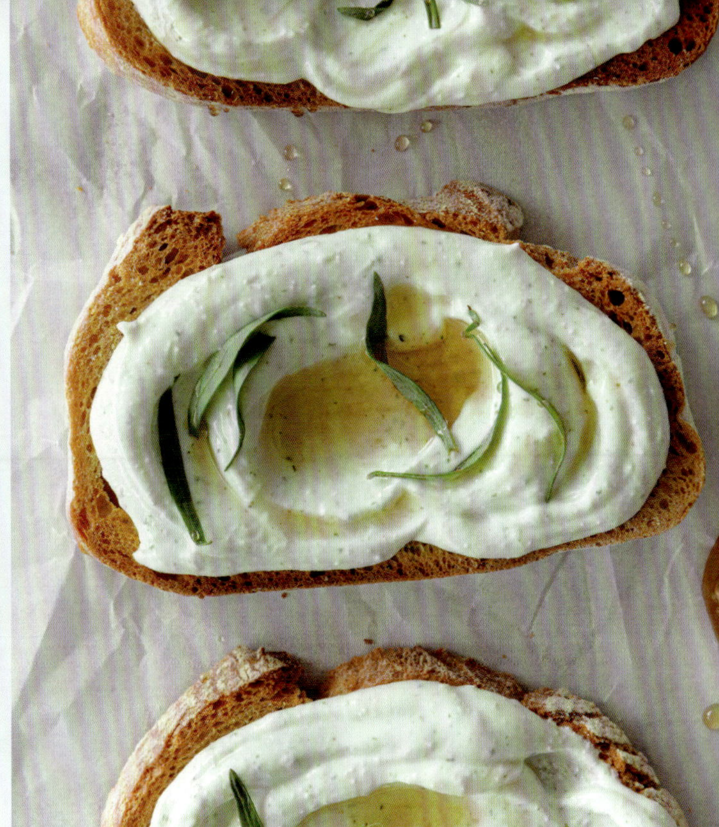

KATIE'S SWEET COTTAGE-CHEESE TOAST

2¼ cups (500g) low-fat cottage cheese
2 tbsp (40g) honey
Juice of ½ lemon
1½ cups (200g) frozen blueberries
4 slices of toasted sourdough bread

1. In a blender, place the cottage cheese, honey, and lemon juice. Blend on high until the mixture is smooth and creamy. Set aside.
2. To a microwave-safe bowl, add the blueberries. Microwave on high for 1 minute, or until the blueberries are warm and saucy.
3. Spread the cottage-cheese mixture evenly over the toast. Top with the warmed blueberries, drizzling the blueberry juices over top for extra flavor. Serve immediately and enjoy.

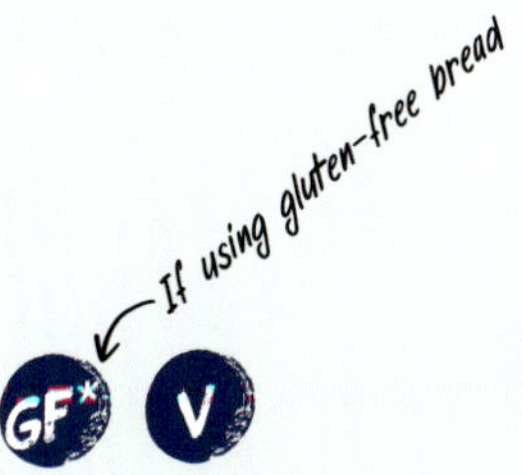

RICOTTA BE KIDDIN' ME SPREAD

2 cups (500g) low-fat ricotta
1 garlic clove
1 tbsp (15ml) olive oil
¼ cup (about 50g) chopped fresh herbs of choice (I use tarragon)
¾ tsp (2.25g) lemon zest
1½ tbsp (23ml) lemon juice
½ tsp (1.5g) salt
¼ tsp (0.75g) black pepper
½ tsp (1.5g) chili flakes
4 slices of toasted sourdough bread

1. In a blender, place the ricotta, garlic, olive oil, fresh herbs, lemon zest, lemon juice, salt, and black pepper. Blend on low until the mixture is smooth and creamy, similar to the texture of cream cheese.
2. Spread the ricotta mixture evenly over the toast. Sprinkle with the chili flakes for extra heat. This spread pairs well with eggs, smoked salmon, or a drizzle of honey for added flavor.

If using gluten-free bread

GF* V

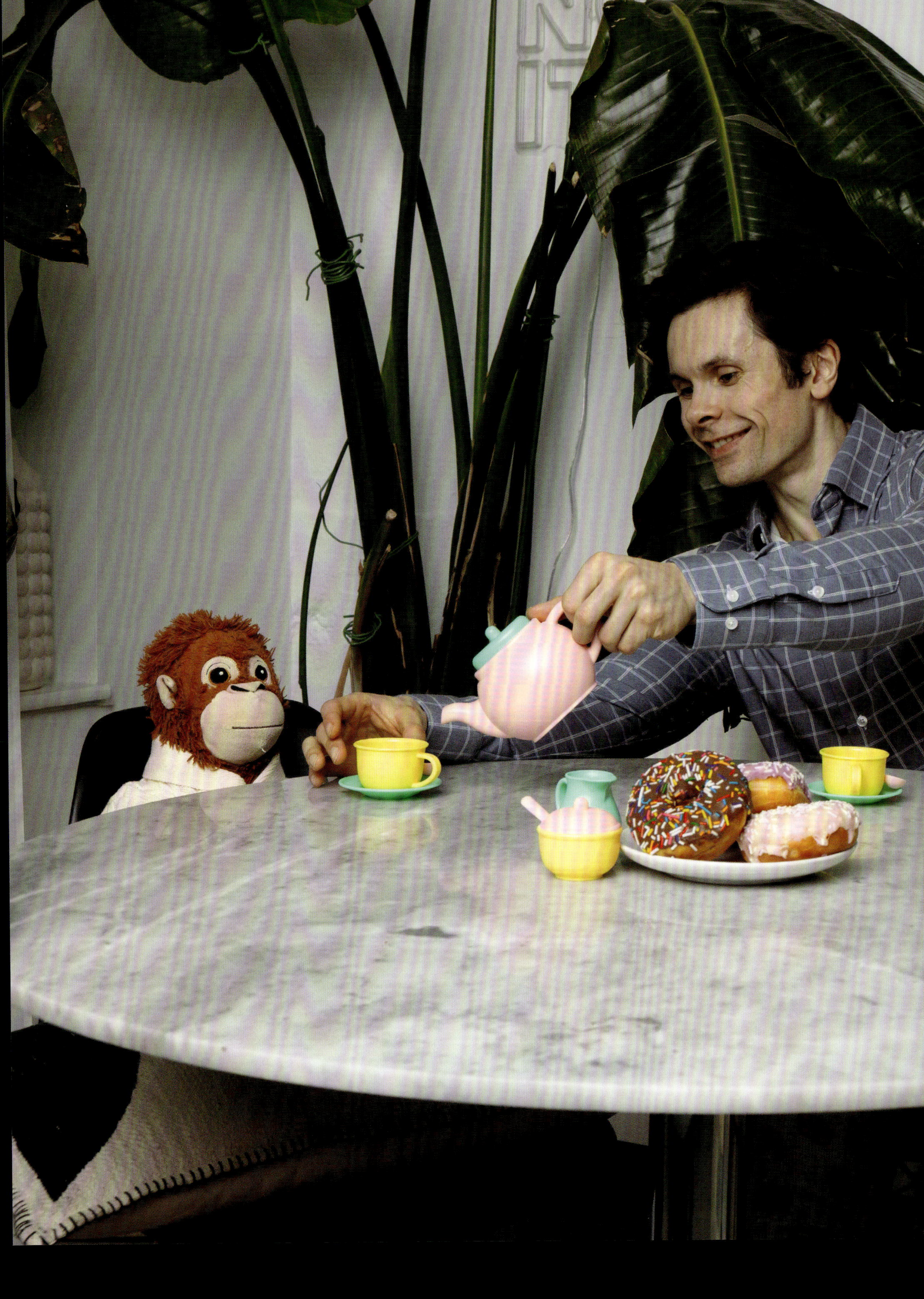

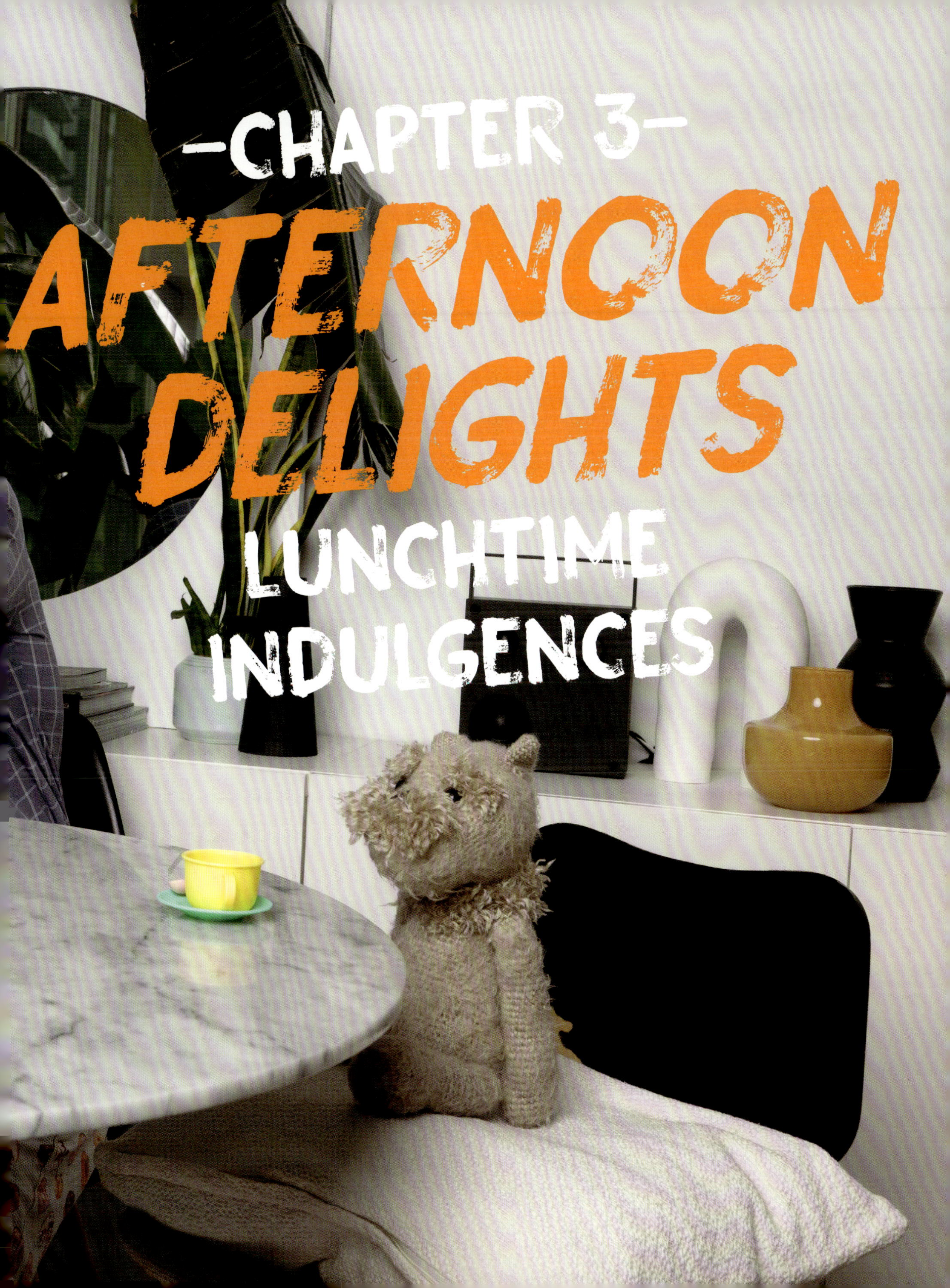

—CHAPTER 3—

AFTERNOON DELIGHTS

LUNCHTIME INDULGENCES

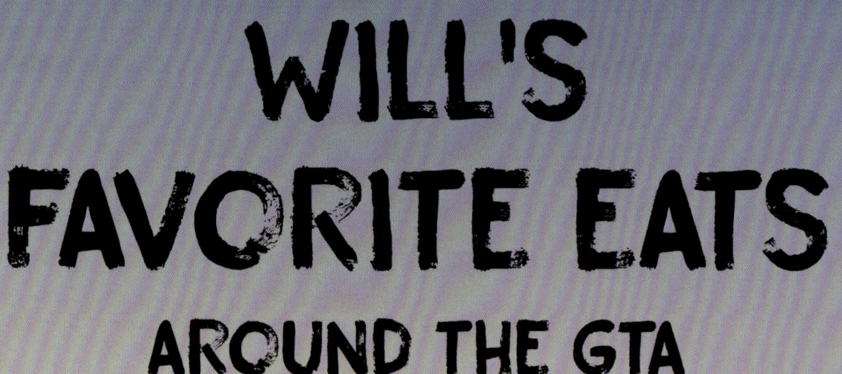

A few things to get straight if you ever visit Toronto: It's the CN Tower, not the Space Needle. You don't need a parka in July. And these are the restaurants (and dishes) you need to try:

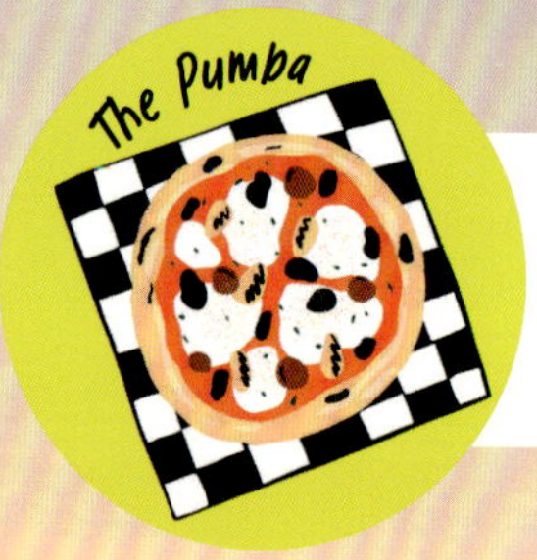

Defina Wood Fired
1485 Dupont St.
Toronto, ON M6P 3S2

All You Knead Bakery
9505 Keele St. Unit #11
Vaughan, ON L6A 1W3

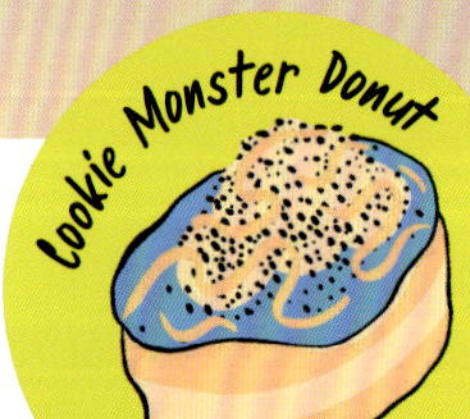

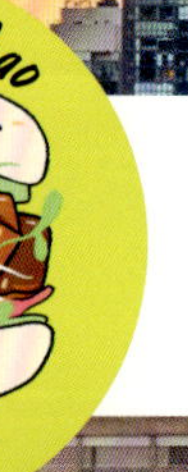

Lee Restaurant
497 Richmond St. W
Toronto, ON M5V 1Y3

Singapore Style Slaw

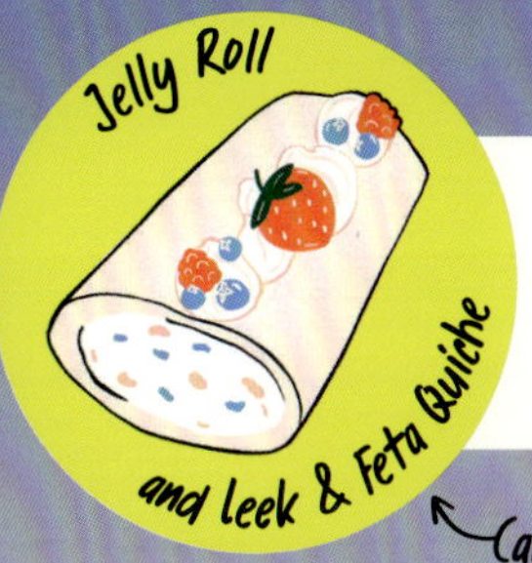

Village Grocer
4476 16th Ave.
Unionville, ON L3R 0M1

(anything from the bakery!)

King Taps
100 King St. W
Toronto, ON M5X 1E1

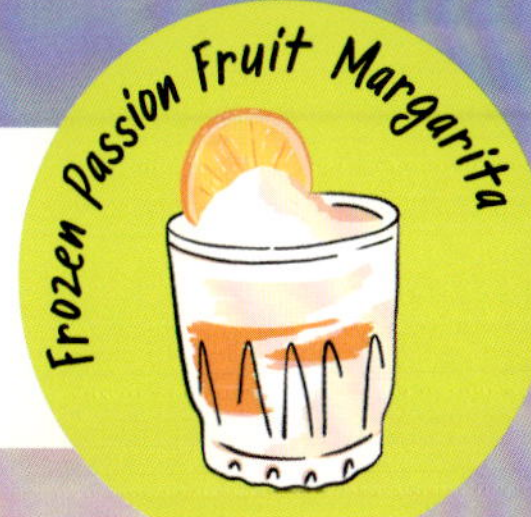

(with a pizza on the side of course)

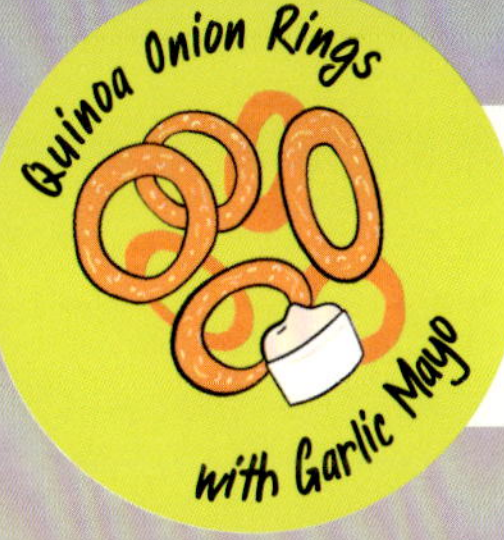

Fresh on Front
47 Front St. E
Toronto, ON M5E 1B3

Unionville Arms
189 Main St Unionville
Unionville, ON L3R 2G8

Grilled Chicken Pizza

Steamed Soup Dumplings

Ding Tai Fung
3235 Hwy 7 #18B
Markham, ON L3R 3P3

Osaka Sushi
5762 Hwy 7
Markham, ON L3P 1A5)

Green Dragon Roll

SPICY CRISPY CHICKEN SANDWICHES

for the chicken:

1 cup (240ml) 1% buttermilk
1½ tsp (4.5g) paprika
1½ tsp (4.5g) garlic powder
1½ tsp (4.5g) salt
1½ tsp (4.5g) pepper
2 chicken breasts, about 8oz (225g) each
1 cup (120g) all-purpose flour
½ tsp (1.5g) onion powder
¼ tsp (0.75g) cayenne pepper

for the Cajun mayo:

¼ cup (60ml) light mayo
¼ cup (60g) nonfat Greek yogurt
1 tsp (5ml) hot sauce
1 tsp (3g) Cajun seasoning
½ tsp (1.5g) garlic powder

for the sandwich:

2 brioche buns
6 slices of extra-crunchy sweet pickle

makes 2 sandwiches / 2 servings

NUTRITION (PER SERVING)

533 calories	**15g** fat
59g protein	**35g** net carbs

The Colonel has his secret recipe, but I think you all deserve to know how best to manipulate your meat at home. Time to grab a couple of chicken breasts, and give 'em a homemade sauce. By the end, you'll have a pair worthy of a Baywatch montage. Some of you might be skeptical about using buttermilk, but despite the name, it actually has the same calories as 1% milk and is packed with more protein and calcium. Buttermilk is also more acidic than regular milk or nut milk, so it really breaks down tough meat and infuses it with more flavor. So, if you like your breasts juicy, buttermilk is your best friend.

1. **To prepare the chicken:** In a large resealable plastic bag, place the buttermilk, 1 teaspoon (3g) of the paprika, 1 teaspoon (3g) of the garlic powder, 1 teaspoon (3g) of the salt, and 1 teaspoon (3g) of the pepper. Seal the bag and shake lightly to combine.
2. To the bag, add the chicken breasts, ensuring they are thoroughly coated in the buttermilk mixture. Let the chicken marinate for at least 2 hours, preferably overnight.
3. To a large bowl, add the remaining ½ teaspoon (1.5g) of the paprika, the remaining ½ teaspoon (1.5g) garlic powder, remaining ½ teaspoon (1.5g) salt, and remaining ½ teaspoon (1.5g) pepper, along with the flour, onion powder, and cayenne pepper.
4. One at a time, remove the chicken breasts from the plastic bag and place them in the flour mixture, evenly coating both sides of each breast.
5. Spray one side of each chicken breast with nonstick cooking spray and place them, sprayed-side up, in the air fryer at 390°F (195°C) for 25 minutes, flipping the chicken halfway through and spraying the top again with nonstick cooking spray.
6. **To make the Cajun mayo:** To a small bowl, add the mayo, Greek yogurt, hot sauce, Cajun seasoning, and garlic powder and stir to combine.
7. **To assemble the sandwiches:** In a skillet over medium-high heat, toast the insides of the brioche buns until golden and crisp. Spread a generous layer of the Cajun mayo on the brioche buns, followed by 3 pickle slices, and finally the chicken breast. Repeat for the second sandwich. Enjoy!

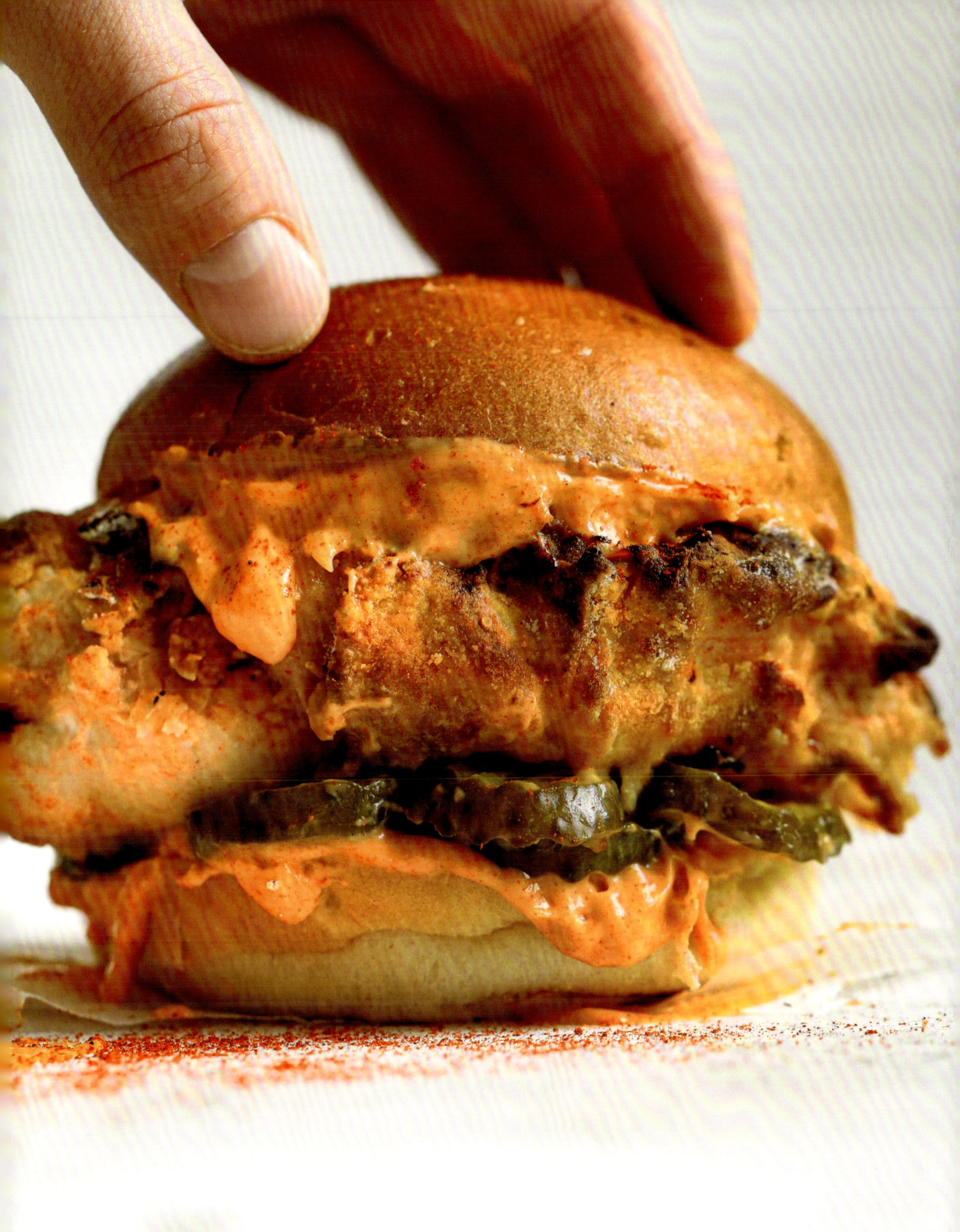

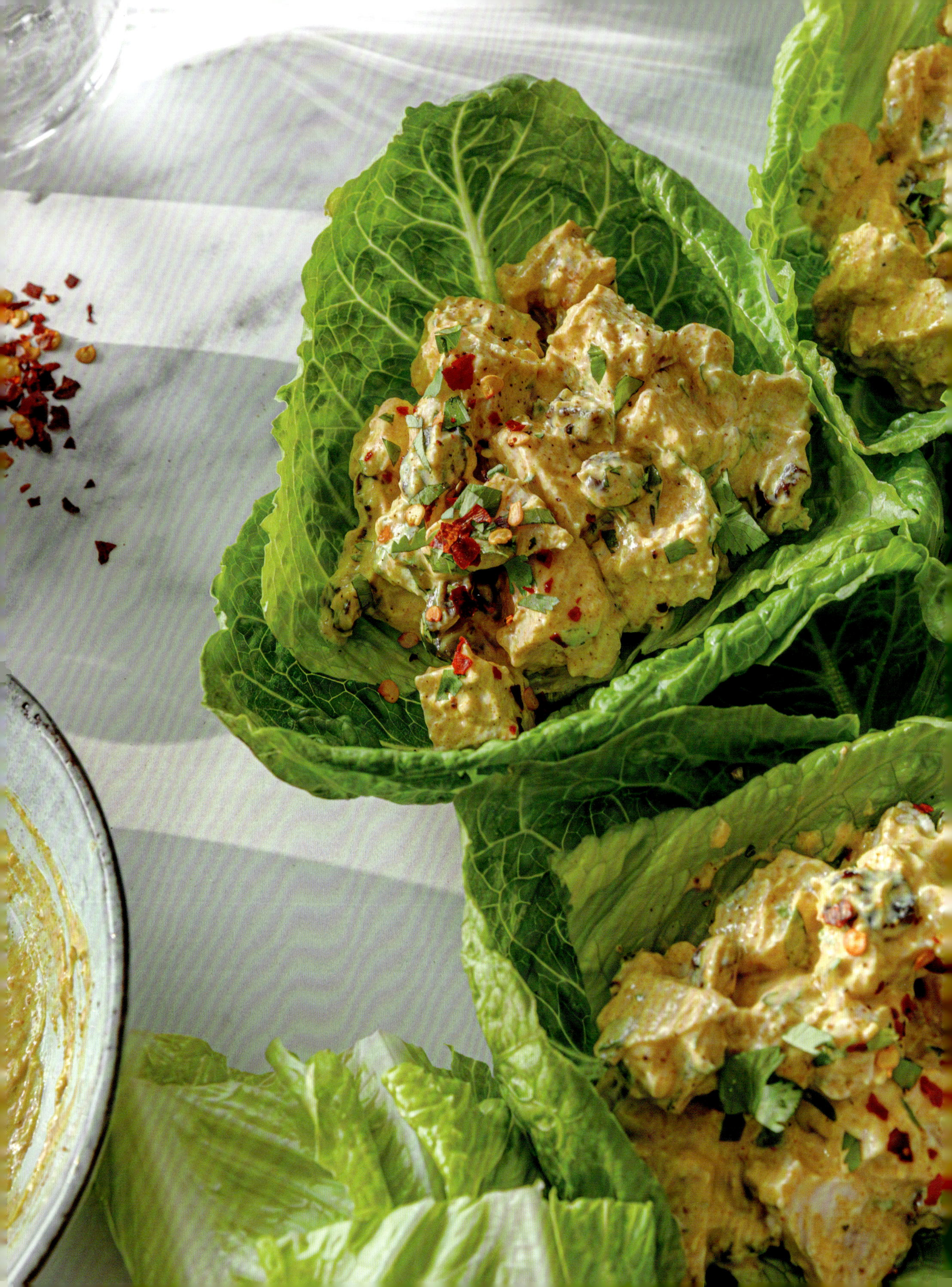

CURRIED CHICKEN LETTUCE WRAPS

- ½ cup (115g) nonfat Greek yogurt
- 1 tsp (3g) curry powder
- 1 tsp (5g) tomato purée or crushed tomatoes
- ¾ cup (100g) diced grilled chicken breast
- 2 tbsp (7.5g) roughly chopped cilantro
- 2 tbsp (20g) raisins
- 3 large romaine lettuce leaves, washed and patted dry
- Salt and pepper, to taste

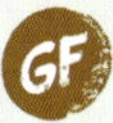

makes 3 wraps / 3 servings

NUTRITION (PER SERVING)

110 calories	**2g** fat
13g protein	**9g** net carbs

Though I'm not usually a fan of wrapping anything up, these lettuce wraps always bring me a pleasurable experience that I'm excited to share with all of you. A top-tier meal-prep option, the curried-chicken mixture is something you can put together quickly, and it will stay fresh in your fridge for 4 to 5 days. If you're extra hungry, make a full meal out of it, and fill a pita or tortilla wrap. If you can't get enough, stand by the fridge and shovel some directly into your mouth. We all do it.

1. To a large mixing bowl, add the Greek yogurt, curry powder, and tomato purée and stir to combine. Add the chicken, cilantro, and raisins and stir well.
2. To each lettuce leaf, add ⅓ of the curried-chicken mixture, season with salt and pepper, wrap it up, and happy snacking!

PECAN CHICKEN SALAD

¼ cup (28g) pecans
½ cup (115g) 2% Greek yogurt
¼ cup (60ml) light mayonnaise
2 tsp (10ml) Dijon mustard
1 tsp (5ml) white wine vinegar
Salt and pepper, to taste
1 lb (450g) grilled chicken breast, chopped
3 stalks of celery, chopped
¼ cup (30g) chopped red onion
¼ cup (15g) roughly chopped fresh parsley
¼ cup (12g) roughly chopped fresh dill

When I think of chicken sandwiches, I think of lots of mayo. Kind of gross, right? Here's a fresher version that won't remind you of stale beer at a college tailgate party. This is a great way to get rid of any extra chicken you have left over from dinner the night before. It works equally well with shredded rotisserie chicken if you want to skip cooking the chicken entirely. Enjoy the salad on its own, or add it to a sandwich or on top of some leafy greens.

1. In a small frying pan over medium-high heat, place the pecans and toast them for 3 to 4 minutes, stirring occasionally, until fragrant and browned. These will burn easily, so keep an eye on them. Once the pecans are toasted, remove them from the heat and finely chop them. Set aside.
2. To a large bowl, add the Greek yogurt, mayo, Dijon mustard, and white wine vinegar and season with salt and pepper. Mix to create a creamy salad dressing.
3. To the dressing, add the chicken, celery, red onion, parsley, dill, and pecans and stir to coat well.

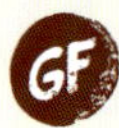

makes 5 servings

NUTRITION (PER SERVING)

190 calories	**10g** fat
31g protein	**4g** net carbs

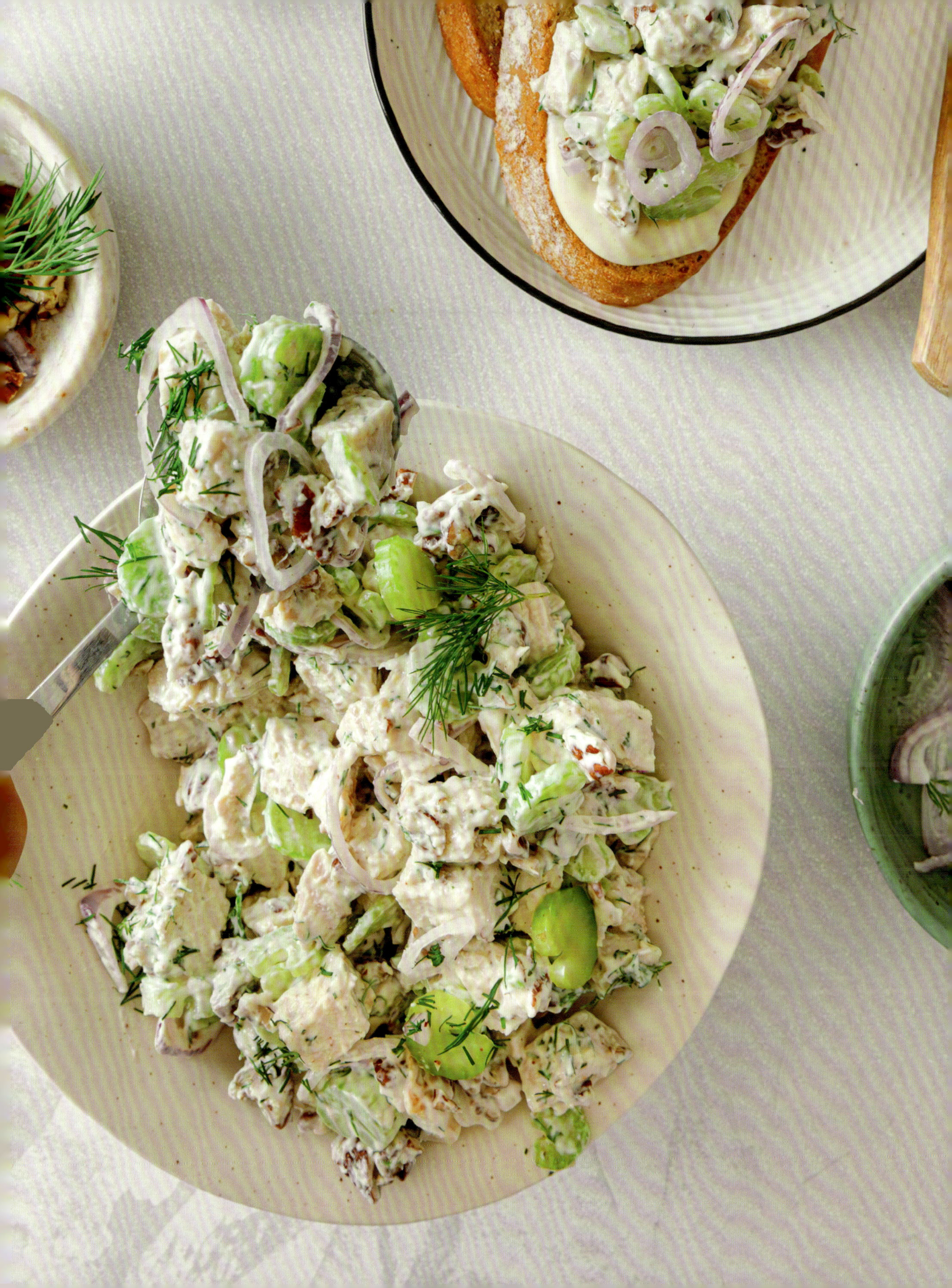

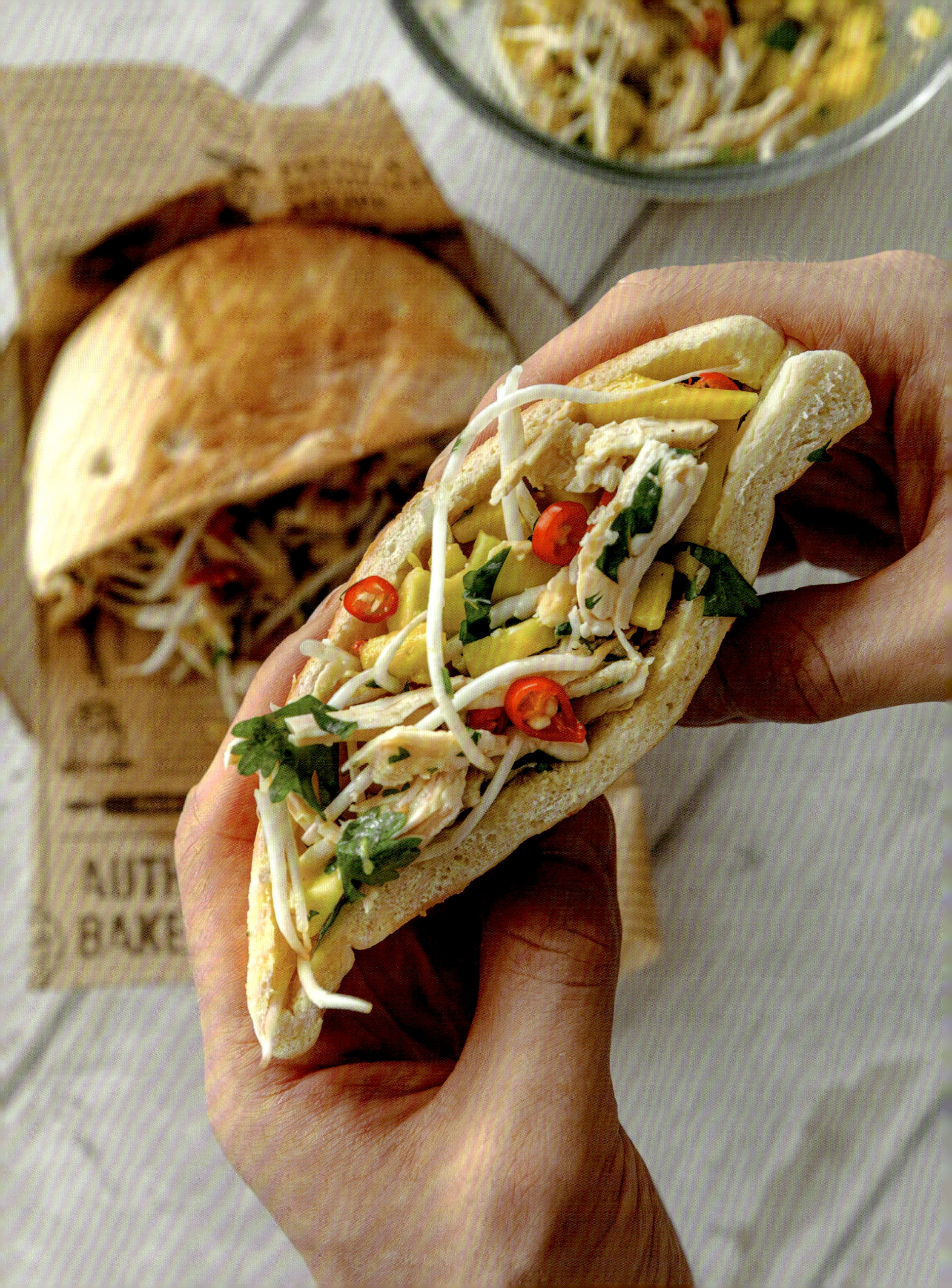

ASIAN MANGO CHICKEN PITA

½ cup (100g) bean sprouts
½ large mango, about 3½oz (100g), thinly sliced
¼ small chile pepper, thinly sliced
¼ cup (15g) cilantro, roughly chopped
5oz (140g) rotisserie chicken breast, shredded
1 tbsp (15ml) sesame-ginger dressing (or other dressing of choice)
1 pita

Packed with protein and low in fat, this perfect postworkout meal is quick and easy yet bursting with flavor, just like me. When you're looking for a good dressing to use for this recipe, try to find something that is roughly 20 calories per tablespoon in order to stay within the macros listed here. Dressings and marinades can be sneakily high calorie, so keep both eyes open.

1. In a large mixing bowl, combine the bean sprouts, mango, chili pepper, cilantro, and chicken breast. Pour the sesame-ginger dressing over top and toss to evenly coat.
2. Heat the pita in the microwave or oven. Once hot, split it open on one side.
3. Stuff the pita with the filling and enjoy leftover filling as a side salad!

makes 1 pita / 1 serving

NUTRITION (PER SERVING)

420 calories | **10g** fat
47g protein | **37g** net carbs

GRILLED VEGETABLE SALAD

for the salad:

1 head of radicchio, cut in half
6–8 asparagus spears
1 portobello mushroom, stem removed
2 endives, ends cut off and guard leaves removed
1 tsp (3g) garlic powder
Salt and pepper, to taste
2–4 tbsp (60g) goat cheese

for the dressing:

½ tsp (250mg) fresh rosemary, chopped
2 tbsp (30ml) grainy mustard
2 tbsp (30ml) balsamic vinegar
2 tbsp (30ml) sugar-free maple syrup
Salt and pepper, to taste

I feel like mixed greens are a little played out, so I made this lettuce-free salad to bring some excitement back to the salad game. Other veggies you can sub that are great on the grill are fennel, bell peppers, zucchini, and, what happens to also be my most used emoji, the eggplant. A great side to complement your meat, or a recipe to double to get a more satisfying meal if you're unfortunately a vegetarian.

1. **To make the salad:** Preheat a barbecue, or if you do not have a barbeque, preheat a grilling pan over medium-high heat.
2. On a baking sheet or large cutting board, lay the radicchio, asparagus, mushroom, and endives and spray the veggies with nonstick cooking spray. Season with the garlic powder and salt and pepper.
3. Place the seasoned vegetables onto the heated barbecue or grilling pan and grill for 3 to 5 minutes, until lightly charred and slightly softened.
4. **To make the dressing:** In a small bowl, combine the rosemary, mustard, balsamic vinegar, and maple syrup and season with salt and pepper. Whisk together to create a thick dressing.
5. Plate the grilled vegetables and pour the dressing over top to create a generous coating.
6. Crumble the goat cheese on top of the grilled vegetables and enjoy!

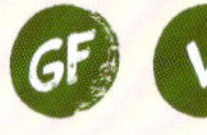

makes 1 salad / 1 serving

NUTRITION (PER SERVING)

383 calories
20g fat
23g protein
25g net carbs

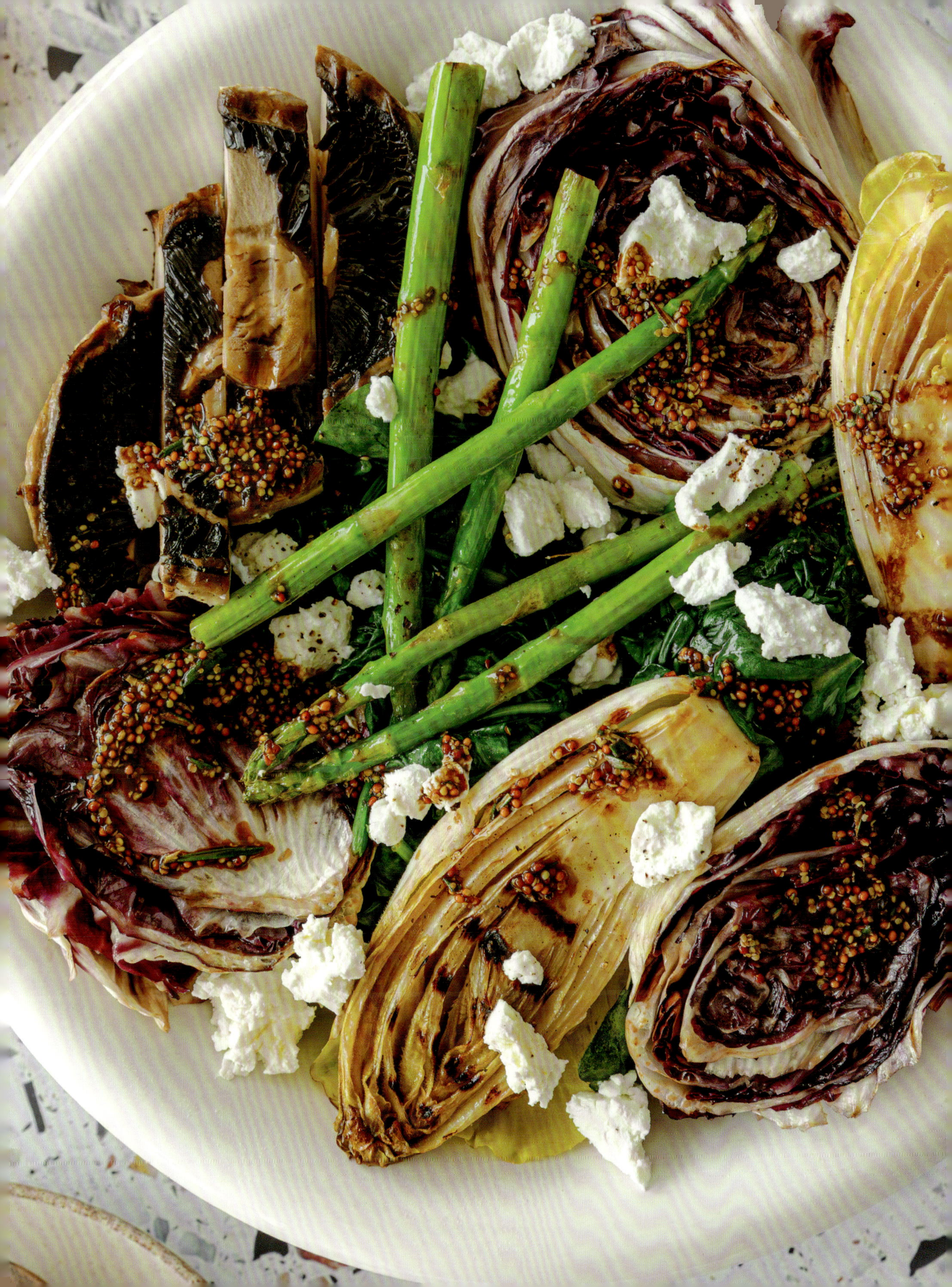

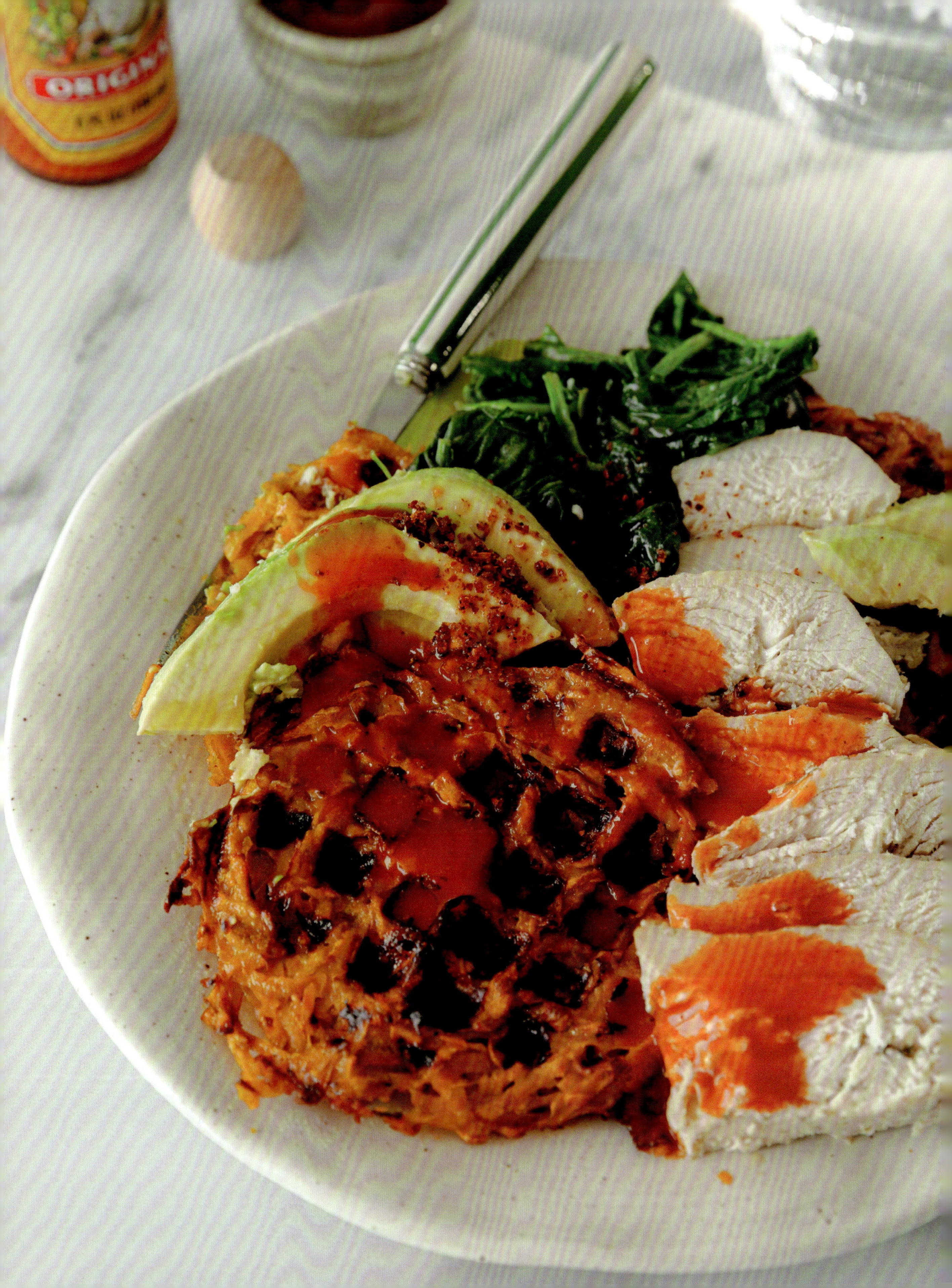

SAVORY SWEET-POTATO CHICKEN AND WAFFLE

- 2 medium sweet potatoes, about 9oz (250g) in total, peeled and shredded
- 1 egg
- 4¼ tbsp (67g) egg whites
- ½ tsp (1.5g) garlic powder
- ½ tsp (1.5g) Tajín seasoning
- ½ tsp (1.5g) salt, plus more to taste
- ¼ tsp (750mg) pepper, plus more to taste
- 1⅔ cup (50g) spinach
- ½ medium avocado (60g), sliced
- 1 grilled chicken breast, about 7oz (200g)
- Hot sauce (optional)

Complex (carbed) Southern belles, these sweet-potato waffles will love anything you top them with, especially some grilled chicken and the explosive juices contained within. The day I created this recipe is the day I discovered Tajín. Although it took me a while to pronounce it properly, I fell in love with its zesty, spicy taste instantly. If you want your meal to really pop with flavor, sprinkle more Tajín over your sliced avocado, and you'll have your own personal fiesta.

1. Preheat a waffle maker.
2. To a large bowl, add the shredded sweet potatoes and press with a paper towel to remove the excess moisture.
3. In a small bowl, whisk together the egg and egg whites. To the shredded sweet potatoes, add the whisked eggs, garlic powder, Tajín, salt, and pepper. Mix until the sweet potato is coated evenly.
4. Spray both sides of the preheated waffle maker with a generous amount of nonstick cooking spray. Scoop an even layer of the sweet potato batter onto the waffle iron and close the lid, letting it cook for 5 to 6 minutes.
5. While the waffle is cooking, heat a small frying pan over medium heat and spray it with nonstick cooking spray. Add the spinach and sauté for 2 to 4 minutes, until wilted. Season with salt and pepper.
6. Once the waffle is cooked through and browned, remove it from the waffle iron, and top with the sautéed spinach, sliced avocado, chicken breast, and hot sauce (if using).

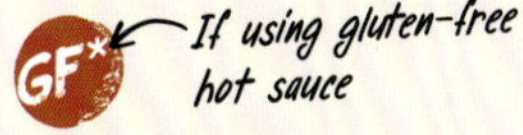

makes 1 serving

NUTRITION (PER SERVING)

675 calories	**16g** fat
76g protein	**56g** net carbs

BBQ PULLED CHICKEN SLIDERS

for the barbecue sauce:

1 (5½oz / 156ml) can tomato paste
¾ cup (180ml) balsamic vinegar
2 tbsp (30ml) low-calorie maple syrup
1 tsp (3g) garlic powder
1 tsp (3g) smoked paprika
Pinch of salt and pepper

for the pulled chicken:

3 chicken breasts, about 18oz (500g) in total

for the coleslaw:

½ medium red cabbage, shredded
½ medium fennel, shredded
¼ cup (15g) roughly chopped parsley
½ cup (120ml) apple cider vinegar
2 tbsp (30ml) olive oil
1 tbsp (15ml) low-calorie maple syrup
Salt and pepper, to taste

for assembly:

6 potato buns, split into halves
12 round slices of pickle

makes 6 sliders / 6 servings

NUTRITION (PER SERVING)

342 calories	**9g** fat
28g protein	**33g** net carbs

I've always said I like my meat pulled, and now you'll know how to give yours a tug for delicious and healthy sliders. It's a top-tier recipe that's equal parts fun to make and fun to eat. If you're a "thighs over breasts" person, I won't stop you. But as long as you keep an eye on your chicken and take it out of the oven before it hits 165°F (74°C), the only thing dry in this kitchen will be the humor in this book.

1. Preheat the oven to 425°F (220°C).
2. **To make the barbecue sauce:** In a medium bowl, whisk together the tomato paste, balsamic vinegar, maple syrup, garlic powder, smoked paprika, and a pinch of salt and pepper.
3. **To make the pulled chicken:** In an oven safe 9 x 9-inch (23 x 23cm) casserole dish, place the chicken breasts. Over the chicken, pour the barbeque sauce to fully coat and massage it into the chicken.
4. Cover the casserole dish with foil and bake for 17 to 20 minutes, until the center of the chicken reaches 155°F (68°C). Once pulled, the residual heat from the oven will bring the chicken to 165°F (74°C).
5. **To make the coleslaw:** While the chicken is baking, to a large mixing bowl, add the cabbage, fennel, and parsley.
6. To create the coleslaw dressing, in a separate small bowl, whisk together the apple cider vinegar, olive oil, and maple syrup and season with salt and pepper. Pour the coleslaw dressing over the cabbage mixture and toss until evenly coated. Set aside.
7. **To assemble:** Once the chicken is cooked, pull it apart using a fork and tongs. Toss the shredded chicken in the remaining barbecue sauce in the casserole dish to fully coat.
8. Place 2 pickle slices on one half of each bun, followed by an even portion of the pulled chicken. Top with the coleslaw and prepare to be amazed.

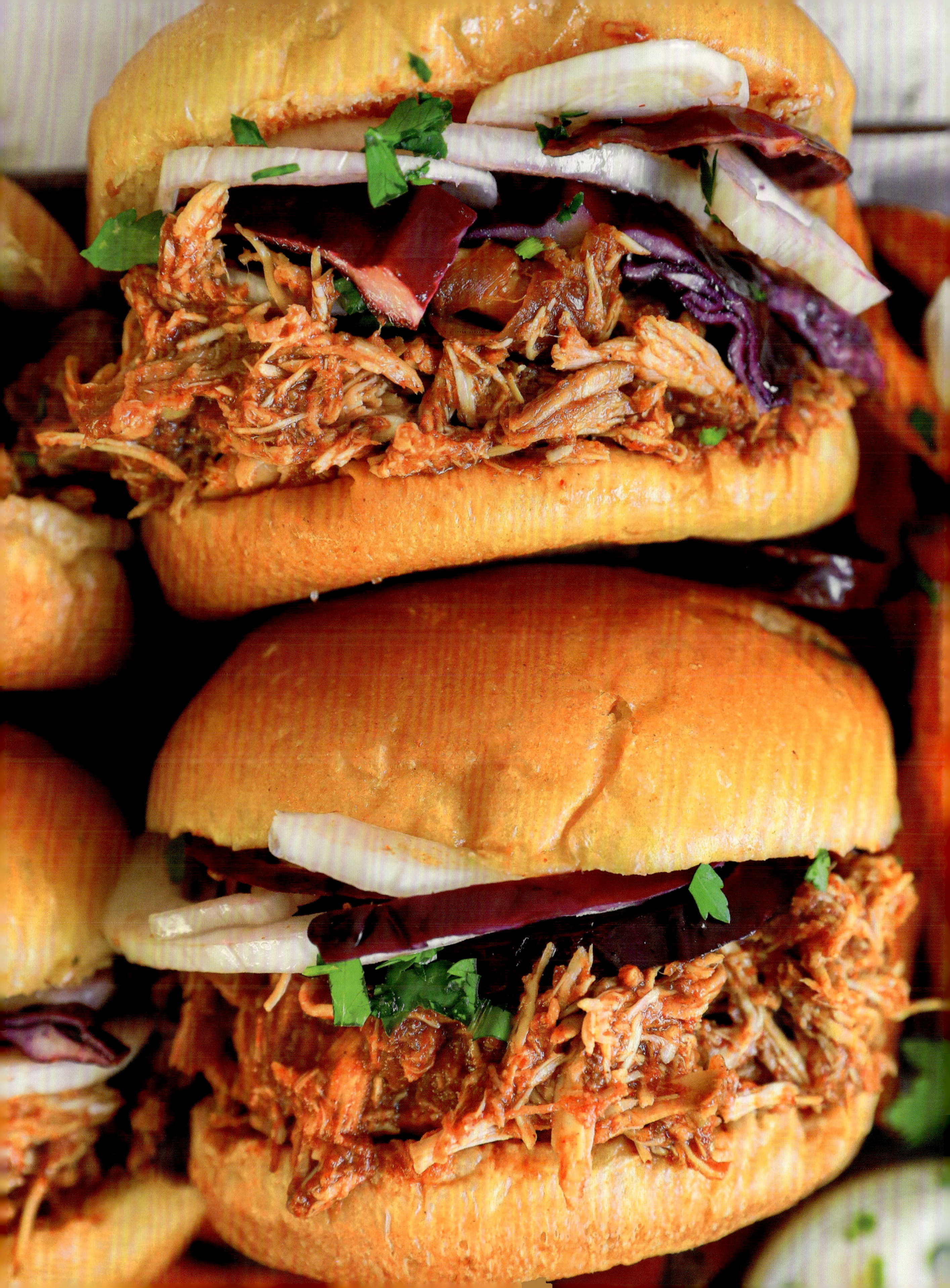

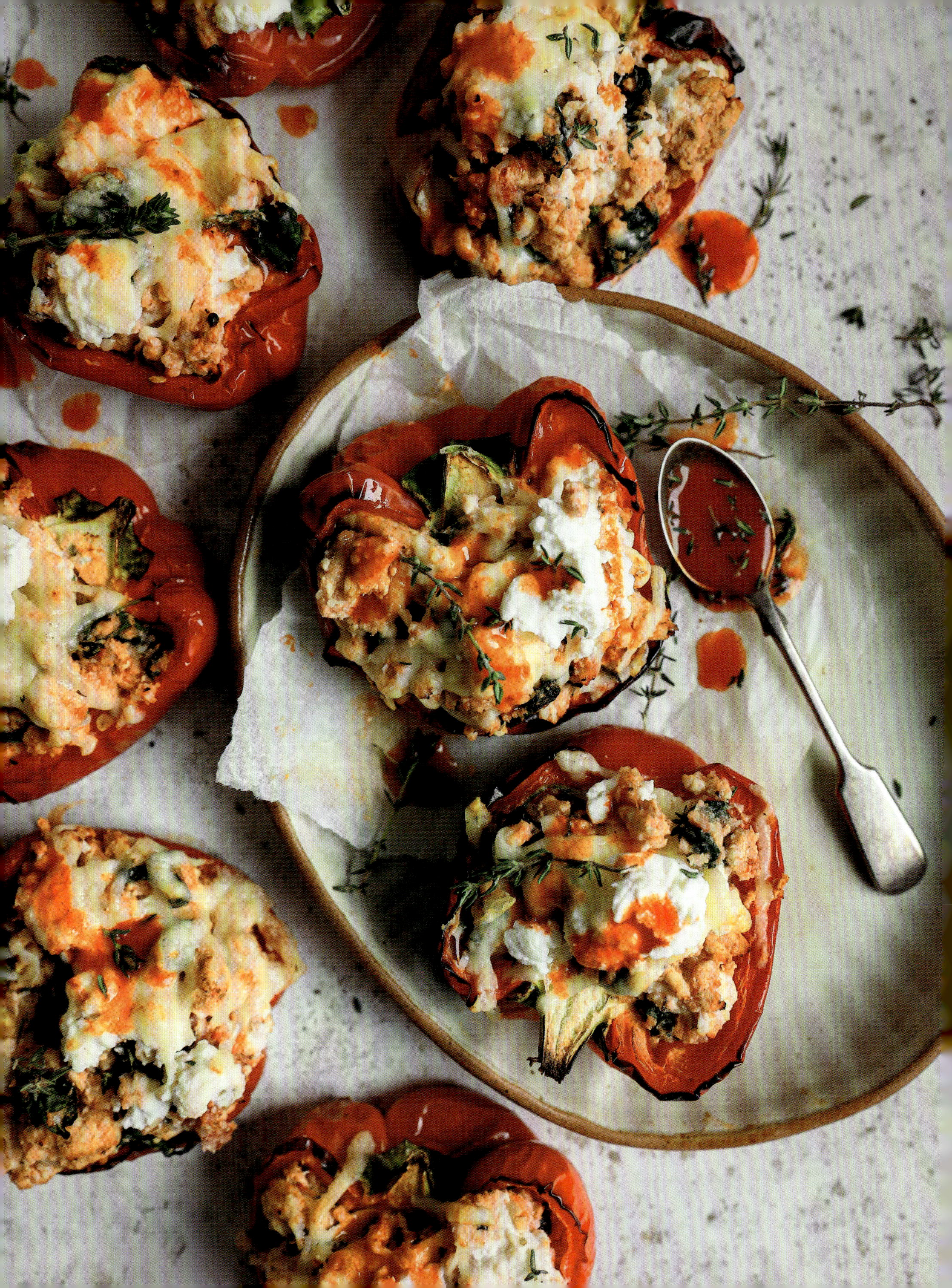

RICOTTA-STUFFED HEALTHY PEPPERS

2 whole bell peppers
½ white onion, sliced
1–2 garlic cloves, roughly chopped
8oz (225g) ground turkey
½ tsp (1.5g) Italian seasoning
½ tsp (1.5g) garlic powder
Salt and pepper, to taste
½ cup (120ml) whole strained tomatoes
1½ cups (100g) frozen cauliflower rice
2 large handfuls of fresh spinach, about 1½ cups (45g)
1 tbsp (6g) Parmesan-and-herb seasoning
¾ cup (186g) low-fat ricotta cheese
½ cup (45g) shredded part-skim mozzarella
Hot sauce (optional)

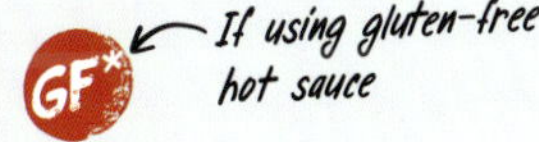

makes 2 stuffed peppers / 2 servings

NUTRITION (PER SERVING)

320 calories	**13g** fat
38g protein	**14.5g** net carbs

A healthy stuffing you can enjoy every night of the week, even if the only dates you're getting are with incognito mode. In my extremely biased opinion, this is one of the best meal-prep recipes of all time—everything you need, neatly packed in a bell-pepper vessel. Depending on the size of your bell peppers, you may end up with a little extra filling. Happy early birthday, and you're welcome. Double or triple the recipe at the start of the week, and these stuffed peppers will stay fresh for up to 5 days in a sealed container in the fridge. To reheat, microwave on high for 2 to 3 minutes, or bake at 425°F (220°C) for 8 to 10 minutes. Happy stuffing!

1. Preheat the oven to 425°F (220°C) convection bake. If you do not have a convection oven, you may need to add a few minutes of baking time.
2. Slice off the tops of the bell peppers and remove the ribs and seeds to hollow them out. In a small baking dish or pan, place the bell peppers upright and set aside.
3. Preheat a large skillet over medium-high heat and spray it with nonstick cooking spray. Once the pan is hot, add the onion and garlic. Sauté for 3 to 5 minutes, stirring often, until softened and translucent.
4. Add the ground turkey, Italian seasoning, and garlic powder and season with salt and pepper. Stir the ingredients together, breaking down the turkey with a spatula or wooden spoon.
5. When the turkey is beginning to brown, add the strained tomatoes. Use a spatula or wooden spoon to break apart the tomatoes and stir to combine.
6. To the turkey mixture, add the cauliflower rice, spinach, and ½ tablespoon (3g) of the Parmesan & herb seasoning. Stir and cook for 2 to 3 minutes, until the spinach has wilted and the turkey is cooked through.
7. Remove the skillet from the heat and add the ricotta, lightly folding it in.
8. Scoop the turkey mixture into both bell peppers, packing the ingredients tightly until both peppers are stuffed.
9. Bake on the middle rack for 15 minutes. Remove from the oven and sprinkle the shredded mozzarella and remaining ½ tablespoon (3g) Parmesan-and-herb seasoning over top. Bake for an additional 15 minutes, or until the cheese is brown and crispy and the peppers are tender. Enjoy with the hot sauce (if using)

TUNA BURGER
WITH PINEAPPLE BUN

¼ white onion, chopped
¼ cup (60g) chopped button mushrooms
½ jalapeño, thinly sliced
Salt and pepper, to taste
1 tuna steak, about 5oz (140g)
½ tsp (1.5g) garlic powder
¼ tsp (750mg) cayenne pepper
2 round slices of pineapple, 1-inch (2.5cm) thick, or 7oz (200g) in total
1 tbsp (15ml) sugar-free walnut maple syrup
1 tsp (6g) pineapple fruit spread
1 tbsp (15g) kimchi
2 thin tomato slices
2 thin avocado slices
1 tsp (1g) roughly chopped cilantro

Bless this mess of a burger that will threaten to stain your entire wardrobe. It has tuna for a delicious and healthy protein, and pineapple for a confusing mix of flavors that'll surprise and reward both you and your significant other. For the best sear, opt for sushi-grade tuna, especially if you like a rare center. Many sushi-grade steaks are flash-frozen at sea to lock in freshness and ensure safety, so be sure to check the freezer section at your grocery store. If using frozen tuna, thaw it fully before searing for the best results.

1. Heat a small frying pan over medium-high heat and spray it with nonstick cooking spray. Add the onion, mushrooms, and jalapeño and sauté for 7 to 9 minutes, until the onion is translucent and the mushrooms are tender. Season the sautéed vegetables with salt and pepper. Remove from the heat and set aside.
2. On both sides of the tuna steak, sprinkle the garlic powder and cayenne pepper and season with salt and pepper.
3. Heat a large grilling pan over medium-high heat and spray it with nonstick cooking spray. Once hot, add the tuna steak and sear each side for 1 to 2 minutes, until the outside is slightly browned but the inside is still pink. Remove from the heat and set aside.
4. Rub the pineapple slices with the walnut maple syrup and add them to the grilling pan. Cook for 2 to 3 minutes per side, until both sides are lightly seared.
5. To construct the burger, place the tuna steak on one pineapple slice, add a layer of the pineapple fruit spread on the tuna, and finish with the kimchi on top.
6. Top with the sautéed vegetables, tomato, avocado, cilantro, and finally, the other pineapple "bun." Knife and fork recommended for this one!

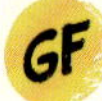

makes 1 burger / 1 serving

NUTRITION (PER SERVING)

349 calories	**7g** fat
38g protein	**32g** net carbs

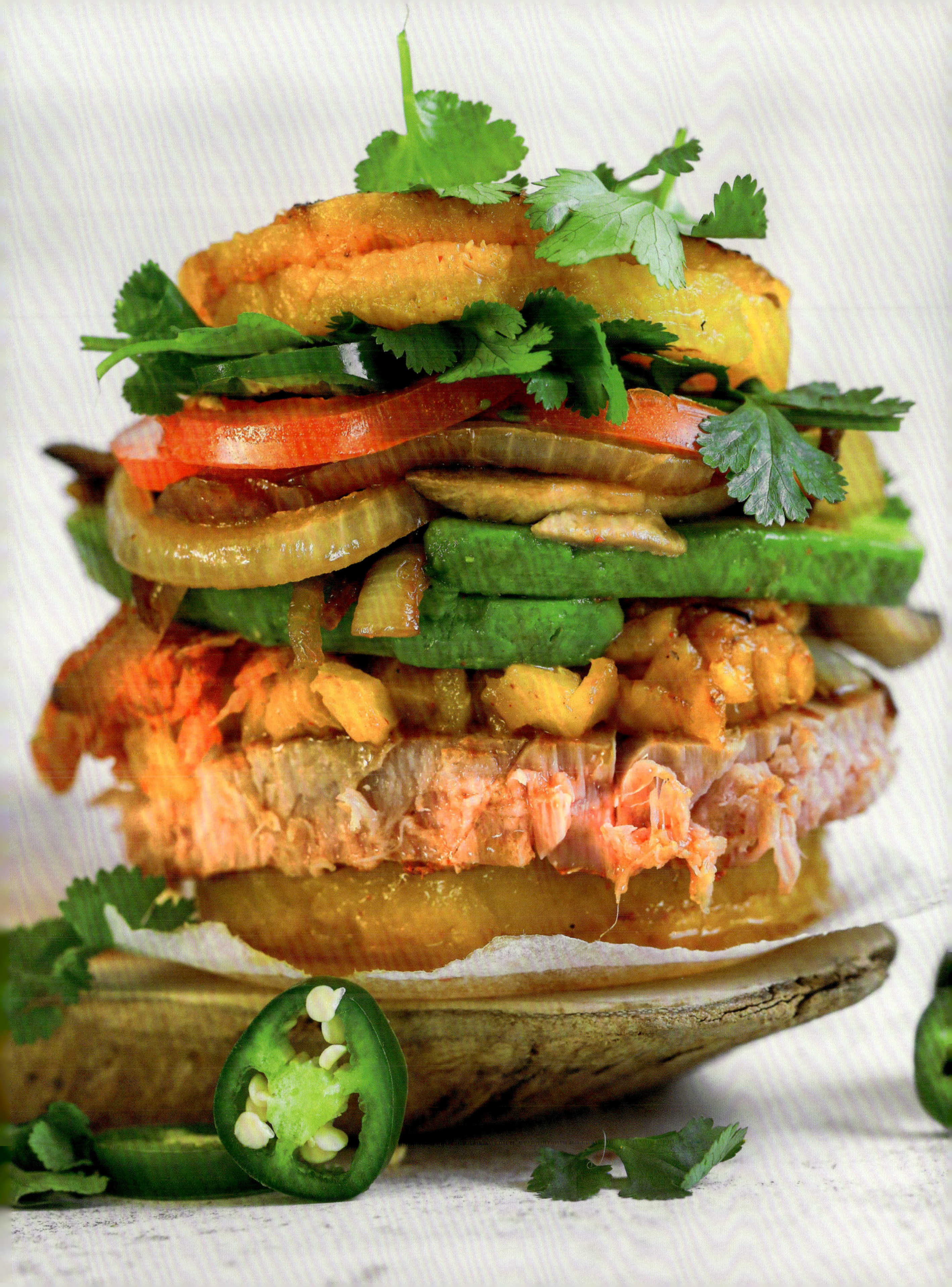

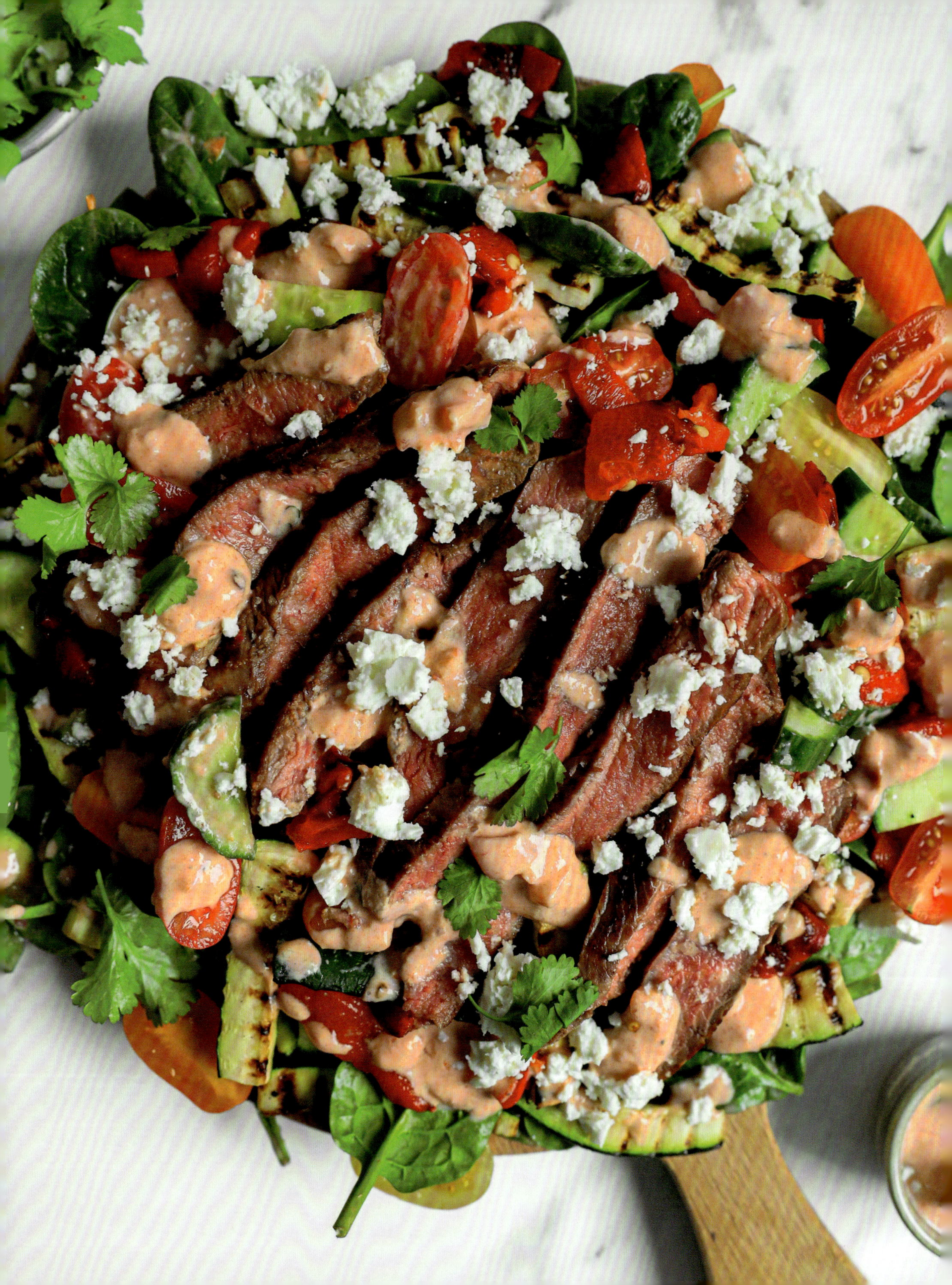

STEAK TACO SALAD

For the steak:

6oz (175g) eye of round steak
Salt, to taste

for the dressing:

6 tbsp (90g) nonfat Greek yogurt
4 tbsp (60ml) salsa
Juice of ½ a lime
½ tsp (1.5g) garlic powder
Salt and pepper, to taste

for the salad:

3⅓ cup (100g) baby spinach
1 medium zucchini, sliced lengthwise and grilled
½ large English cucumber, sliced into half moons
⅔ cup (100g) grape tomatoes
½ cup (30g) roughly chopped cilantro
½ roasted red bell pepper, diced
½ cup (60g) feta cheese, crumbled

It's like Chipotle, but you spend your night enjoying it from the couch instead of the bathroom. This high-protein salad packs bold flavors, crisp veggies, and a creamy, tangy dressing, all topped with juicy grilled steak. Eye of round is a lean cut, so cooking it quickly and letting it rest for at least 10 minutes is key to keeping it tender before slicing. Always slice against the grain for the most tender bites. As for grilling the zucchini, spray both sides with nonstick cooking spray, and season with salt and pepper. Cook on a preheated grill pan or barbeque over medium-high heat for 3 to 4 minutes per side, until grill marks appear and the zucchini is tender but not mushy.

1. **To make the steak:** Preheat a grilling pan over medium-high heat and spray it with nonstick cooking spray. Once the pan is hot, add the steak, season with salt, and grill for 2 to 3 minutes. Flip the steak and grill for an additional 2 to 3 minutes. Keep flipping until the steak reaches your desired level of doneness (130°F / 54°C for medium rare), then remove from the heat and set aside to rest.
2. **To make the dressing:** To a small bowl, add the Greek yogurt, salsa, lime juice, and garlic powder and season with salt and pepper. Stir to create a creamy dressing.
3. **To make the salad:** To a large bowl, add the baby spinach as the salad base. Top with the grilled zucchini, cucumber, grape tomatoes, cilantro, and roasted red bell pepper.
4. Thinly slice the steak into strips ½-inch (1cm) thick, and place them on top of the salad.
5. Pour the dressing over the salad and top with the crumbled feta cheese.
6. Toss until everything is evenly coated with the dressing and dig in.

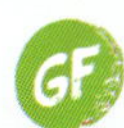

makes 1 salad / 1 serving

NUTRITION (PER SERVING)

625 calories	**24g** fat
69g protein	**33g** net carbs

TURKEY MEATBALL SUBS

for the meatballs:

1 lb (450g) ground turkey
½ cup (60g) zucchini, shredded and drained of moisture
1 egg
2 garlic cloves, minced
1 tbsp (9g) onion powder
1 tbsp (9g) dried oregano
1 tbsp (9g) salt
Pepper, to taste

for the sauce:

11 oz (325ml) strained tomatoes
1 tbsp (3.75g) fresh basil, chopped
½ tsp (1.5g) garlic powder
½ tsp (1.5g) onion powder
¼ tsp (750mg) chili flakes (optional)
Salt and pepper, to taste

for the subs:

2 sub rolls, 6 inches (15cm) each, split in half
⅔ cup (60g) shredded part-skim mozzarella cheese

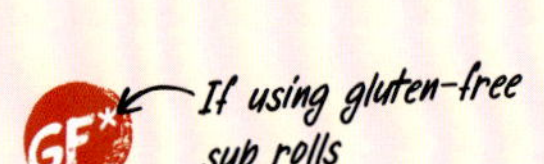

makes 2 subs / 2 servings

NUTRITION (PER SERVING)

849 calories	**32g** fat
66g protein	**68g** net carbs

Don't tell Nonna about this recipe—she'll never be convinced anything could be healthier than the dishes coming out of her kitchen. When it comes to handling your meat, don't pack the balls too tightly—keeping them loose makes them tender instead of dense. Embrace the perfectly imperfect shape. These meatballs are also a great meal-prep option; if you want to give your buns a day off, enjoy them over pasta, roasted veggies, or straight off the plate. You can store the meatballs and sauce together in a sealed container in the fridge for 4 to 5 days. To reheat, microwave on high for 1½ to 2 minutes, and they're good as new.

1. **To make the meatballs:** Preheat the oven to 400°F (200°C). Line two baking sheets with parchment paper.
2. To a large mixing bowl, add the ground turkey, zucchini, egg, garlic, onion powder, oregano, and salt and season with pepper. Using your hands, knead the ingredients together until evenly combined.
3. Form the meat mixture into golf-ball-size meatballs. On one of the prepared baking sheets, evenly space out the meatballs.
4. Bake the meatballs on the top rack for 15 minutes. Flip the meatballs and bake for an additional 5 minutes.
5. **To make the sauce:** While the meatballs are baking, to a medium saucepan, add the strained tomatoes, basil, garlic powder, onion powder and chili flakes (if using) and season with salt and pepper. Simmer for 10 to 12 minutes, until the sauce starts to bubble and thicken.
6. **To make the subs:** Toast the sub rolls in the oven until they're lightly golden and crispy around the edges. To construct the sub, spread the tomato sauce on the bottom layers of the bun, then evenly distribute the turkey meatballs. Top the meatballs with more tomato sauce and the mozzarella.
7. On the second prepared baking sheet, lay out the subs open face. Broil until the cheese is melted. Keep an eye on these, as they can burn quickly.
8. Remove the subs from the oven, place the top buns on the sandwiches, and *buon appetito*!

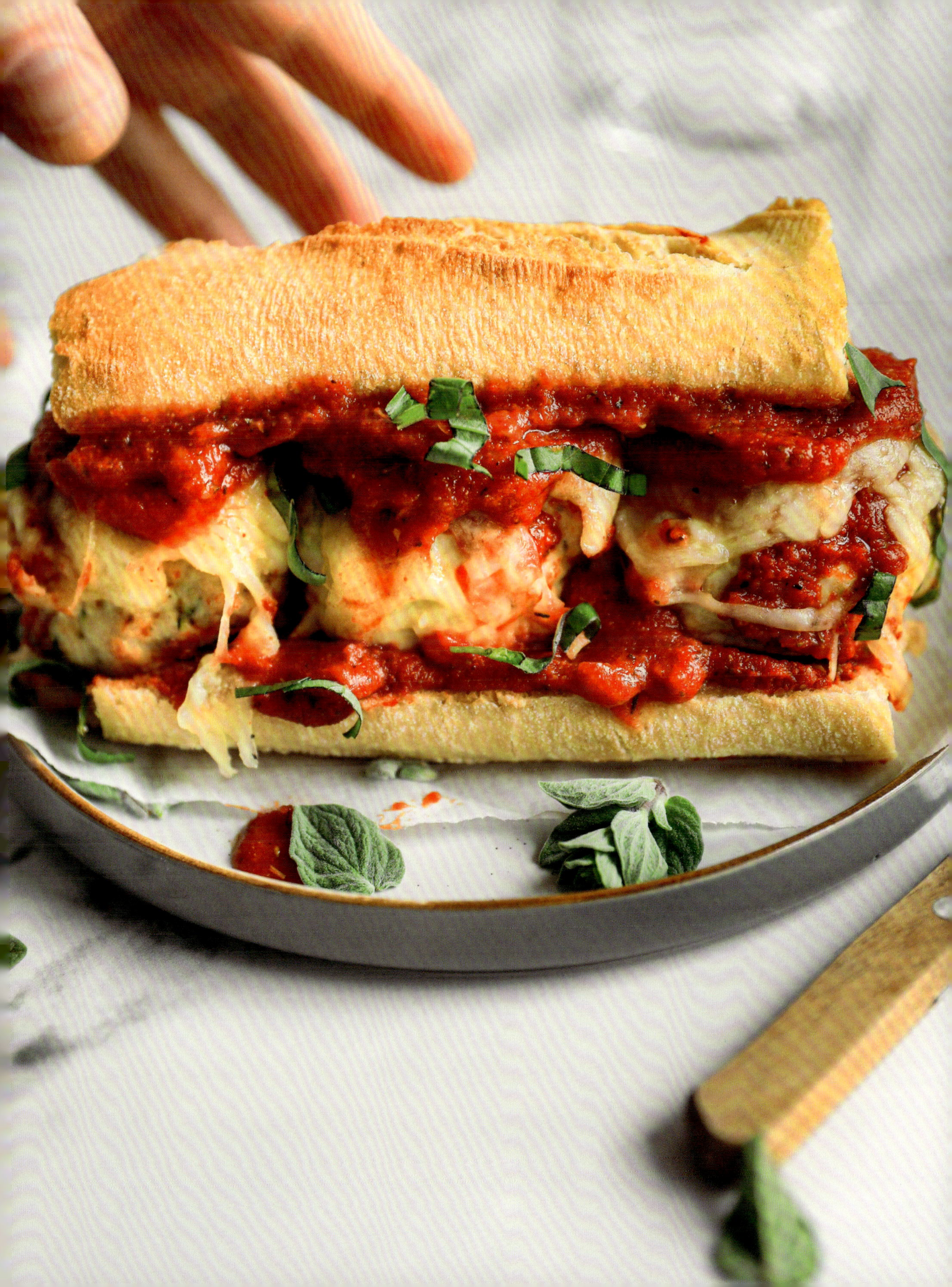

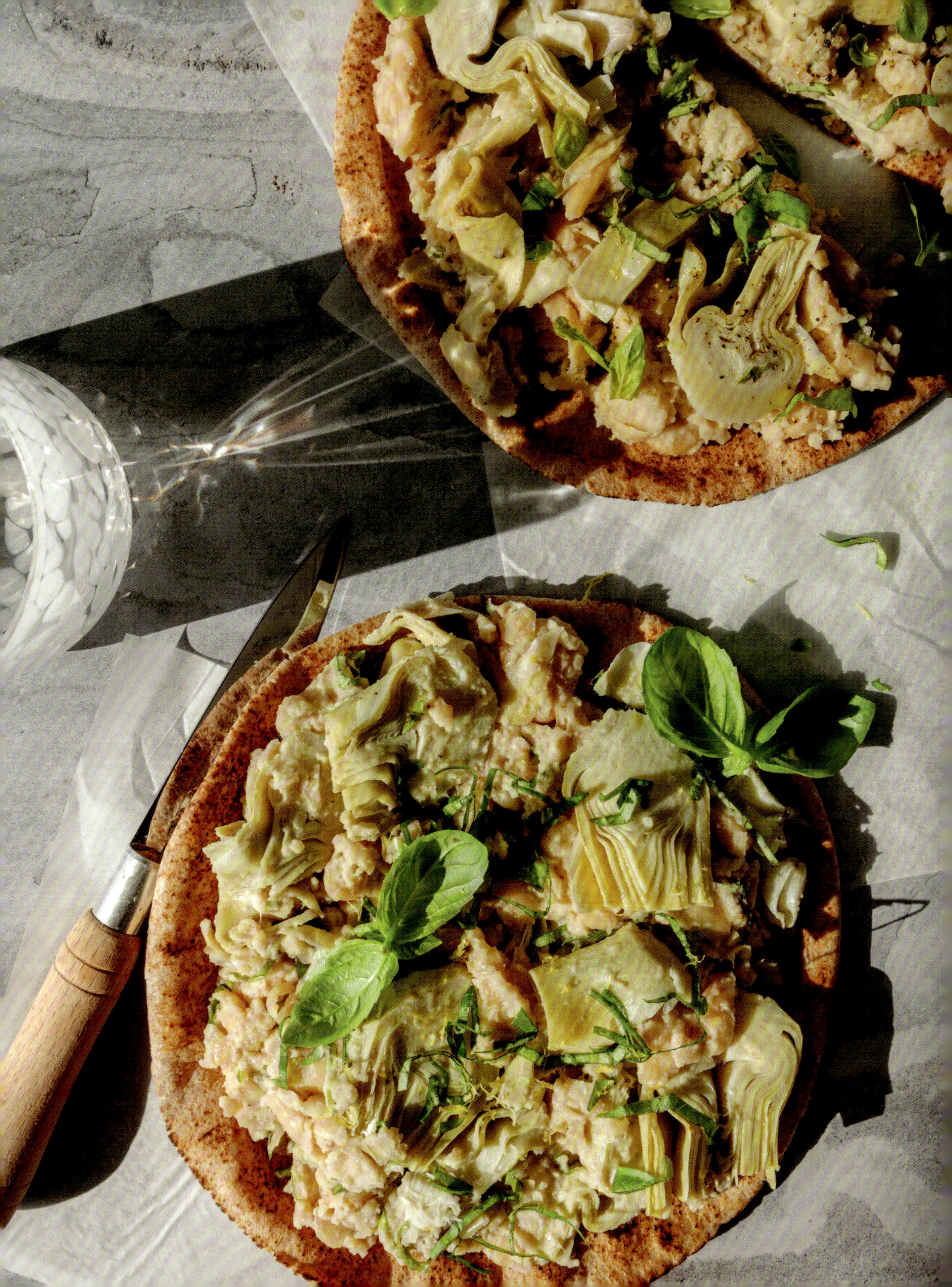

WHITE BEAN AND ARTICHOKE FLATBREAD

14oz (400g) can white beans, rinsed and drained
1 garlic clove, roughly chopped
½ cup (30g) fresh basil, roughly chopped
1 large tortilla or pita, about 60g
1 heaping cup (about 180g) canned artichoke hearts in water, drained and diced
Juice of 1 lemon
Salt and pepper, to taste

If she says she only dates vegans, whip up this plant-based recipe to sweep her off her feet. You won't have to pretend it tastes good. While I use white beans in this recipe, this is an inclusive cookbook. Feel free to substitute them for black beans, red beans, lentils, or anything that tickles your fancy. The tortilla is up to you, but if you're tracking macros, aim for one under 130 calories—bonus points if it's high-protein. If you're not in the mood to share, just wrap the bean filling in a tortilla, grill it over medium heat for 1 to 2 minutes per side, and boom—you've got yourself a vegan burrito.

1. Preheat the oven to 450°F (230°C).
2. To a food processor or blender, add the white beans, garlic, and half (15g) of the basil. Pulse until almost smooth, with some chunks remaining for texture.
3. On a baking sheet, place the tortilla or pita and bake for 2 to 3 minutes, until it's toasted and the edges crisp.
4. To a large bowl, add the artichoke hearts and lemon juice and season with salt and pepper.
5. To the bowl, add the bean mixture and stir to combine.
6. Scoop a thick layer of the artichoke-bean mixture evenly on the tortilla and top with the remaining basil.
7. Slice into as many pieces as desired and enjoy!

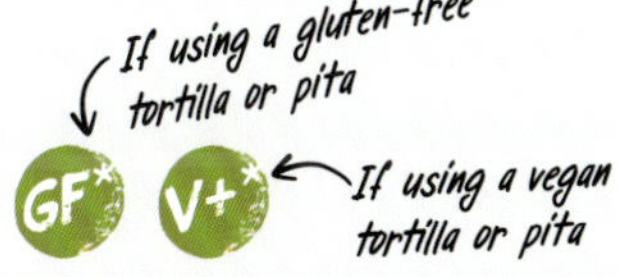

makes 1 flatbread / 1 serving

NUTRITION (PER SERVING)

367 calories | **2.5g** fat
27g protein | **59g** net carbs

SHAWARMA CHICKEN

1 tsp (3g) salt
1 tsp (3g) paprika
1 tsp (3g) cumin
1 tsp (3g) garlic powder
1 tsp (3g) onion powder
½ tsp (1.5g) cinnamon
¼ tsp (750mg) allspice
½ tsp (1.5g) turmeric
½ tsp (1.5g) curry powder
⅛ tsp (1.5g) cayenne
½ cup (115g) nonfat Greek yogurt
1 tbsp (15ml) olive oil
1 lb (450g) chicken breasts, chopped into bite-size pieces

Nothing says "last night was wild" like waking up to a half-eaten shawarma on your nightstand. If drunk you and sober you agree on anything, it's that shawarma is always the right choice. When it comes to meal prep, this chicken is a must-add protein option to your monthly rotation. It stays juicy and fresh for 4 to 5 days in the fridge as long as it's stored in an airtight container. When you're ready to eat, just microwave for 2 to 3 minutes. Enjoy it on its own, stuffed in a pita, or served over rice.

1. In a large mixing bowl, combine the salt, paprika, cumin, garlic powder, onion powder, cinnamon, allspice, turmeric, curry powder, and cayenne. Mix until the spices are evenly distributed.
2. Add the yogurt and olive oil and stir until a thick, pasty marinade forms.
3. Add the chicken to the bowl and stir until the pieces are fully coated in the marinade. Cover the bowl with plastic wrap and refrigerate for at least 5 hours. For best results, marinate overnight.
4. When ready to cook, heat a medium frying pan over medium-high heat and spray it with nonstick cooking spray. Once hot, add the marinated chicken and cook for 5 to 7 minutes, or until the chicken is golden and cooked through to at least 165°F (74°C) with no pink remaining. Enjoy!

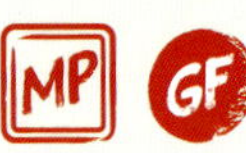

makes 2 servings

NUTRITION (PER SERVING)

324 calories	**10g** fat
57g protein	**1.5g** net carbs

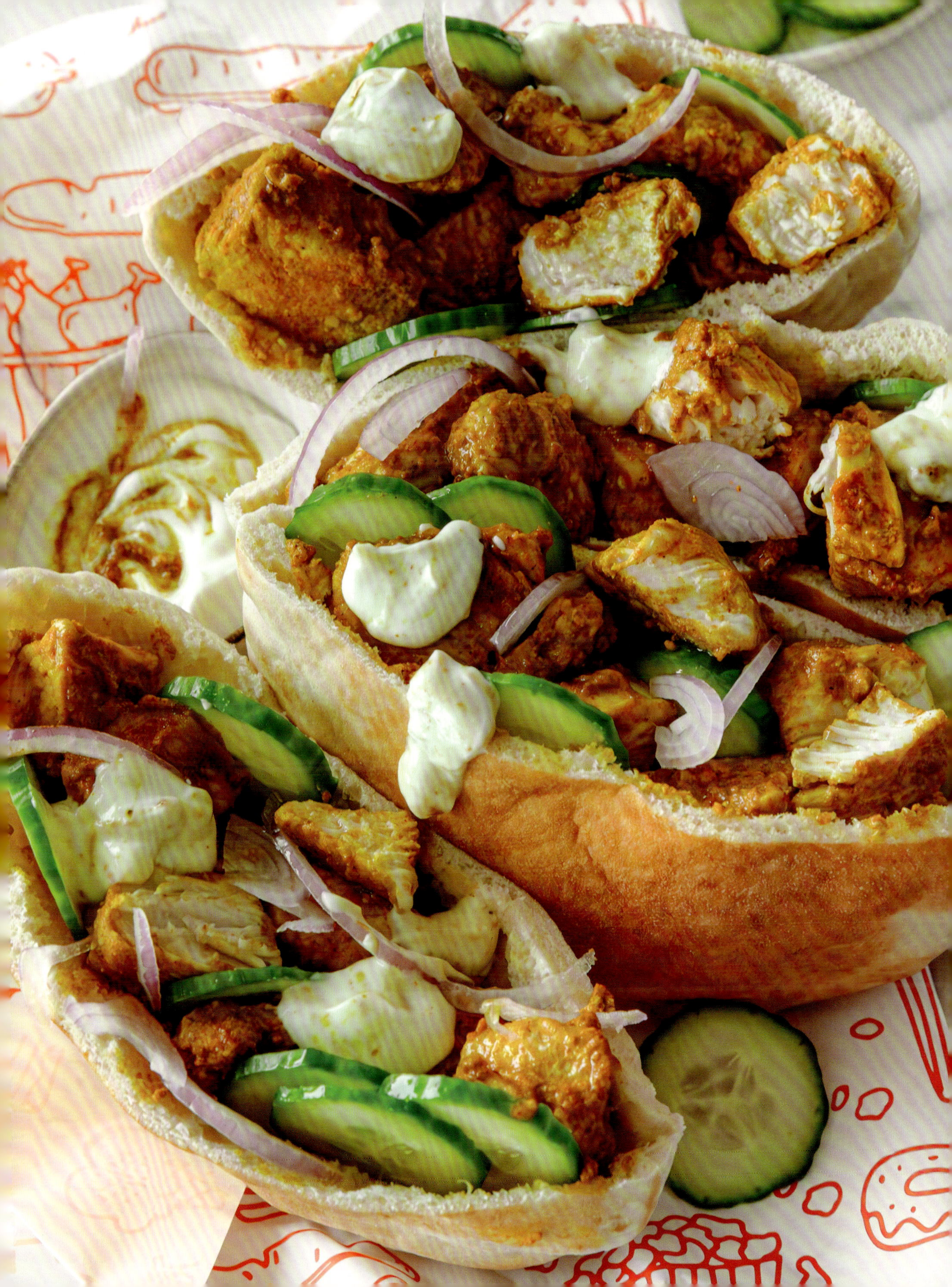

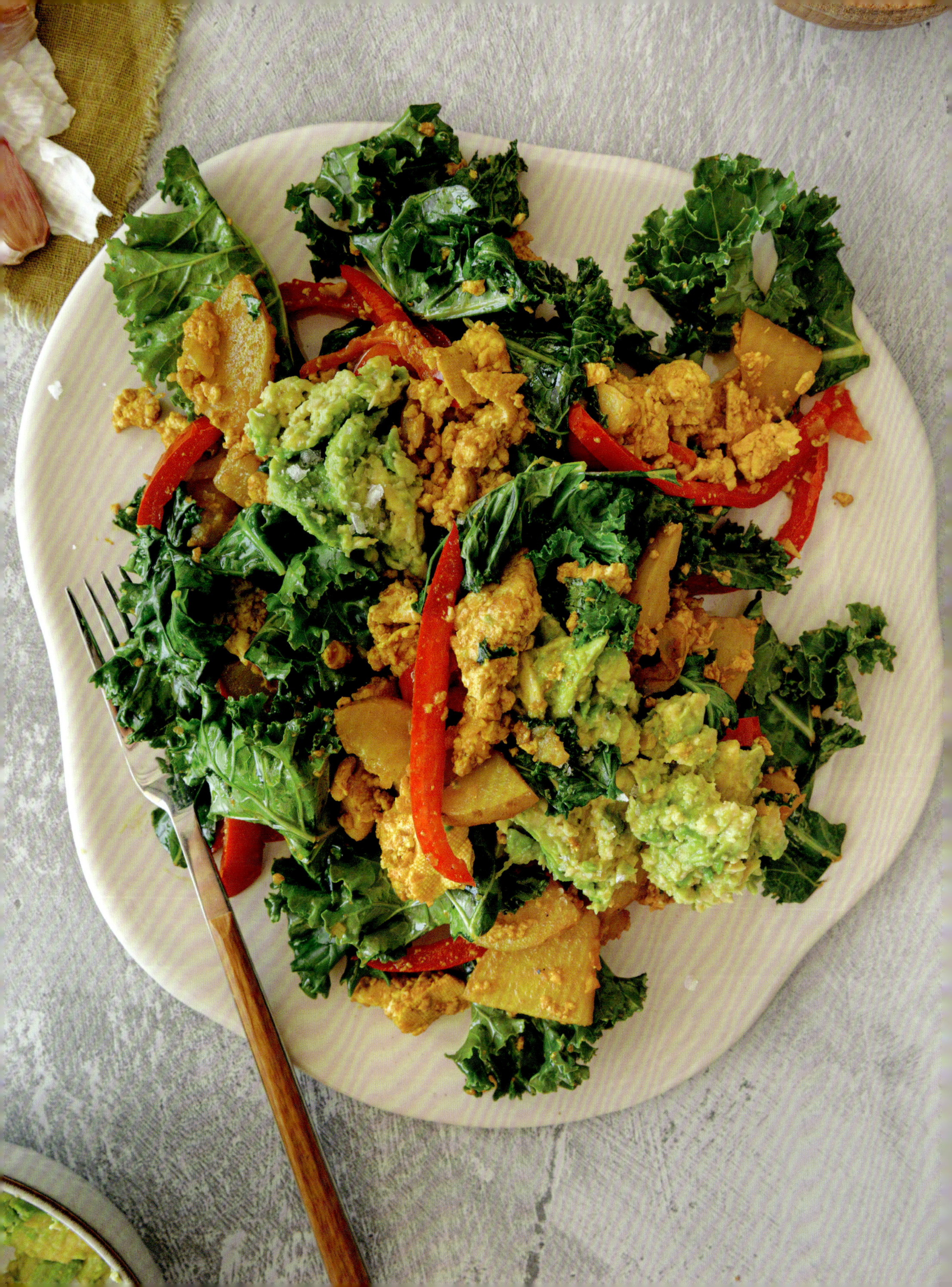

TOFU VEGGIE SCRAMBLE

1 large russet potato
½ cup (75g) bell pepper, thinly sliced
2 garlic cloves, diced
1 lb (450g) firm tofu, drained and pressed
1½ cups (100g) kale, roughly chopped
¼ cup (60ml) soy sauce
¼ cup (36g) nutritional yeast
1 tsp (3g) turmeric
1 tsp (3g) cumin
2 tsp (6g) garlic powder
½ avocado, mashed

If you think tofu is bland, that just means you cooked it wrong. Luckily, I've done the hard work for you, so follow this recipe, and try not to ruin it. Tofu holds more water than a conspiracy theorist's underground bunker, so you gotta press it. Wrap it in paper towels, slap something heavy on top (a pan or a stack of cookbooks—whatever works), and let it sit for 15 to 30 minutes. Less water = crispier tofu, and crispy tofu = actual flavor absorption, so don't skip this step.

1. Using a fork, poke holes in the potato. Microwave the potato on high for 5 to 6 minutes. Remove it from the microwave and let it cool for 5 minutes, then chop into bite-size chunks.
2. Heat a large frying pan over medium-high heat and spray it with nonstick cooking spray. Add the potato, bell pepper, and garlic and sauté for 4 to 5 minutes, stirring occasionally, until the peppers soften.
3. Using your fingers, crumble the tofu into the pan so it resembles scrambled eggs. Stir together to combine and let cook for an additional 3 to 5 minutes, until the tofu begins to crisp.
4. Add the kale and cook for 2 minutes to let it wilt down.
5. Add the soy sauce, nutritional yeast, turmeric, cumin, and garlic powder and stir to coat the contents of the pan. Cook for an additional 3 to 5 minutes.
6. Remove from the heat and top with the mashed avocado before dividing the mixture between two plates and serving.

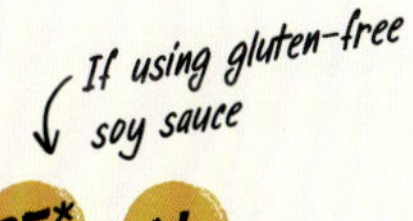

makes 2 servings

NUTRITION (PER SERVING)

462 calories	**17g** fat
31g protein	**46g** net carbs

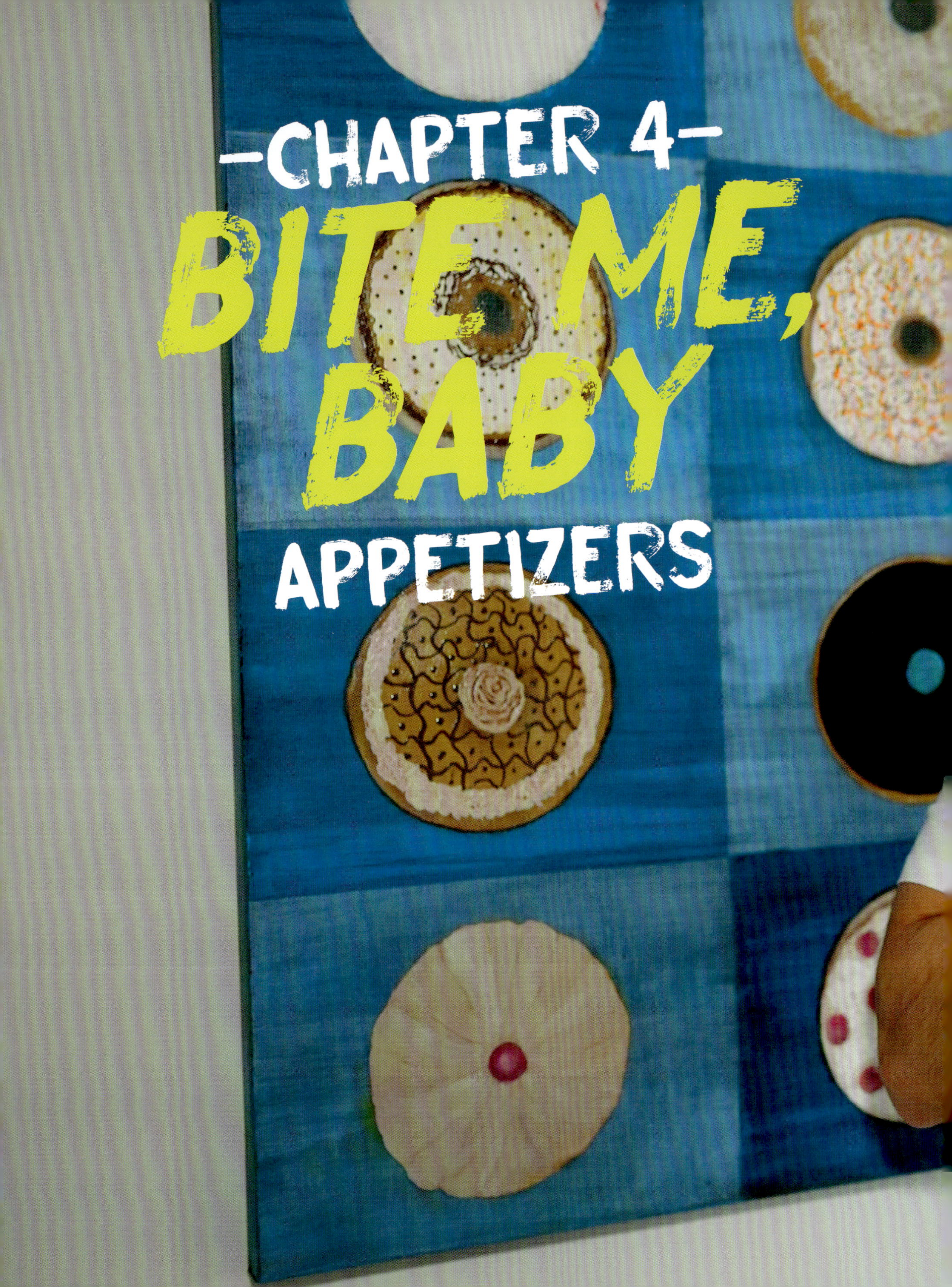

—CHAPTER 4—

BITE ME, BABY

APPETIZERS

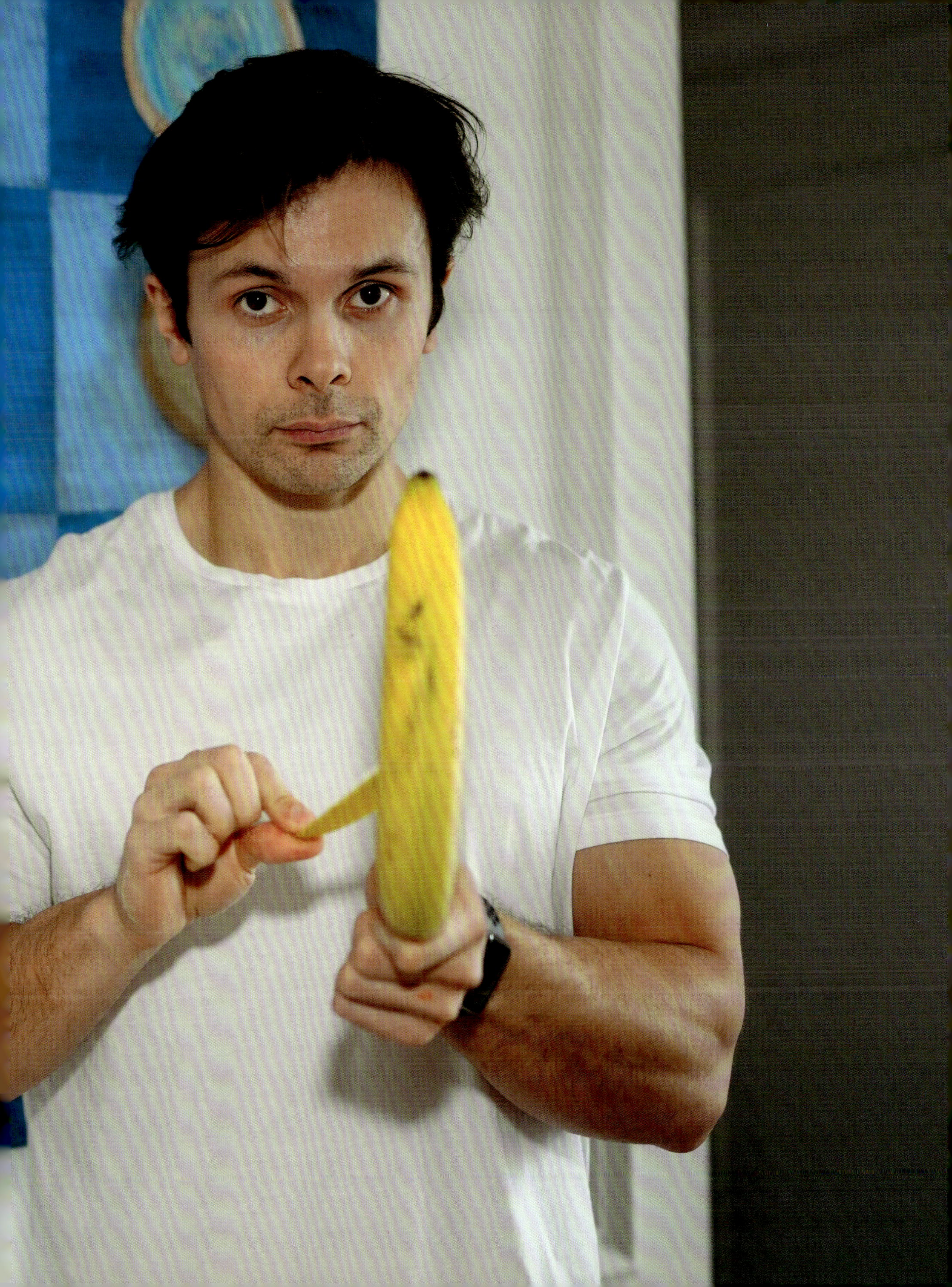

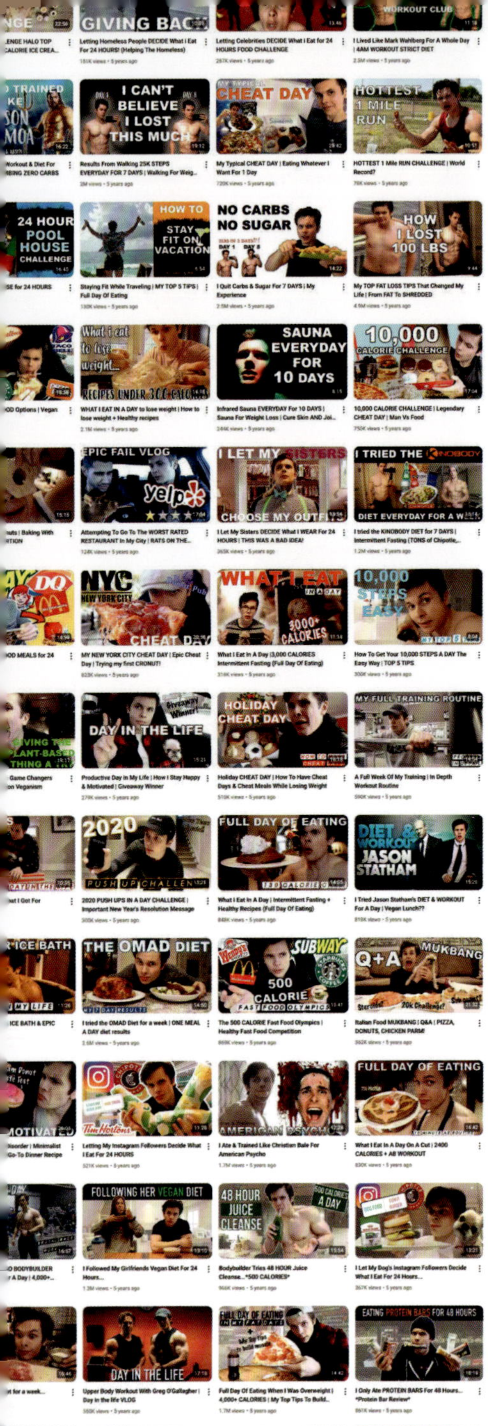

YOUTUBE Q&A

WITH WILL

I started my YouTube channel with a camera, a dog, some questionable ideas, and absolutely no clue what I was doing. Fast-forward to today, and somehow, it's turned into my full-time job—one that involves eating copious amounts of food, pushing my body to its limits, and embarrassing myself on the internet (all in the name of content). It's been a ridiculous, incredible journey, and I wouldn't trade it for anything. Here's a look behind the scenes.

1. **The video I'm most proud of is** my powerlifting competition.
2. **The hardest video I've ever filmed was** training at North America's highest gym **because** my body wasn't used to being that high up.
3. **The craziest challenge I've ever attempted was** walking 100,000 steps in a day, **and if I could do it again**, I wouldn't (lol). I've suffered from knee pain ever since.
4. **The biggest "pinch me" moment of my YouTube career was when** I realized people were watching for me and not necessarily the idea. It's allowed me to be in line more with the content I truly want to make.
5. **If I could collab with anyone in the world, it would be** John Mayer **because** he's my celebrity crush and seems like an interesting guy.
6. **One video idea I had but never filmed was** a 30,000-calorie challenge, **because** I didn't want to do too much damage to my body.
7. **The most unexpected thing I learned from YouTube is** simplicity is key.
8. **The video that almost broke me was** the altitude gym.

9. **The biggest risk I took on my channel was** reducing video frequency, **and it paid off because** it's allowed me to enjoy the process of creating again, and I think people are seeing that through what they're watching. Nothing feels forced, and it's sustainable.

10. **If I could redo one video with what I know now**, it wouldn't be one, but a few. During the pandemic, I traveled to the States to shoot a ton of videos, and they all performed horribly. Looking back, they were all too personal and didn't have broad appeal. I should've planned more with concepts.

11. **The YouTube milestone that meant the most to me was** hitting 100k subscribers **because** it showed me I was capable of doing this as a career, and Ollie was still around.

12. **One behind-the-scenes struggle people don't see is** planning unique content week after week. Coming up with ideas is a full-time job itself.

13. **The moment I realized YouTube could be my full-time job was** when I got my first paycheck back in December 2019, and it was higher than my personal-training monthly salary.

14. **If I could give my day one YouTube self one piece of advice, it would be** try to keep the fun in it at all times. Sometimes when it becomes a business, you lose the joy. It's not that serious, so remember why you started it.

15. **The weirdest thing I've ever done for a video is . . .** lol, this one is too crazy to answer without it being a page of its own . . .

16. **The moment I laughed the hardest while filming was when** filming with Chef Andre Rush.

17. **Ten years from now, I hope people remember my channel for** being a place where an average guy wasn't afraid to try things out, even if it meant looking ridiculous along the way. I never wanted to take myself too seriously, but I always believed in showing up, putting in the work, and making progress, especially in the gym. More than anything, I hope my channel feels like a space where people can laugh, learn, and feel like they have a friend they've never met, someone who makes the journey a little more fun and a little less intimidating.

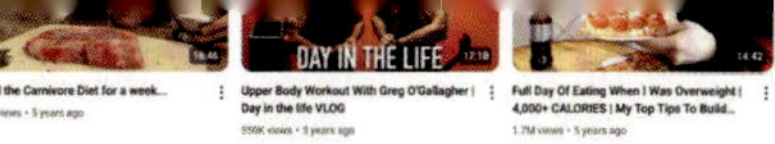
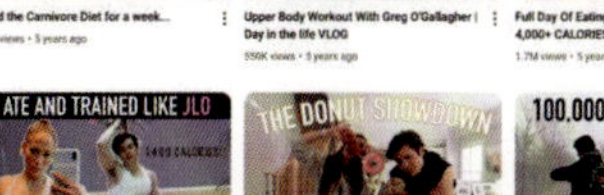
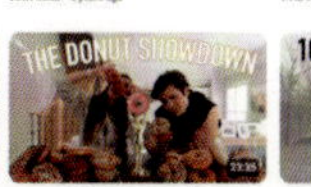
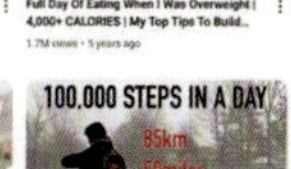
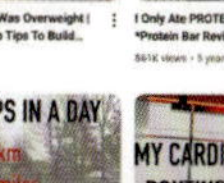
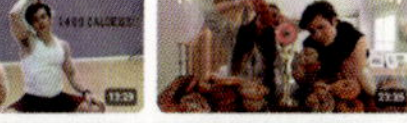
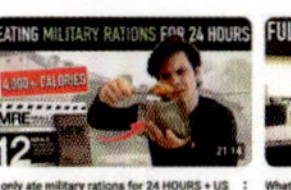
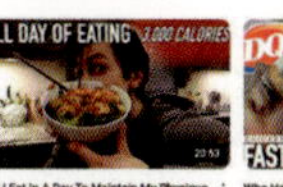
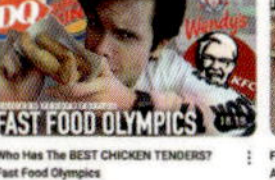
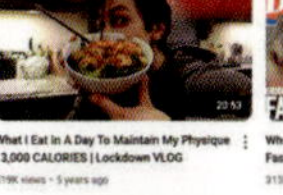
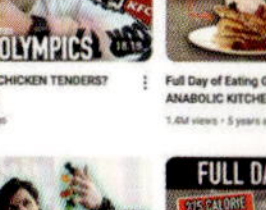
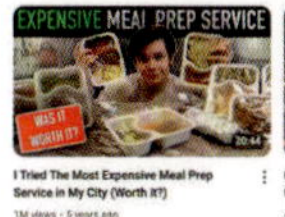
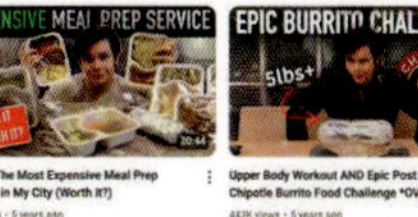
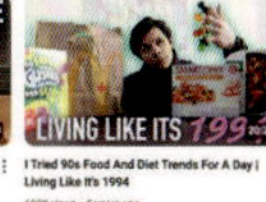
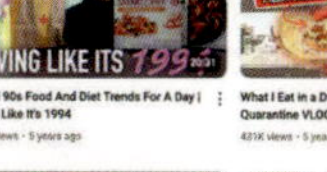
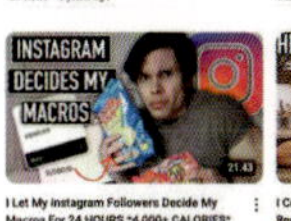
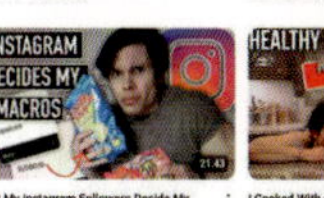
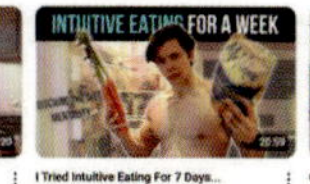
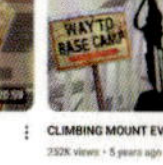
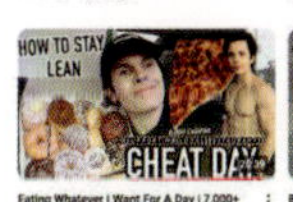
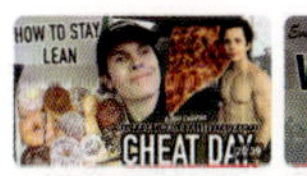
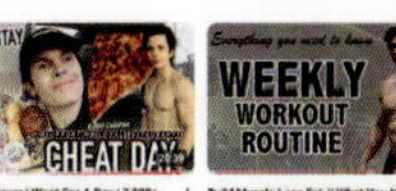
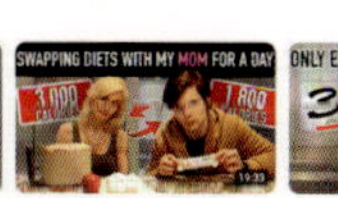
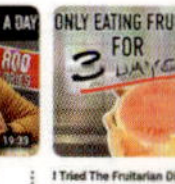
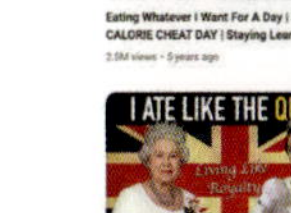
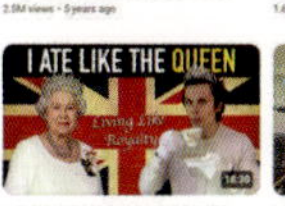
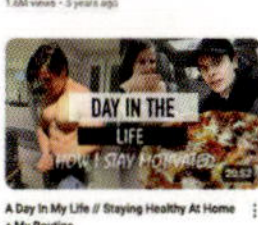
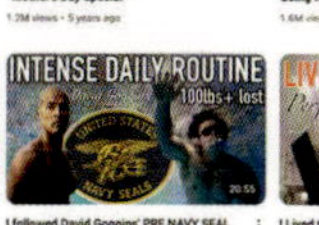
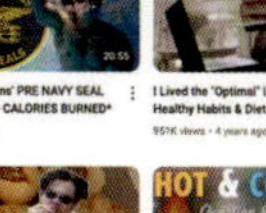
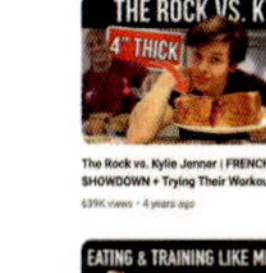
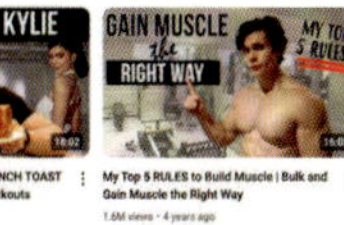
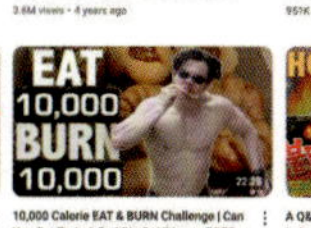
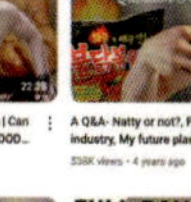
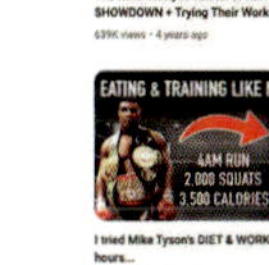
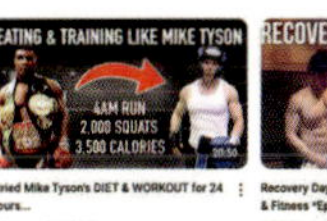
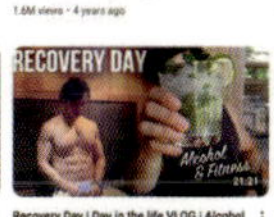
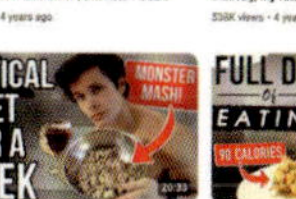
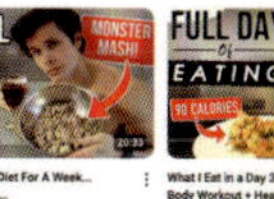
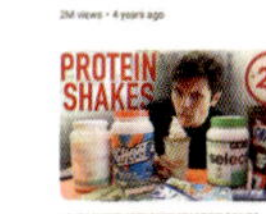
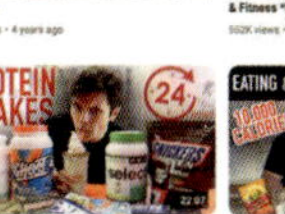
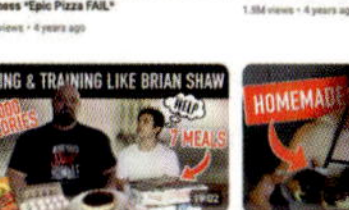
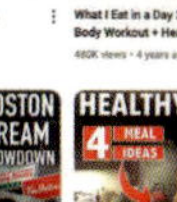
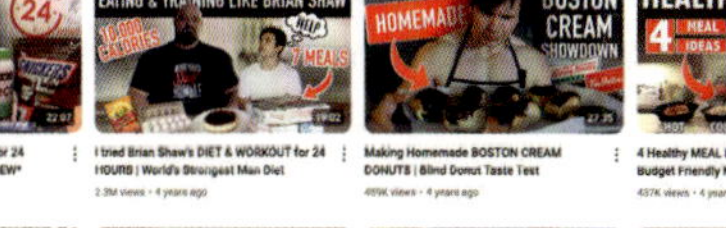
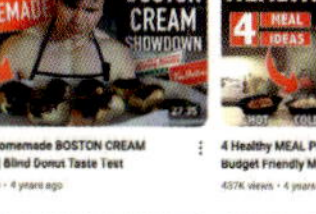
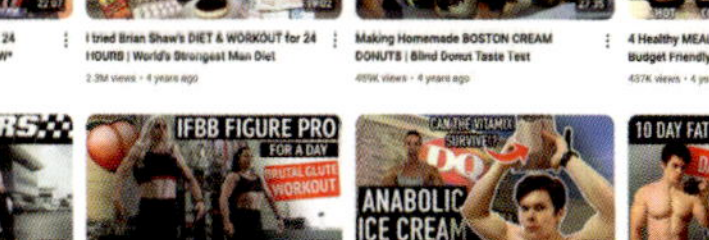
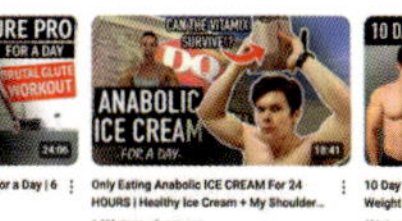
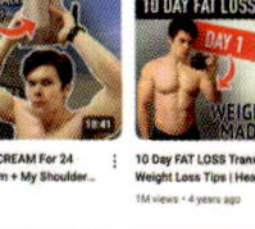
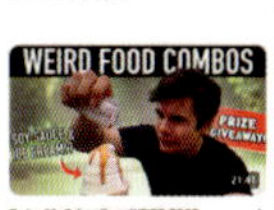
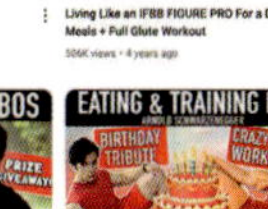
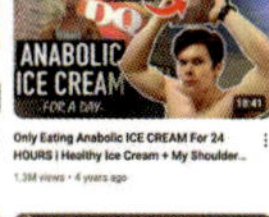
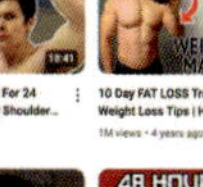
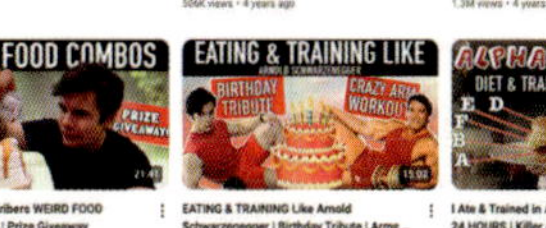
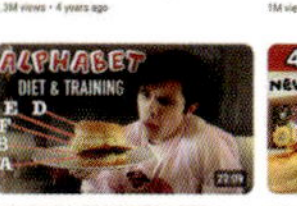
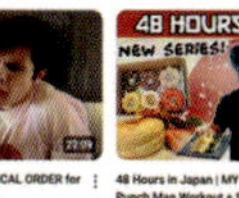
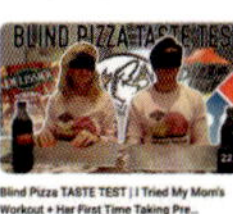
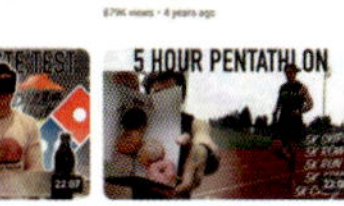
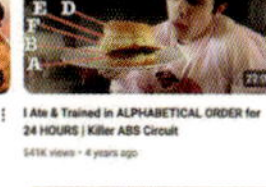
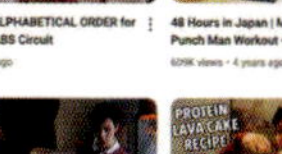
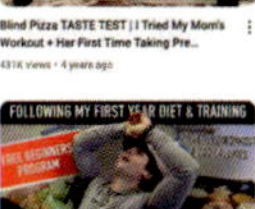
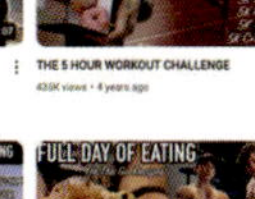
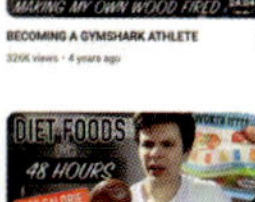
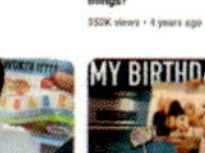
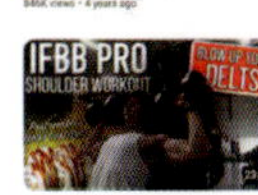
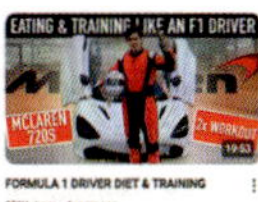
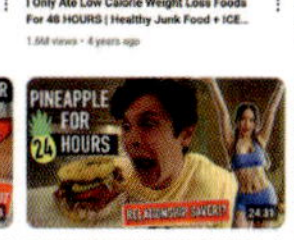
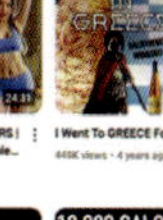
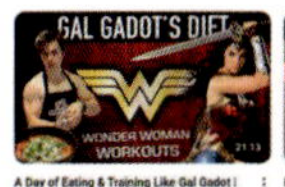
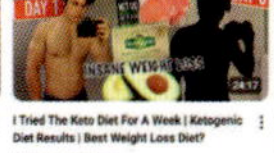
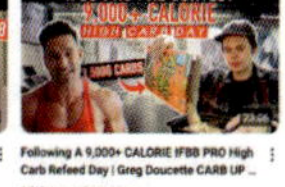
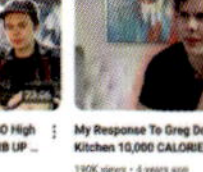

ZUCCHINI BOATS

2 medium zucchinis
1 tsp (3g) Italian seasoning
1 tsp (3g) garlic powder
Salt and pepper, to taste
2 turkey sausages, about 188g in total, casings removed
½ cup (120ml) strained tomatoes
⅔ cup (80g) shredded low-fat cheddar cheese

My second favorite way to enjoy a zucchini, these boats are quick and easy to make, and you'll devour them even quicker. The zucchini is just a canvas for you to fill with your mind's desires, and I certainly encourage that. Season your meat with curry powder, mix in some sautéed spinach for a little extra fiber, or add a drizzle of your favorite low-calorie condiment—pretend you're in your first year of college, and experiment a little. If you are meal prepping this recipe, I recommend taking the zucchinis out of the oven after 15 minutes so they stay firm. Store in a sealed container in the fridge for up to 4 days, and to reheat, bake in the oven at 375°F (190°C) for 8 minutes, until the cheese bubbles.

1. Preheat the oven to 350°F (180°C). Line a baking sheet with parchment paper.
2. Cut off the ends of both zucchinis, then cut each zucchini in half lengthwise. Using a spoon, scoop out and discard the seeds and some of the flesh of the zucchinis to create the "boat" shape.
3. On the prepared baking sheet, place the zucchini boats with the insides facing up. Season the insides of the zucchini boats with the Italian seasoning, garlic powder, and salt and pepper. Set aside.
4. Preheat a medium frying pan over medium-high heat and spray it with nonstick cooking spray. Once hot, add the turkey sausages, using a spatula to break them apart into a crumble. Cook for 4 to 5 minutes, until slightly browned and cook through.
5. Add the strained tomatoes and season with additional salt and pepper. Stir to combine.
6. Once heated through, scoop the turkey sauce mixture evenly into the zucchini boats, and top with the cheese.
7. Bake for 25 minutes, until the cheese is golden and crispy and the zucchinis have softened.

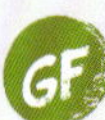

makes 4 zucchini boats / 2 servings

NUTRITION (PER SERVING)	
230 calories	**10g** fat
24.5g protein	**10.5g** net carbs

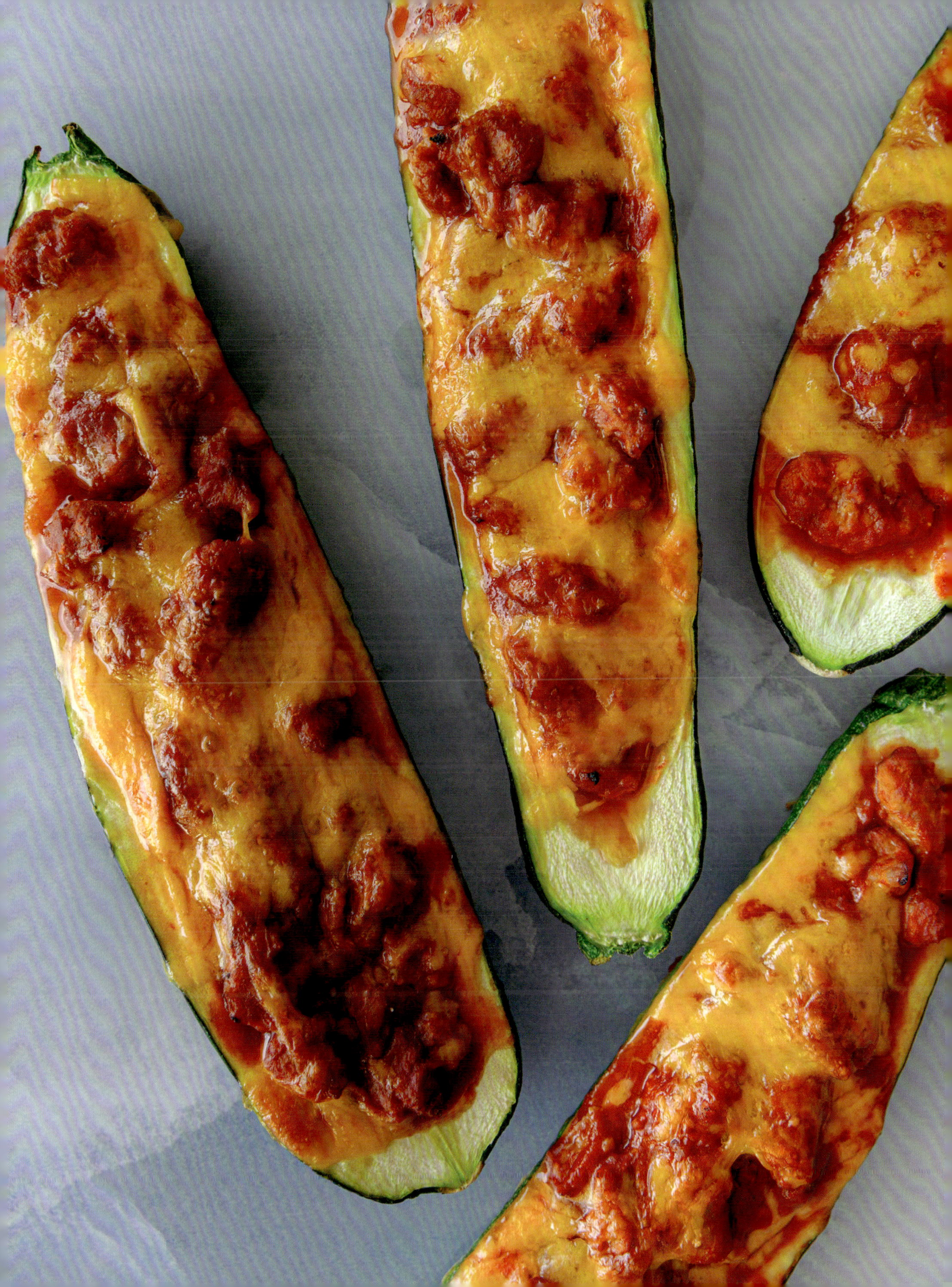

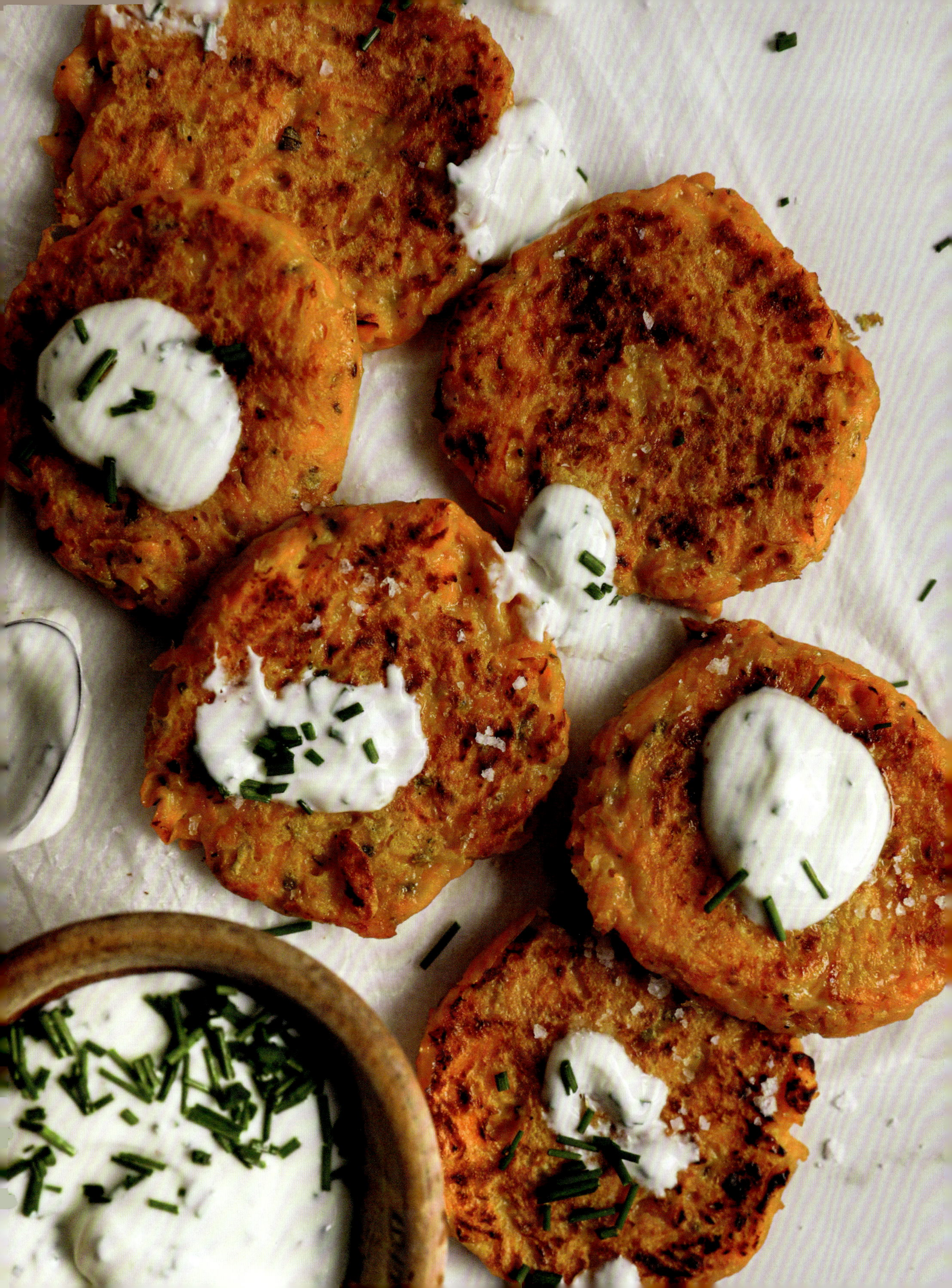

BUTTERNUT SQUASH FRITTERS

- 2½ cups (about 300g) lightly packed butternut squash, peeled and shredded
- ⅓ cup (40g) coconut flour
- 1 egg, lightly beaten
- ½ tsp (1.5g) garlic powder
- 1½ tbsp (10g) fresh sage, minced
- 1 tsp (3g) dried thyme
- Salt and pepper, to taste
- Nonfat Greek yogurt, for topping (optional)
- Chopped chives, for topping (optional)

Hi everyone—Victoria here. I've tried hundreds of Will's recipes over the years, and guess what? These are my top pick. The thyme and fresh sage transport you straight to Thanksgiving dinner but are far lighter and healthier. Don't skimp out on the Greek yogurt garnish either—it adds a nice freshness, and some protein too. These fritters will be your new obsession! No fresh herbs? No problem. You can swap in dried herbs, but since they're more concentrated, use only about ⅓ of the amount called for with the fresh alternatives to keep the flavor balanced.

1. To a large bowl, add the butternut squash, coconut flour, egg, garlic powder, sage, and thyme. Season with salt and pepper and mix until combined.
2. Heat a large frying pan over medium-high heat and spray it with nonstick cooking spray. With a spoon, scoop the squash mixture into small round balls and place them in the pan, using a spatula or the palm of your hand to flatten them lightly.
3. Fry the fritters for 3 minutes, until the bottom is golden brown and crisp. Flip and cook for an additional 3 minutes.
4. Enjoy the fritters on their own, or top with the Greek yogurt and chives (if using).

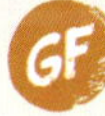

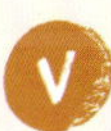

makes 6 fritters / 6 servings

NUTRITION (PER SERVING)

52.5 calories　**1.8g** fat
2.5g protein　**6.6g** net carbs

QUICK-BAKE FALAFEL

1 (14oz / 400g) can chickpeas, drained and rinsed
3 garlic cloves, roughly chopped
¼ cup (15g) roughly chopped parsley
¼ cup (28g) chopped yellow or red onion
1 tbsp (15ml) olive oil
2 tbsp (30ml) lemon juice
1 tsp (3g) cumin
1 tsp (3g) ground coriander
¾ tsp (225mg) cayenne powder
Salt and pepper, to taste
3 tbsp (30g) flour of choice (I use brown rice flour)
1 tsp (5g) baking soda

You'll never feel awful with this falafel. Pop a couple of these balls in your mouth to find the rainbow on a rainy day. Your falafel experience is entirely up to you—keep it classic in a salad or pita, get creative and use them as vegan meatballs, or go full chaos mode and turn the batter into falafel waffles (highly recommended). Meal preppers, take note: Store cooked falafel in a sealed container in the fridge for 3 to 4 days, then bake at 375°F (190°C) for 5 to 8 minutes to crisp them back up. For a light tahini dressing to drizzle over top of your falafel, mix together ¼ cup (60ml) tahini, ¼ cup (60ml) water, 1 tbsp (15ml) lemon juice, and season with salt and pepper.

1. Preheat the oven to 375°F (190°C). Line a baking sheet with parchment paper.
2. To a food processor, add the chickpeas, garlic, parsley, onion, olive oil, lemon juice, cumin, coriander, and cayenne powder and season with salt and pepper. Pulse until chunky and combined. It is important not to overblend the ingredients.
3. Add the flour and baking soda. Using a spoon, combine well, then form the mixture into 5 equal falafel balls and place them on the prepared baking sheet.
4. Bake for 30 to 32 minutes, flipping halfway, until they are crispy and slightly golden.

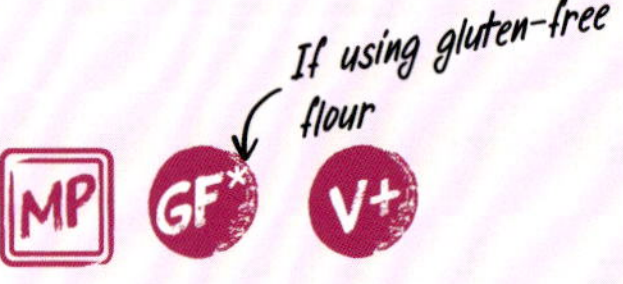

makes 5 servings

NUTRITION (PER SERVING)

145 calories	**5g** fat
6g protein	**19g** net carbs

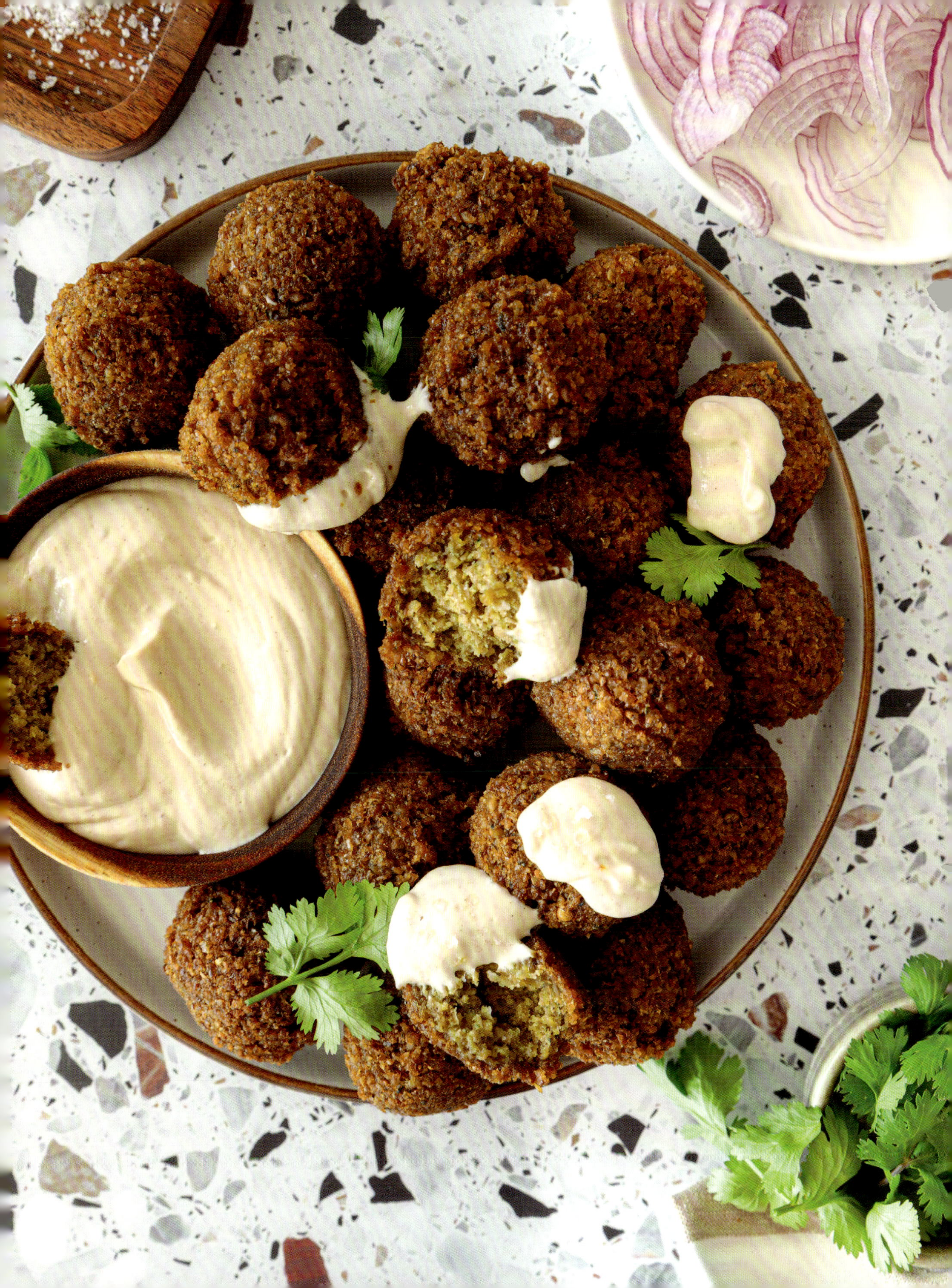

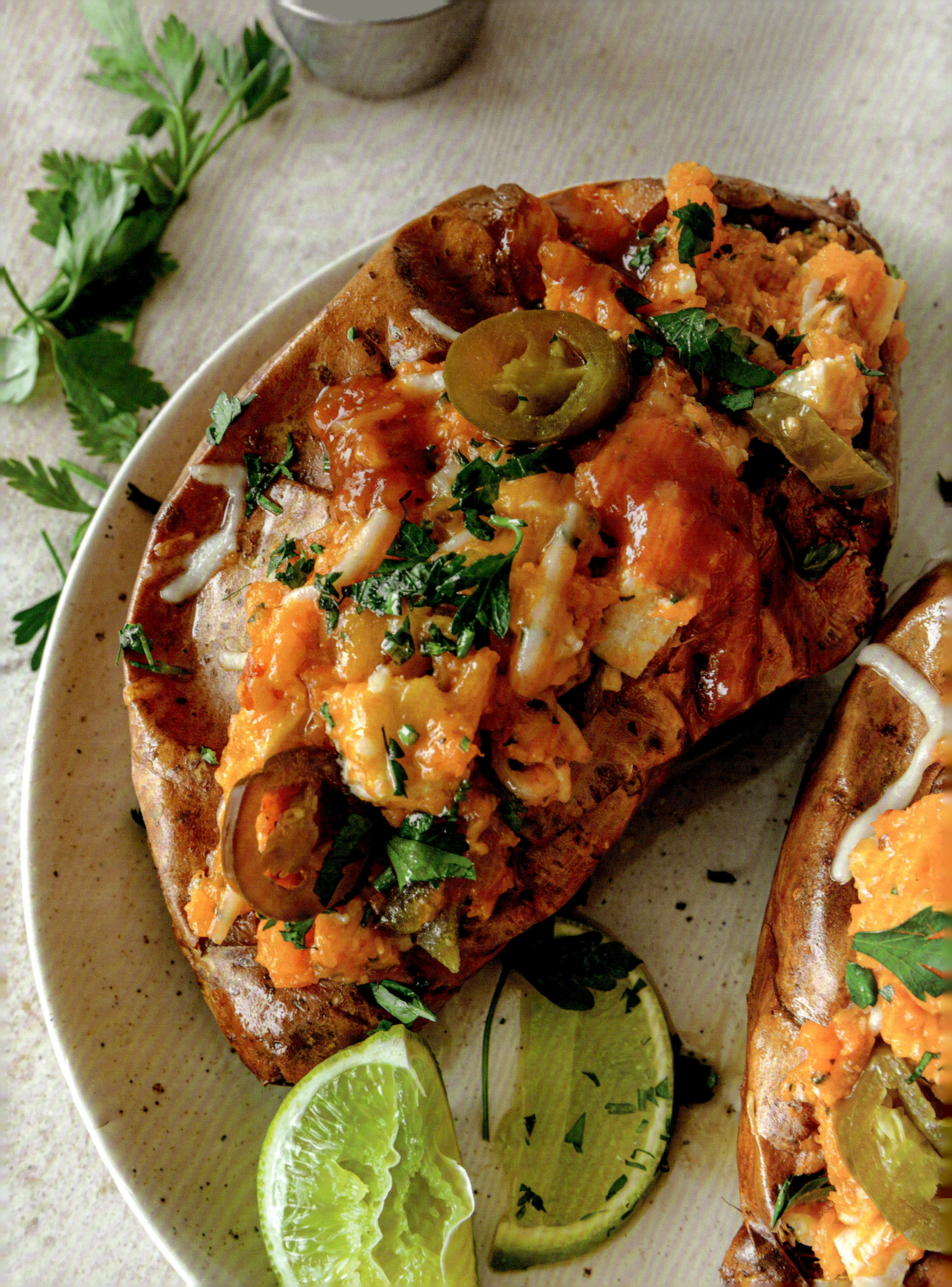

MEXICAN TWICE-BAKED STUFFED SWEET POTATO

- 1 large sweet potato, washed and scrubbed
- 1 chicken breast, about 8oz (225g), cooked and chopped
- 1 tbsp (15g) pickled jalapeños, diced
- ½ cup (30g) cilantro, roughly chopped
- 1½ tbsp (23ml) salsa
- ½ tsp (1.5g) chipotle-pepper powder
- ¼ cup (30g) shredded Tex-Mex cheese
- Salt and pepper, to taste

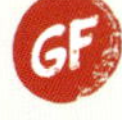

makes 2 stuffed potato halves / 2 servings

NUTRITION (PER SERVING)

445 calories
6.5g fat
43.5g protein
53g net carbs

Few things in life are as fun as getting baked and getting stuffed, and today you'll be doing both, treating these lucky sweet potatoes to the time of their lives. A fantastic meal-prep option, make one for each day of the week, and they'll stay fresh in the fridge for up to 5 days. When hunger strikes, just microwave for 2 to 3 minutes, and voilà—gourmet meal faster than making toast. To keep this dish interesting, I like to switch up the international cuisine inspiration. For an Italian twist, mix in roasted red peppers, roasted garlic, oregano, basil, tomato sauce, and mozzarella. What creative combo will you come up with?

1. Preheat the oven to 400°F (200°C).
2. Using a fork, poke holes in the sweet potato to help release moisture and allow the sweet potato to crisp up in the oven. Wrap it in foil and place it either directly on the oven rack or on a baking sheet. Bake for 45 minutes, or until the sweet potato is tender when poked with a fork. Leave the oven on.
3. Cut the sweet potato in half lengthwise and scoop the insides out into a bowl. On a baking sheet, set aside the sweet potato skins.
4. To the bowl with the sweet potato insides, add the chicken breast, jalapeños, cilantro, salsa, chipotle-pepper powder, and half (⅛ cup / 15g) of the cheese and season with salt and pepper. Using a fork, fold the ingredients together.
5. Pile the sweet-potato mixture back into the sweet-potato skins and sprinkle the remaining ⅛ cup (15g) cheese on top.
6. Bake for 15 minutes, until the cheese is crispy and golden.

CAULIFLOWER AND LEEK SOUP

1 medium head of cauliflower, chopped
2 leeks, chopped
1 celery stalk, chopped
1 garlic clove, chopped
1 shallot, chopped
1 tsp (3g) nutmeg
1 bay leaf
Salt and pepper, to taste
4 cups (1L) vegetable broth

If you read only one headnote in this book, make it this one: WASH YOUR LEEKS. These sneaky little guys are dirt hoarders. To clean them properly, slice off the root end, cut them in half lengthwise, and run each piece under cold water, making sure to rinse between the layers. Take your time, unless you enjoy the surprise crunch of dirt in your food. Turn this dish into a complete meal by adding some protein bread for dipping—because sometimes, food should feel like a hug. There's just something very comforting about a hot bowl of soup . . . a rare soothing sensation for my throat.

1. Heat a large stock pot over medium-high heat and spray it with nonstick cooking spray. Once hot, add the cauliflower, leeks, celery, garlic, shallot, nutmeg, and bay leaf and season with salt and pepper. Stir together and sauté for 5 to 7 minutes, until the vegetables begin to soften.
2. To the pot, add the vegetable broth. Bring it to a boil, then reduce the heat to low and simmer for 20 to 30 minutes, until all the vegetables are soft enough to purée.
3. Remove and discard the bay leaf. Using a blender or immersion blender, purée the ingredients until smooth.
4. Add more seasoning to taste, and enjoy.

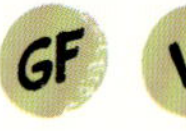

makes 3 servings

NUTRITION (PER SERVING)

115 calories	**1g** fat
6g protein	**18g** net carbs

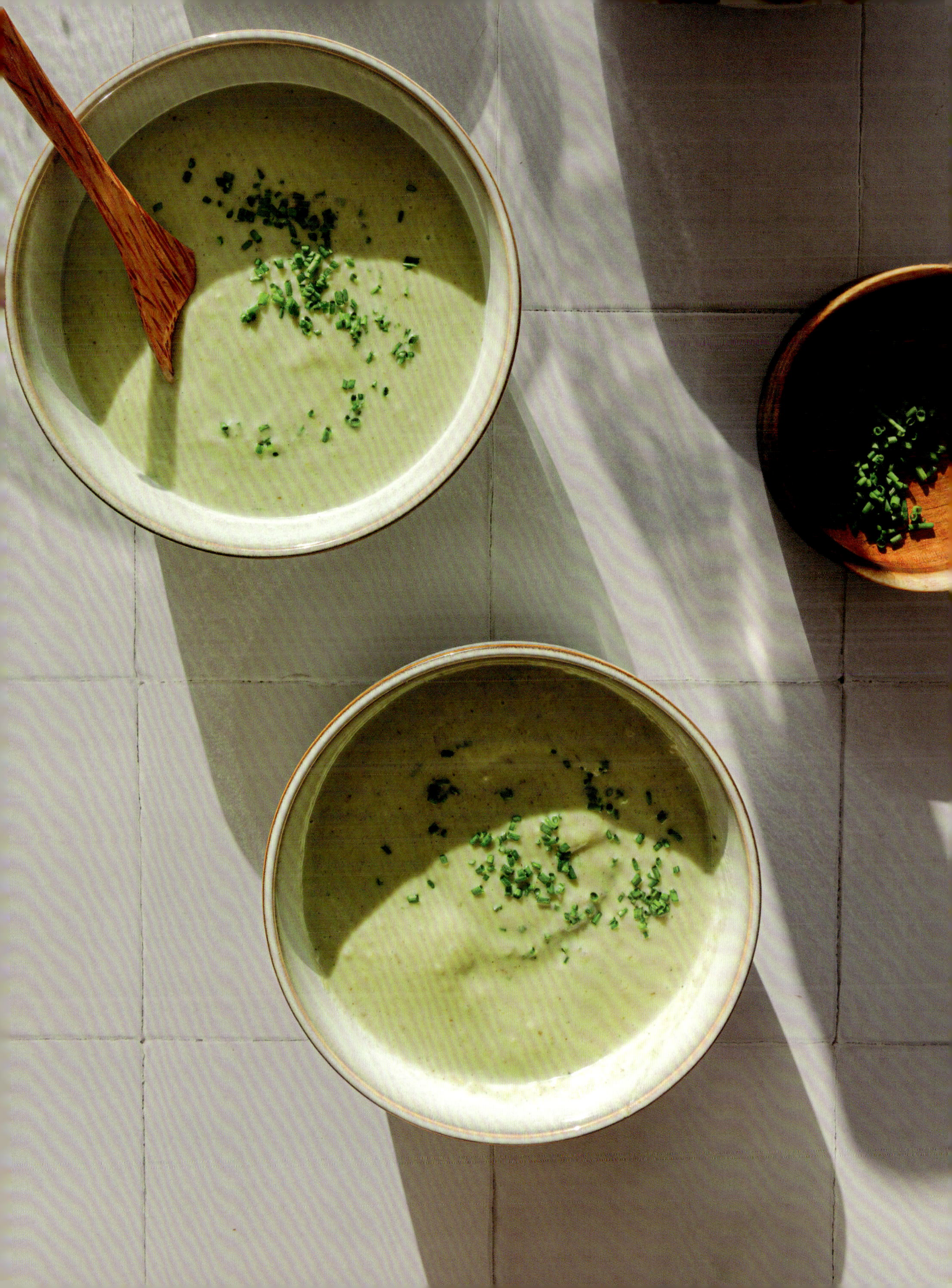

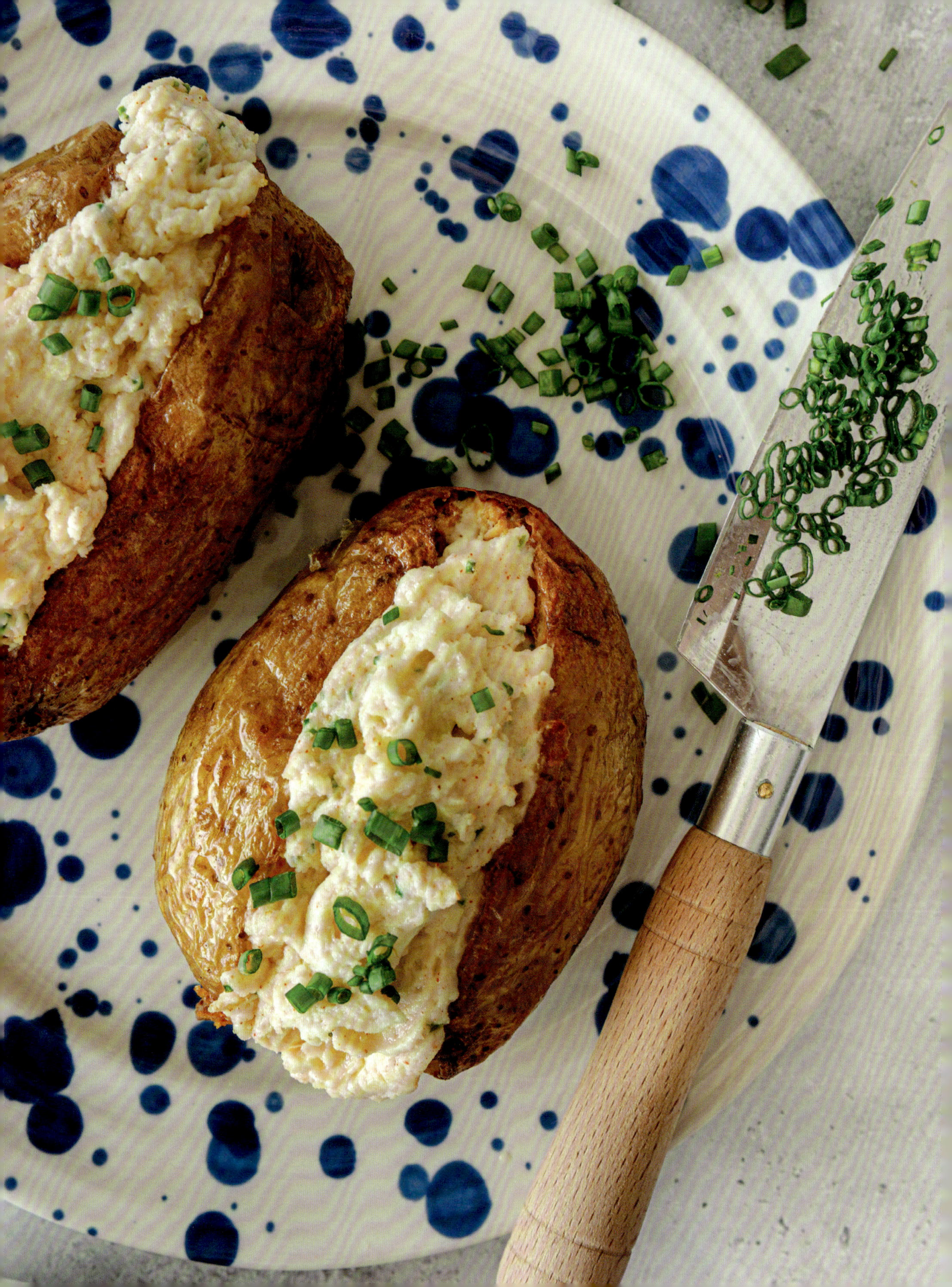

ENHANCED TWICE-BAKED POTATO

1 large russet potato, washed and scrubbed
¼ cup (60g) nonfat Greek yogurt
½ oz (16.7g) slice of Laughing Cow Light cheese
½ tsp (1.5g) garlic powder
¼ tsp (750mg) Cajun seasoning
1 stalk of green onion, diced
Salt and pepper, to taste

Enhancing your baked potato is just like adding some extra "herbs" to your batch of brownies. It will leave you smiling ear to ear and hungry for more. The key to getting that perfectly fluffy inside is baking the potato fully until it's soft enough to scoop easily (don't rush it). Using Greek yogurt instead of sour cream adds protein while keeping it creamy, and Laughing Cow cheese melts seamlessly for a velvety texture. If you have an extra big potato and the inside's seeming kind of dry, just add a bit more Greek yogurt, and you're golden. For extra crispiness, bake the stuffed potatoes on the top rack, or give them a quick broil at the end.

1. Preheat the oven to 400°F (200°C). Line a baking sheet with parchment paper.
2. On the prepared baking sheet, place the potato. Using a fork, poke holes in the potato at least 10 times. Bake for 45 to 55 minutes, until the potato is soft on the inside. Alternatively, there are lots of microwave hacks out there, so feel free to use those. As long as the potato is soft and can be scooped out, it's fine.
3. Cut the potato in half lengthwise and scoop the insides out into a bowl. Set aside the potato skins on the same baking sheet.
4. To the bowl with the potato insides, add the Greek yogurt, cheese, garlic powder, Cajun seasoning, and green onion and season with salt and pepper. Stir to combine.
5. Scoop the potato mixture back into each half of the potato skins and bake for 8 to 10 minutes, until the tops get crispy.

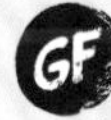

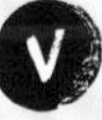

makes 1 baked potato / 1 serving

NUTRITION (PER SERVING)

373 calories	**2g** fat
15g protein	**71g** net carbs

CHICKEN SUMMER ROLLS

- 3 sheets of rice paper, 8 inches (20cm) each
- 1 cup (42.5g) spring mix or other salad greens, roughly chopped
- ½ cup (125g) fresh mint, roughly chopped
- ¼ cup (15g) fresh cilantro, roughly chopped
- ½ English cucumber, roughly chopped
- 3½ tbsp (30g) avocado, chopped
- 1 chicken breast, about 6oz (175g), grilled

These rolls are so good, you'll want to swallow them whole. But for liability reasons, I recommend chewing, or at least having someone familiar with your throat nearby. The key to success? Don't oversoak the rice paper—dip it in warm water for just 5 seconds so it stays pliable without getting too sticky. Rolling takes some practice, so think of it like wrapping a burrito, but with extra patience. For meal prep, store the rolls in an airtight container with a damp paper towel on top to keep them from drying out. They'll stay fresh for up to 2 days, making them a great grab-and-go option. Just don't forget your favorite dipping sauce.

1. Fill a large bowl with warm water. Into the warm water, dip one sheet of the rice paper, making sure it's fully submerged. Hold under water for 5 seconds.
2. Remove the rice paper from the water and place it on a cutting board or flat surface. Down the center of the rice paper, place a small handful of mixed greens, leaving 1 inch (2.5cm) of space at each end for folding.
3. Place some mint, cilantro, and cucumber on top of the spring mix. Add about a third (10g) of the avocado over top, followed by a third (about 60g) of the chicken.
4. Delicately roll the rice paper around the filling, making sure not to pull too hard. It takes some practice—think burrito.
5. Repeat steps 1 to 4 to make two more summer rolls.
6. Enjoy the summer rolls on their own or serve with your favorite Asian-style dipping sauce.

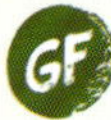

makes 3 rolls / 3 servings

NUTRITION (PER SERVING)

90 calories	**2g** fat
10g protein	**8g** net carbs

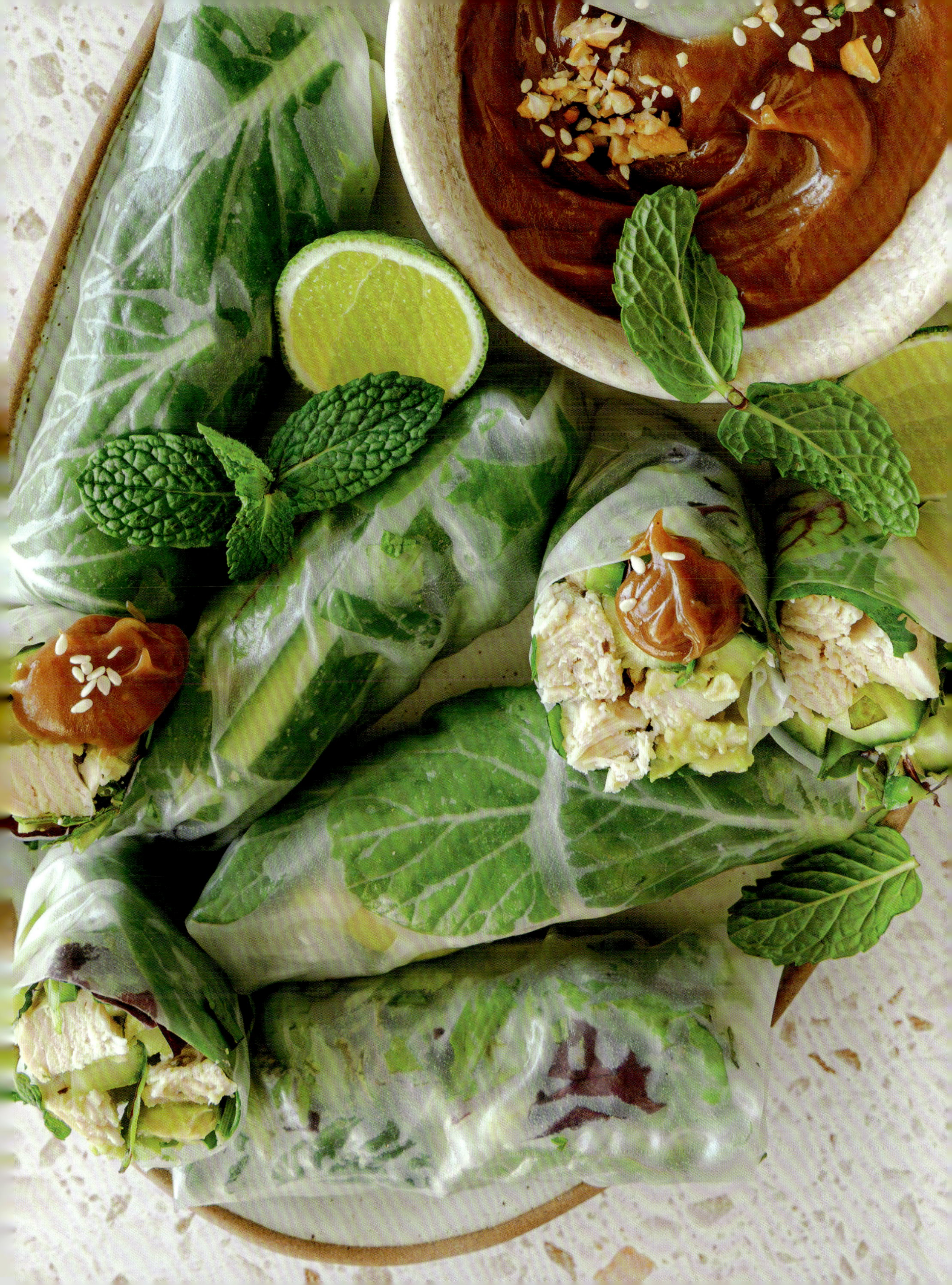

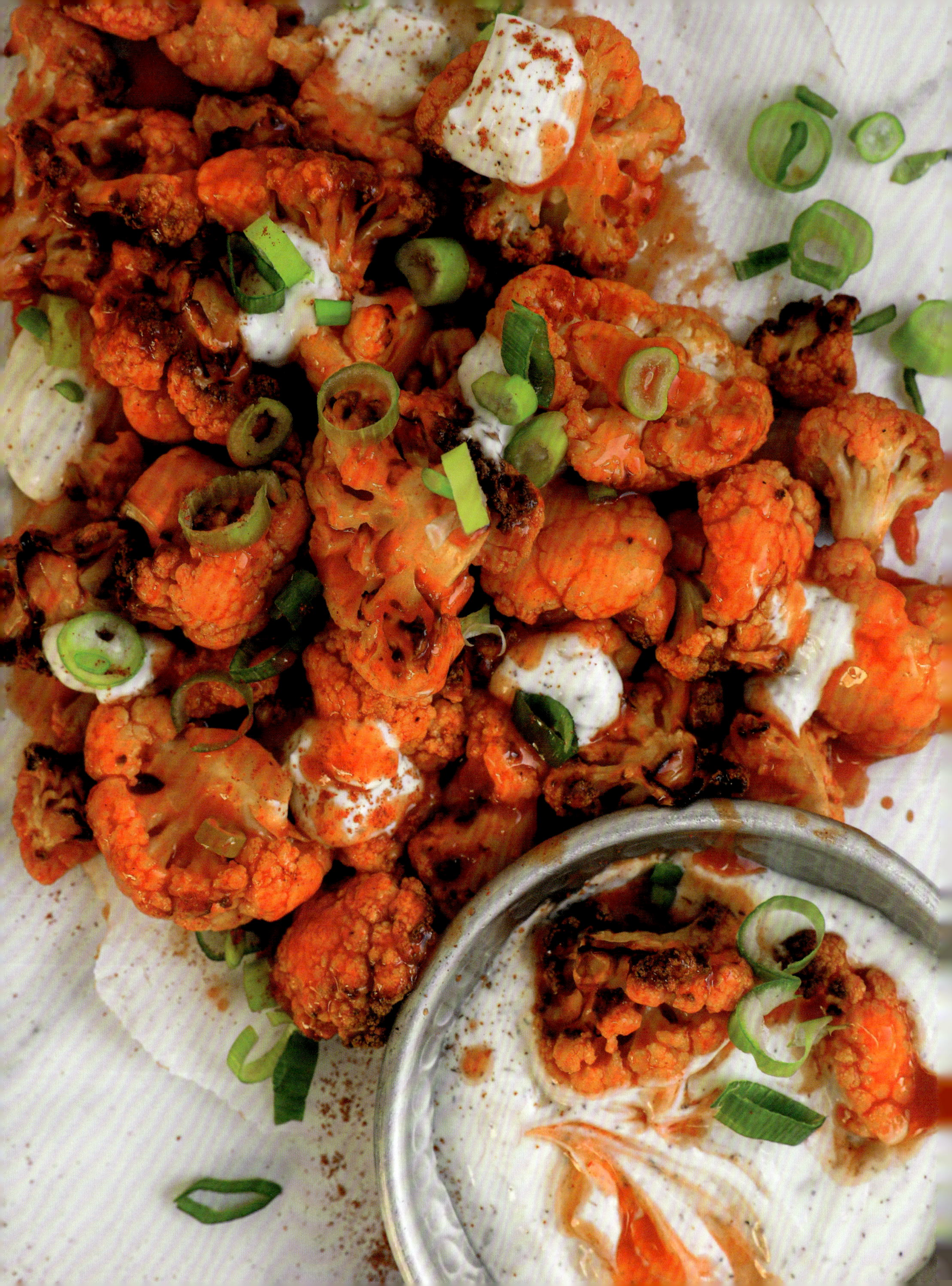

BUFFALO CAULIFLOWER BITES

for the cauliflower bites:

- 1 large head of cauliflower, cut into bite-size pieces
- 1 egg, beaten
- 1 tsp (3g) garlic powder
- 1 cup (120g) almond flour
- ½ tsp (1.5g) salt
- 1 tsp (3g) onion powder

for the buffalo sauce:

- 1 cup (240ml) Frank's RedHot Original
- ½ cup (120ml) low-sodium vegetable broth
- ⅓ cup (38g) raw cashews
- ¼ cup (60ml) white vinegar
- ½ tsp (1.5g) garlic powder
- ½ tsp (1.5g) onion powder

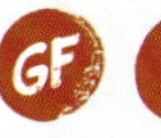

makes 4 servings

NUTRITION (PER SERVING)	
197 calories	**13g** fat
9g protein	**10g** net carbs

You might miss the big game because all your attention will be on these delicious Buffalo bites. They're still a sad excuse for chicken wings, but in the world of Buffalo-related things, it's a top-tier recipe. The secret to getting these crispy? Space them out on the baking sheet—if they're too close, they'll steam instead of bake. For the Buffalo sauce, blending cashews into the mix gives it a rich, creamy texture without needing butter. And the final broil is key. It locks in the flavor and adds that perfect char, but watch closely so they don't burn. Serve with your favorite dip and prepare for zero leftovers.

1. **To make the cauliflower bites:** Preheat the oven to 425°F (220°C). Line a baking sheet with parchment paper.
2. To a large resealable plastic bag, add the cauliflower and beaten egg. Seal the bag and shake to fully coat the cauliflower.
3. To a medium bowl, add the garlic powder, almond flour, salt, and onion powder and stir to combine. To the bag with the cauliflower, add the powder mixture. Reseal and shake until the cauliflower is evenly coated.
4. On the prepared baking sheet, lay the coated cauliflower evenly so the pieces do not overlap. Bake for 22 to 25 minutes, until the edges are brown.
5. **To make the buffalo sauce:** While the cauliflower bakes, to a blender, add the Frank's RedHot, vegetable broth, cashews, vinegar, garlic powder, and onion powder. Blend until smooth.
6. When the cauliflower is done cooking, transfer it to a large bowl, pour the Buffalo sauce over top, and toss until completely coated.
7. Set the oven to broil. Return the cauliflower to the baking sheet and bake on the top rack for 5 minutes. Keep an eye on these because they can burn quickly under the broiler.
8. Remove the cauliflower from the oven and serve on its own, with any remaining Buffalo sauce, or with your favorite dipping sauce.

WARM ROOT-VEGETABLE SALAD

for the salad:

½ tbsp (8ml) coconut oil
2¼ cups (250g) butternut squash, peeled and sliced into thick fries
2¼ cups (250g) daikon radish, peeled and sliced into thick fries
1½ cups (250g) rutabaga, peeled and sliced into thick fries
2 cups (250g) zucchini, sliced into thick fries
Salt and pepper, to taste
3 cups (90g) spinach
1 grilled chicken breast, about 8oz (225g)

for the tahini dressing:

2 tbsp (30g) tahini
Juice from ½ lemon
½ tsp (1.5g) cayenne pepper
½ tsp (1.5g) cumin
Salt and pepper, to taste

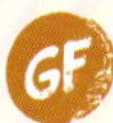

makes 2 servings

NUTRITION (PER SERVING)

415 calories
13.5g fat
31.5g protein
42g net carbs

Hi, readers, it's Katie! This is the first recipe William and I made together, nonstop . . . for months. It's not only tasty but is a nostalgic recipe for us. It's great as a salad, but also in a wrap or on a bed of rice. The key to getting perfectly tender veggies? Cut them into uniform pieces so they cook evenly, and don't rush the simmer—20 to 25 minutes ensures they soften without becoming mushy. I hope you love it as much as we do!

1. **To make the salad:** Heat a large pot over medium-high heat and add the coconut oil.
2. Meanwhile, in a separate pot over high heat or with a kettle, bring 1½ cups (360ml) of water to a boil.
3. To the pot with the coconut oil, add the squash, radish, rutabaga, and zucchini and season with salt and pepper. Stir until the vegetables are lightly coated in the coconut oil.
4. Add the boiling water. Cover with the lid and reduce the heat to low to simmer. Cook for 20 to 25 minutes, allowing the vegetables to soften.
5. **To make the tahini dressing:** While the vegetables are simmering, to a small bowl, add the tahini, 2 tablespoons (30ml) water, the lemon juice, cayenne pepper, and cumin. Season with salt and pepper and stir to combine. Set aside.
6. Once the vegetables have softened and a small amount of broth is left at the bottom of the pot, remove it from the heat.
7. To plate, evenly distribute the spinach in two bowls and top with the simmered vegetables and grilled chicken breast. Finish with a drizzle of the tahini dressing.

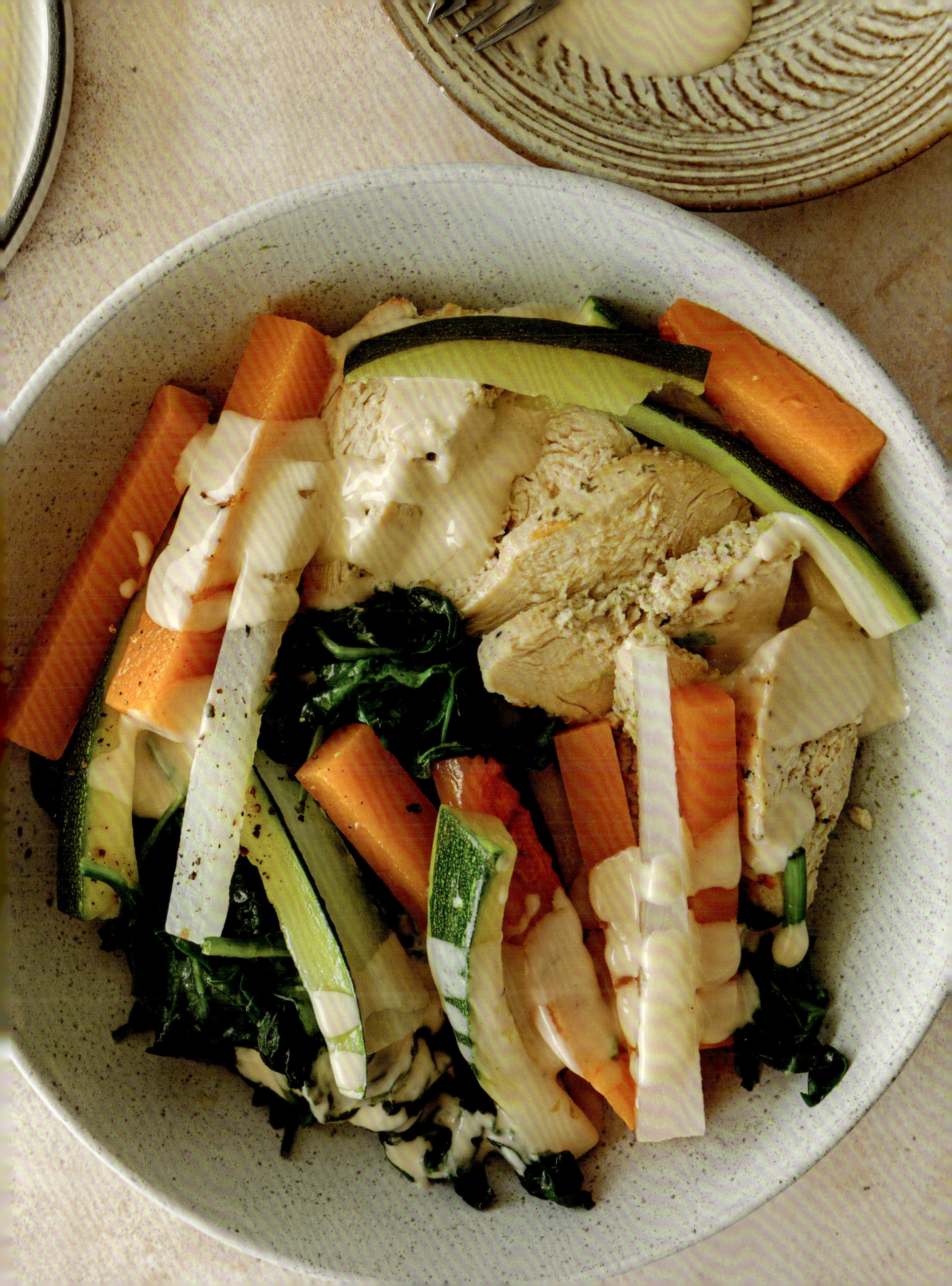

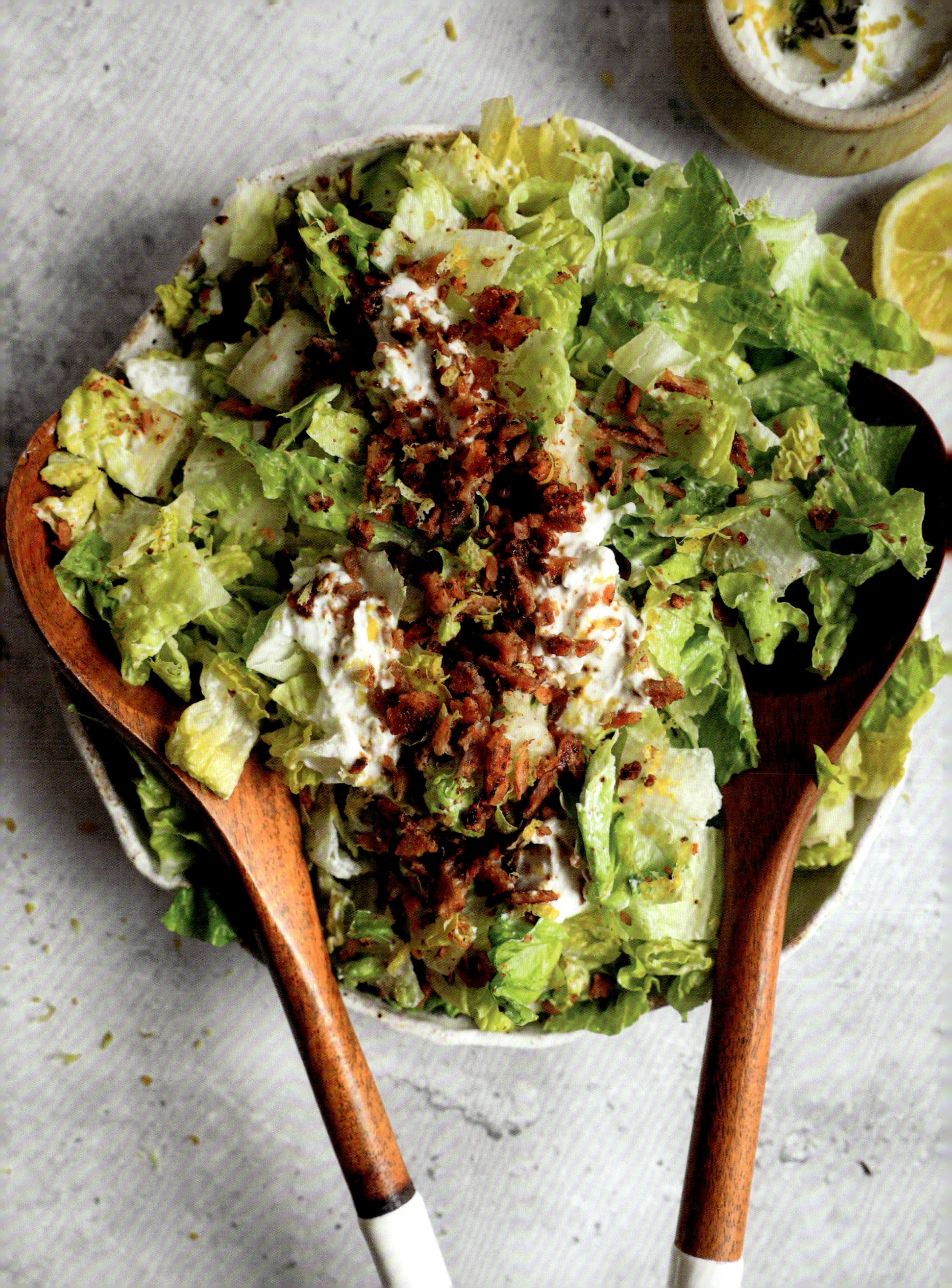

HEALTHY CAESAR SALAD

for the Greek yogurt "Caesar" dressing:

½ cup (100g) nonfat Greek yogurt
Juice of 1 medium lemon
½ tsp (1.5g) garlic powder
½ tsp (1.5g) onion powder
½ tsp (1g) Parmesan-and-herb seasoning
Pinch of salt and pepper

for the salad:

7 cups (300g) romaine lettuce, chopped
2 strips of chicken bacon, cooked and diced

Hail Caesar! Here's a staple-cut recipe of mine, a twist on the classic that'll still deliver a familiar creamy experience while keeping calories low and volume high. If you think all Caesar salads are healthy just because they're salads . . . I don't even know what to say to you. Traditional Caesar dressing is basically a charcuterie board in liquid form—loaded with eggs, anchovies, cheese, and oil. But like turning water into wine, I've pulled off a miracle here, swapping in smarter ingredients that deliver the same bold flavor while actually supporting your gains.

1. **To make the Greek yogurt "Caesar" dressing:** To a large bowl, add the Greek yogurt, half of the lemon juice, the garlic powder, onion powder, and Parmesan-and-herb seasoning. Season with salt and pepper and stir to combine.
2. Add in the rest of the lemon juice and stir until the mixture resembles a creamy salad dressing.
3. **To make the salad:** To a large bowl, add the romaine lettuce and chicken bacon and toss with the Greek yogurt "Caesar" dressing to coat. That's it!

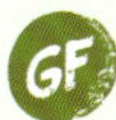

makes 1 salad / 1 serving

NUTRITION (PER SERVING)

165 calories	**4g** fat
18g protein	**15g** net carbs

TUNA-STUFFED AVOCADOS

- 1 lime
- 1 medium avocado, sliced in half lengthwise and pitted
- ½ cup (30g) cilantro, roughly chopped
- 1 red bell pepper, roughly chopped
- 1 Roma tomato, or a small handful of grape tomatoes, roughly chopped
- 1 jalapeño, diced
- 2 (5oz / 140g) cans white tuna, drained and flaked
- Salt and pepper, to taste

Since this generation will never be able to afford their dream home, you might as well look the best out of your four roommates by splurging on the avocado for this meal. Depending on how high you pile your stuffed avocados, you might have some extra filling. Consider it a little bonus from me to you. For an even creamier texture, mix in a heaping tablespoon of Greek yogurt, and dig in.

1. On a cutting board, roll out the lime to soften it and cut it in half. Into a large bowl, squeeze the juice from both halves.
2. Into the bowl, scoop out the insides of the avocado. Set the avocado shells aside.
3. Add the cilantro, bell pepper, tomato, jalapeño, and white tuna. Season with salt and pepper.
4. Using a fork, mash all the ingredients together until evenly combined into a clumpy mixture. Do not overmix! It should be chunky.
5. Scoop the tuna-avocado mixture back into the avocado shells. Serve and enjoy!

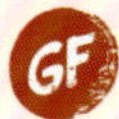

makes 1 serving

NUTRITION (PER SERVING)

413 calories	**13g** fat
59g protein	**15g** net carbs

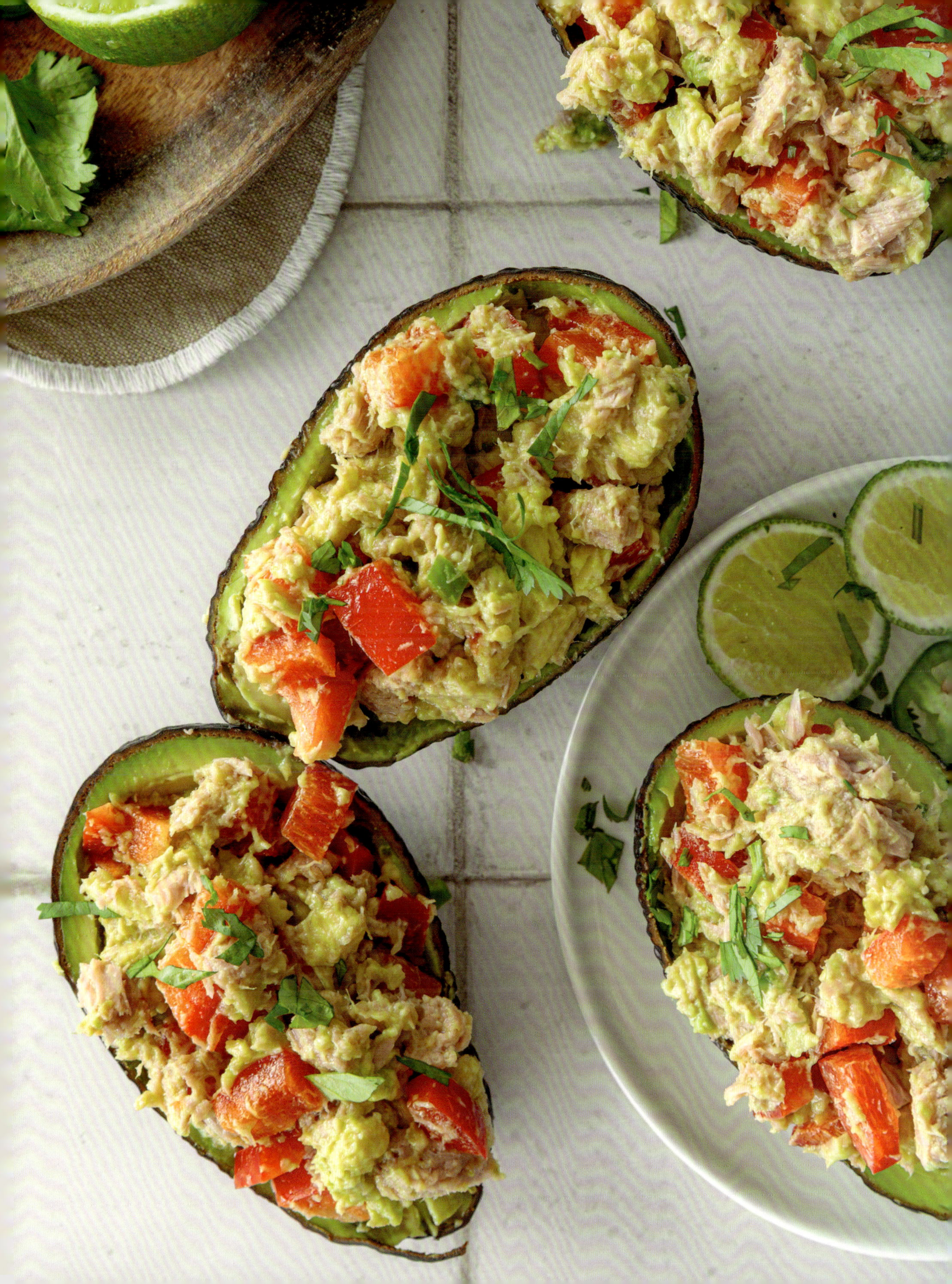

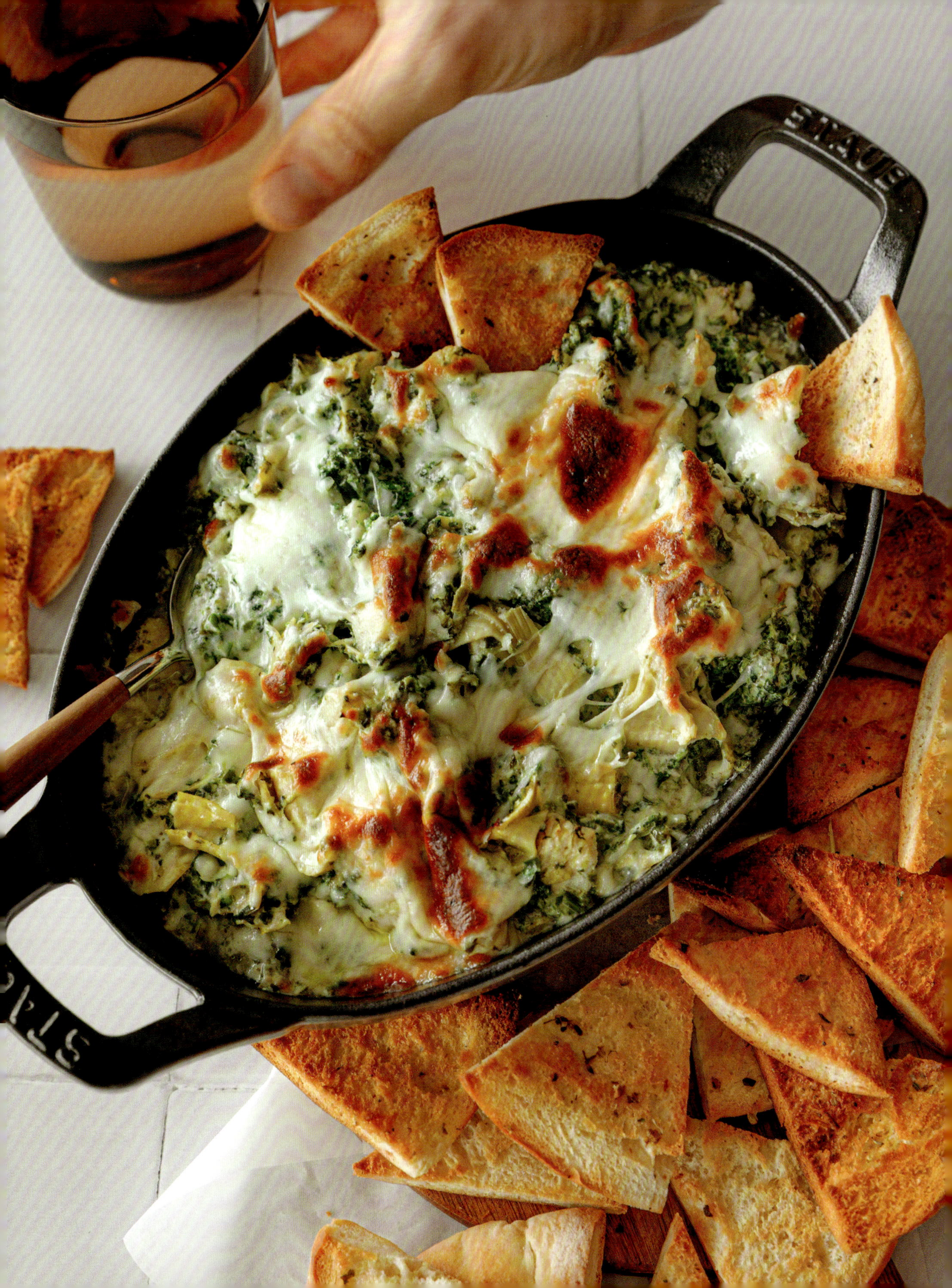
STAUB

ANABOLIC SPINACH ARTICHOKE DIP
WITH PITA CHIPS

- 1 (14oz / 400g) can quartered artichoke hearts, drained and chopped
- 2 garlic cloves, finely chopped
- 10oz (300g) frozen spinach, thawed and drained
- 1 cup (230g) nonfat Greek yogurt
- Juice of ½ lemon
- 1 cup (90g) shredded part-skim mozzarella cheese
- ⅓ cup (40g) grated Parmesan cheese
- Salt and pepper, to taste
- 2½ tbsp (38ml) olive oil
- ½ tsp (1.5g) garlic powder
- 1 tsp (3g) dried rosemary
- 4 whole-wheat pitas, each cut into 8 triangular pieces

Fueling my gains *and* my memories, this recipe is in honor of one of my favorite appetizers as a kid, back when I would down them so fast my parents feared I'd be putting the choke in artichoke. Drain your spinach and artichokes really well. Excess moisture can make the dip watery instead of thick and gooey. If you like a little extra kick, try adding a pinch of red pepper flakes or a squeeze of lemon juice to brighten up the flavors.

1. Preheat the oven to 350°F (180°C). Line a baking sheet with parchment paper.
2. In a large bowl, mix together the artichoke hearts, garlic, spinach, Greek yogurt, lemon juice, ¾ cup (67.5g) of the mozzarella, and the Parmesan. Season with salt and pepper.
3. Transfer the mixture to a medium oven-safe casserole dish or bowl and sprinkle an even layer of the remaining mozzarella cheese on top.
4. Bake for 20 to 25 minutes, until the top is golden brown and the dip is heated through.
5. While the dip is baking, in a large bowl, add the olive oil, garlic powder, and rosemary and season with additional salt and pepper. Stir well to combine. Add the pita triangles to the bowl and toss to coat in the olive oil mixture.
6. On the prepared baking sheet, lay the pita chips. Bake for 8 to 10 minutes, until crispy.
7. Serve the dip in the dish it was baked in, along with the crispy pita chips. Dip and enjoy.

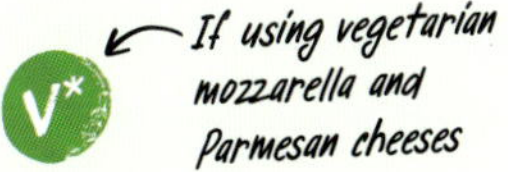

makes 4 servings

NUTRITION (PER SERVING)

494 calories	**23g** fat
29g protein	**36g** net carbs

PINEAPPLE SALSA

1½ cups (210g) pineapple, diced
½ jalapeño, diced
¼ cup (15g) chopped cilantro
¼ cup (28g) chopped red onion
¼ cup (37.5g) chopped red bell pepper
Juice of 1 lime
Salt and pepper, to taste

This salsa is more refreshing than an afternoon of puppy yoga, and more versatile than Christian Bale. Eat it on its own, with tortilla chips, on your favorite protein, or even as a curry topping. The possibilities are endless! For this recipe, picking the right pineapple is key. Look for one that is golden yellow, is slightly soft when squeezed, and smells sweet at the base. If it has a green shell or has no scent, it's probably underripe.

1. To a large bowl, add the pineapple, jalapeño, cilantro, onion, bell pepper, and lime juice. Season with salt and pepper.
2. Toss the ingredients to combine into a salsa.

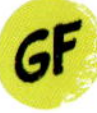

makes 2 servings

NUTRITION (PER SERVING)

82 calories	**0g** fat
1g protein	**18g** net carbs

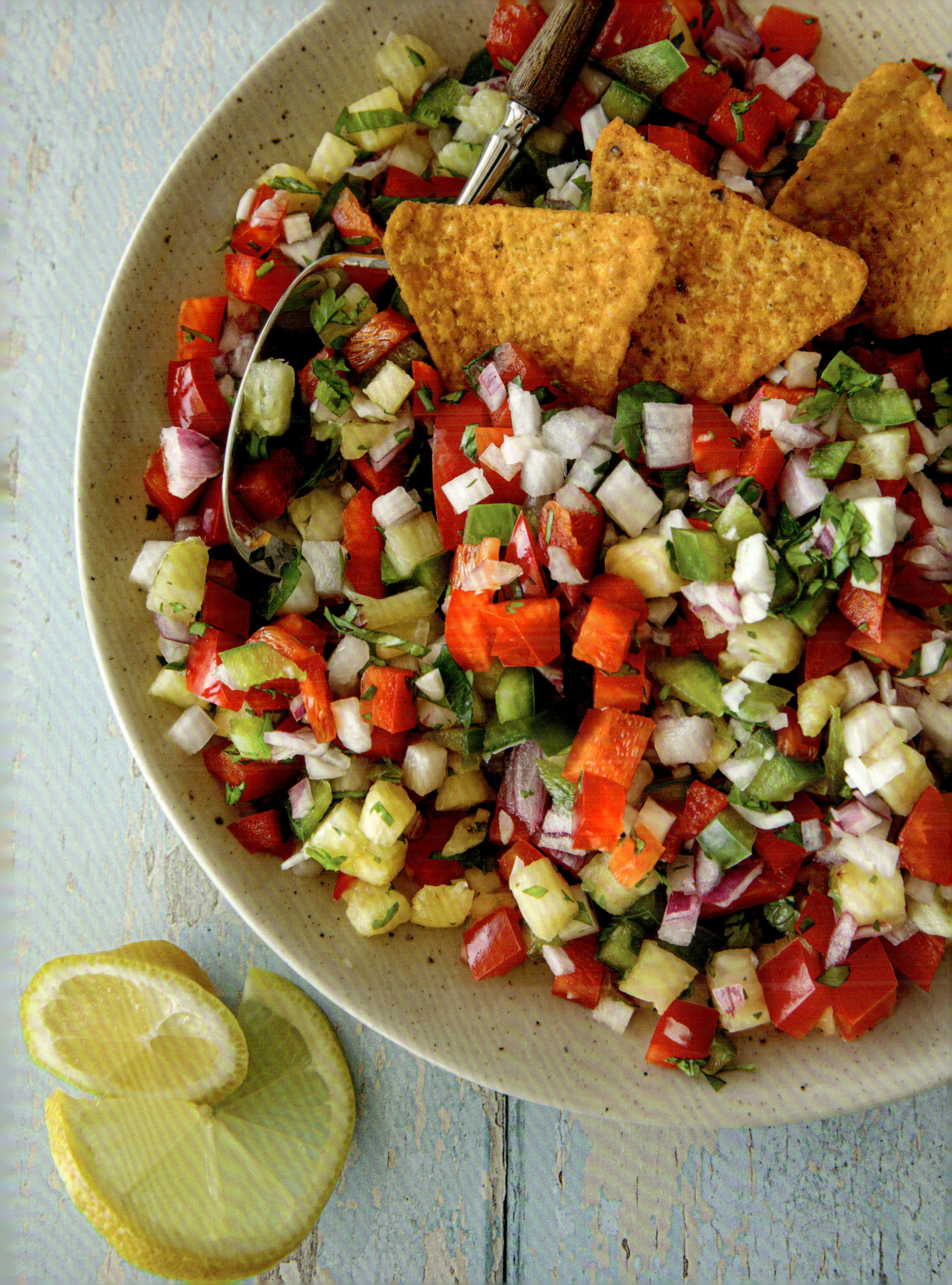

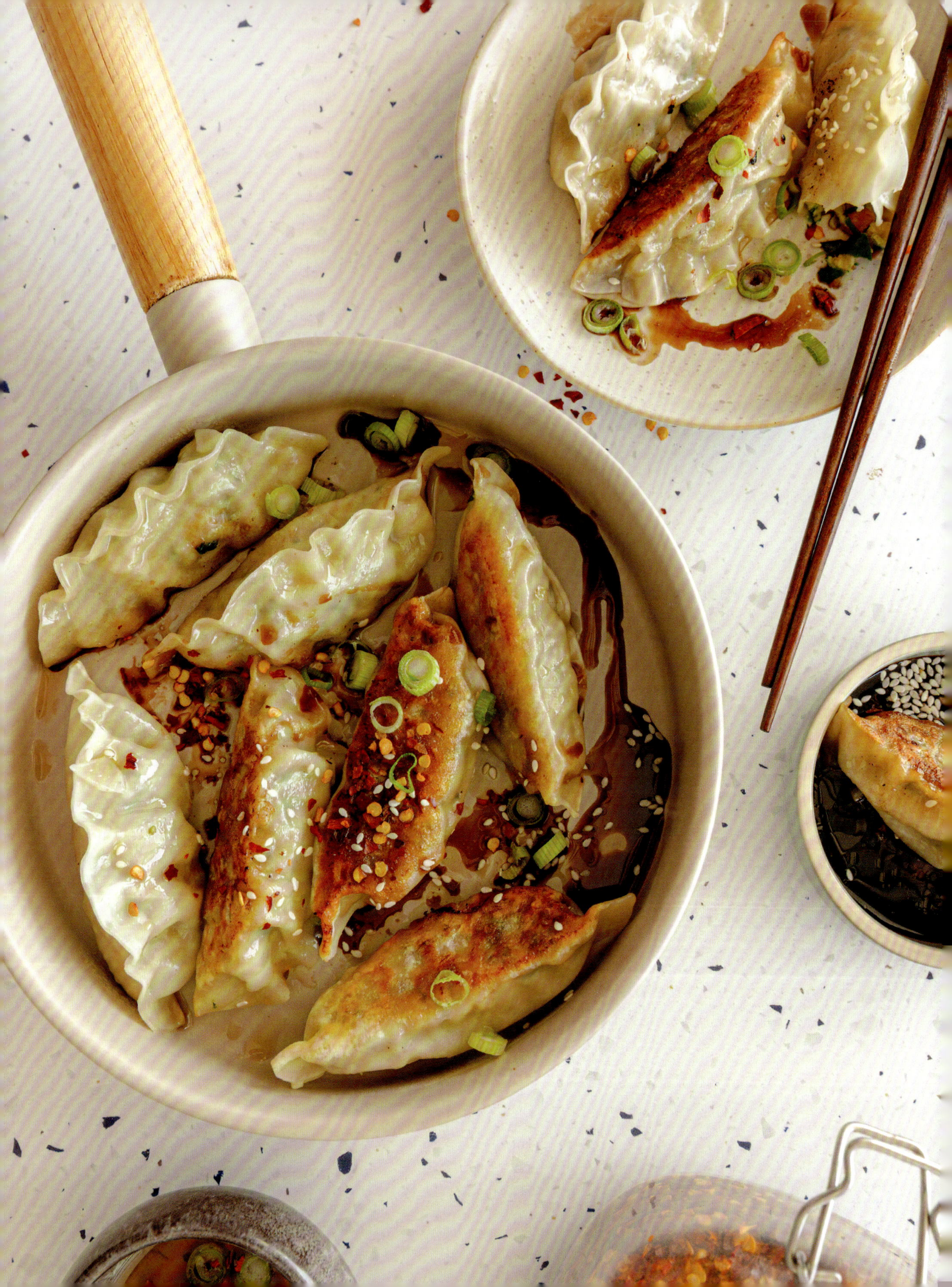

CHICKEN POTSTICKERS

- 1-inch (2.5cm) knob of fresh ginger, diced
- 1 garlic clove, finely diced
- 1 cup (100g) cabbage, finely chopped
- 2 stalks of green onion, diced
- Pinch of salt
- 8oz (225g) extra-lean ground chicken
- 1¼ tbsp (23ml) soy sauce
- ½ tsp (2.5ml) sesame oil
- 20 circular dumpling wrappers

These chicken potstickers will do more than stick to your pan—they'll help you stick to your macros goals. The magic is in keeping the filling moist but not watery—let the cabbage mixture cool completely before mixing it with the chicken to avoid excess liquid. When pan-frying, make sure the potstickers aren't touching, so they crisp up properly instead of steaming into a dumpling disaster. Serve them with soy sauce, chili crisp, or even a side of smug satisfaction, because, yes, you just made homemade potstickers.

1. Line a baking sheet with parchment paper and set aside.
2. Place a medium frying pan over medium heat and spray it with nonstick cooking spray. Add the ginger and garlic and sauté for 30 seconds, until fragrant.
3. Add the cabbage and green onion. Season with a pinch of salt and cook for 5 to 6 minutes, until the cabbage becomes translucent. Remove from the heat and allow the mixture to cool.
4. In a large mixing bowl, combine the ground chicken, cooled cabbage mixture, soy sauce, and sesame oil. Mix until evenly combined.
5. Fill a small bowl with water. Take one dumpling wrapper and dip the outer edge into the water, leaving the center dry. In the center of the wrapper, place about 1 tablespoon of filling. Fold the wrapper over the filling and pinch the edges tightly to seal, ensuring the filling is evenly distributed. Place the potsticker on the prepared baking sheet. Repeat with the remaining wrappers and filling.
6. Heat a large frying pan over high heat and spray it generously with nonstick cooking spray. Arrange half of the potstickers in the pan in a single layer, ensuring they do not overlap. Cover the pot with the lid and sear for 2 to 3 minutes, until the bottoms are golden brown.
7. Carefully open the lid and pour in ¼ cup (60ml) water. Be cautious, as it may splatter! Close the lid, reduce the heat to medium, and cook for an additional 5 to 6 minutes.
8. Remove the lid and cook for another 2 to 3 minutes, or until the water evaporates and the bottoms are crisp. The internal temperature should reach 165°F (74°C). Repeat with the second half of the potstickers. Allow to cool slightly before serving. Enjoy!

makes 20 potstickers / 4 servings

NUTRITION (PER SERVING)

245 calories	**5g** fat
16g protein	**33.5g** net carbs

-CHAPTER 5-

FEEDING THE FAMILY

MAINS

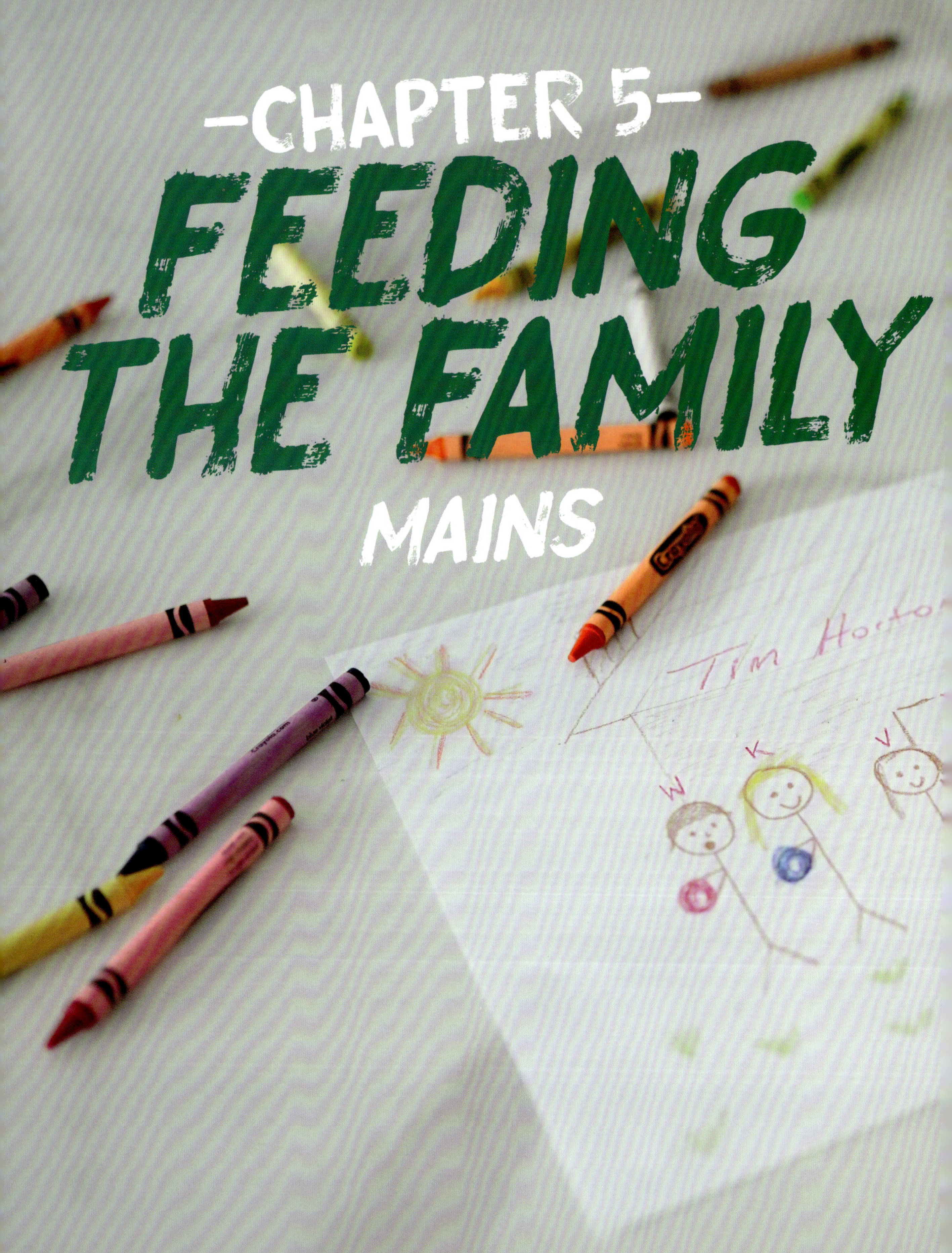

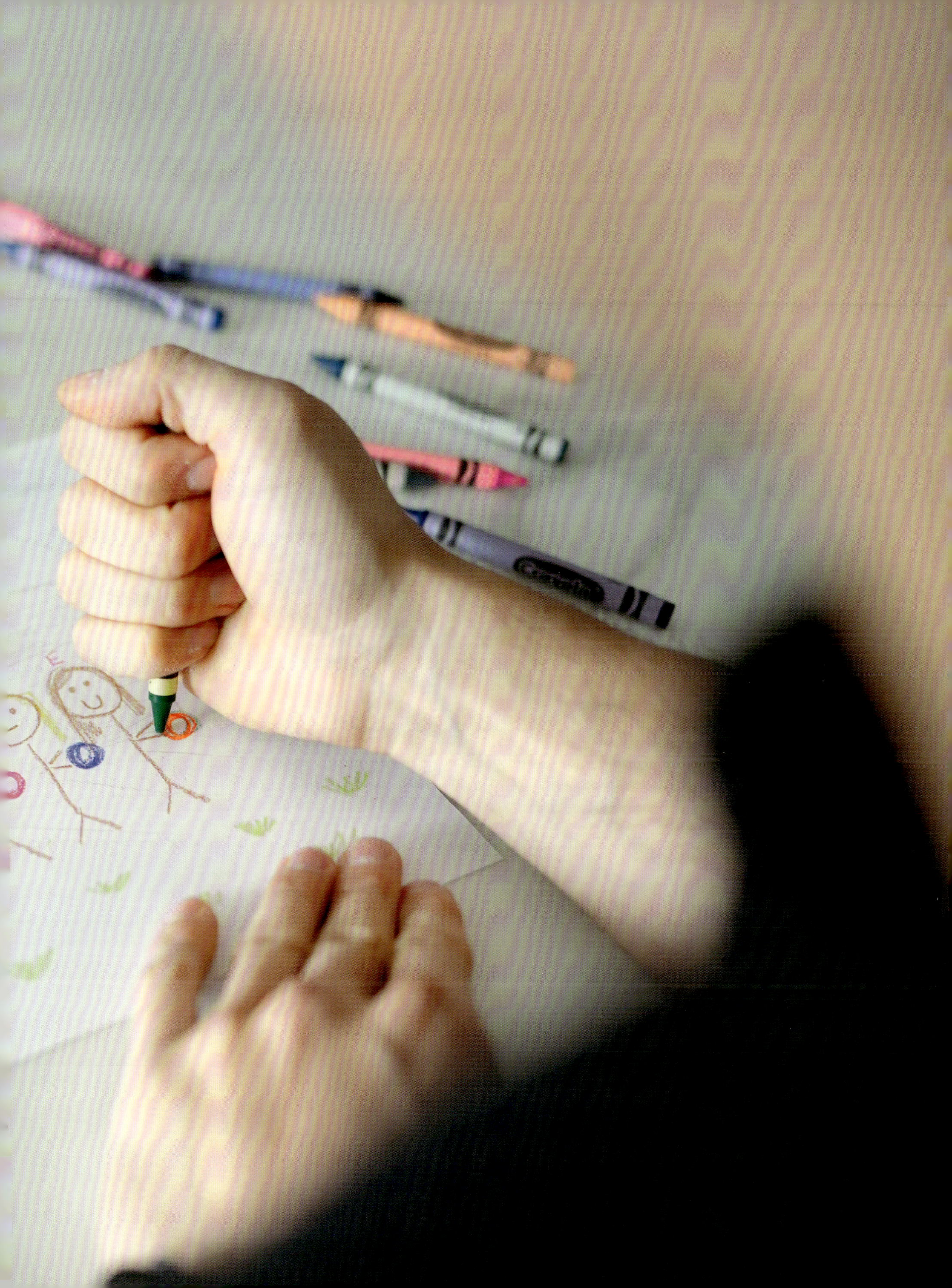

The whole Tenny gang with our old dog, Arthur.

The giver of good genetics herself, Mama Tenny.

Ollie's homecoming in July 2005.

Showing Grandma Tenny my best toothless smile.

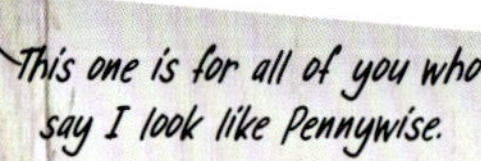

This one is for all of you who say I look like Pennywise.

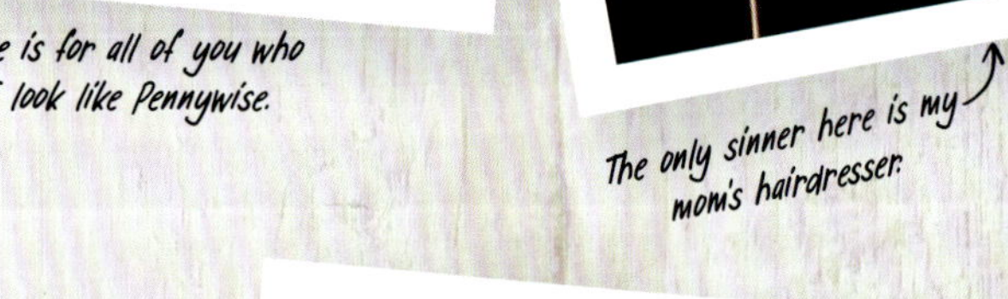

The only sinner here is my mom's hairdresser.

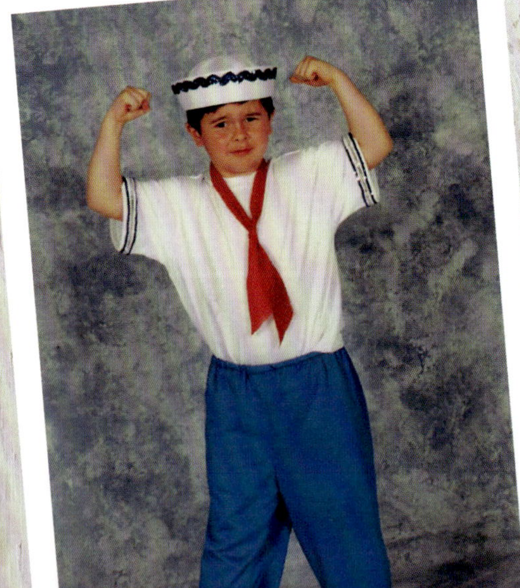

Natty or not?

Just your typical middle child.

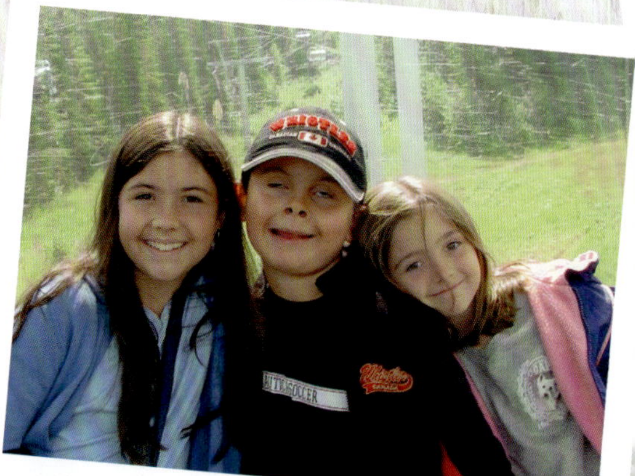

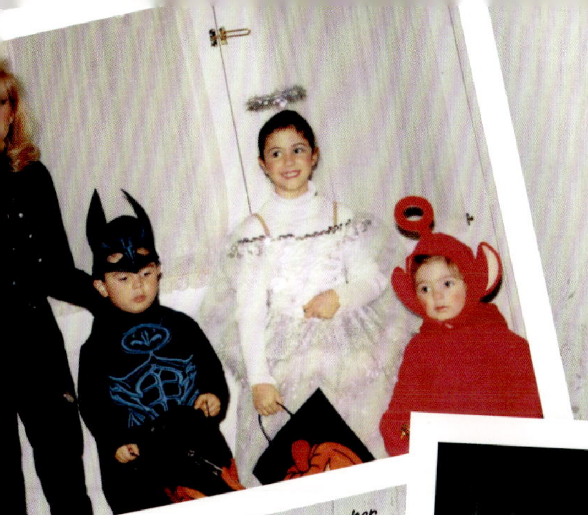

Deep in thought, trying to remember which houses give out the full-size chocolate bars.

When my mom told us we couldn't get McDonald's because we had food at home.

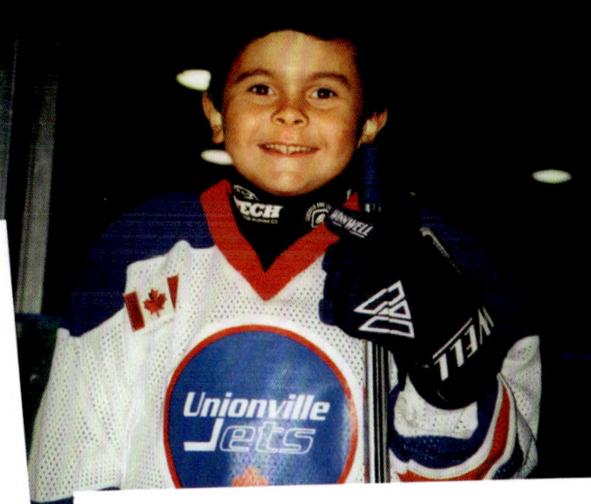

Hoping my smile will keep me out of the penalty box.

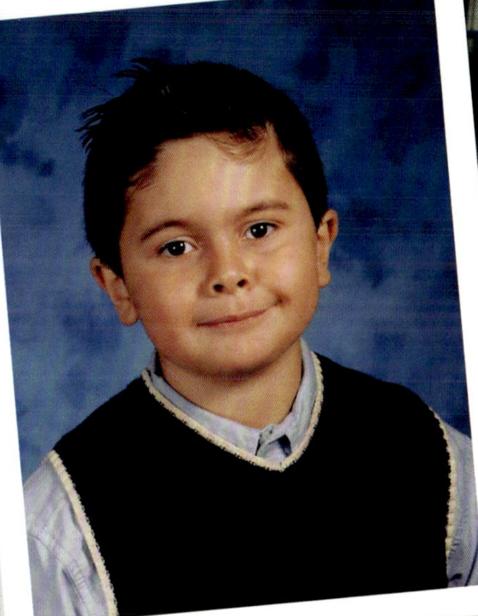

I nailed the "passing a random stranger on the street" smile for school picture day, don't you think?

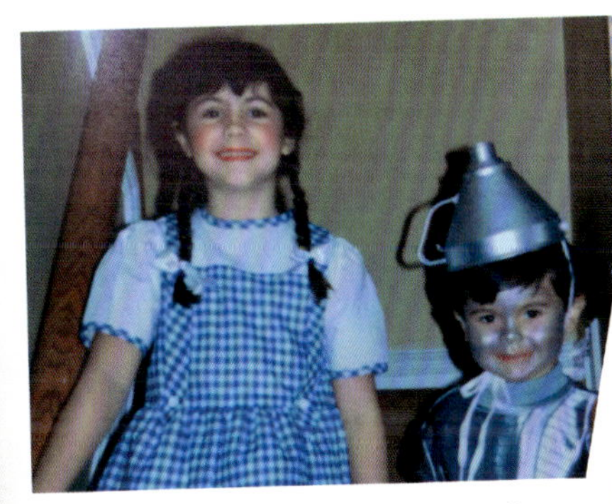

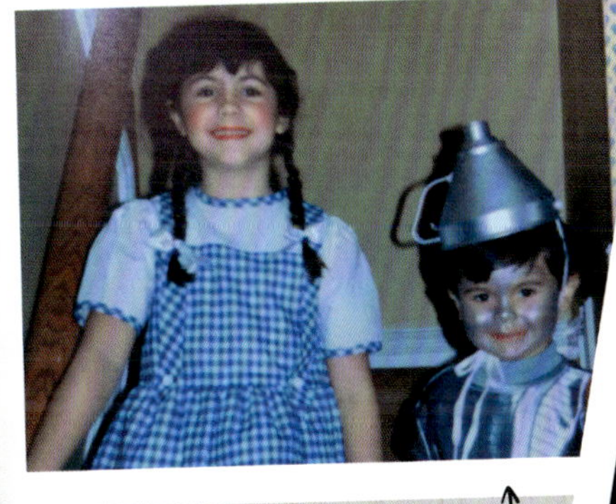

If I only had a heart.

When I was a baby, you could rely on me for one thing—my face was always covered in food.

My sister often dressed me up as Sailor Moon, but I couldn't care less when food was on the table.

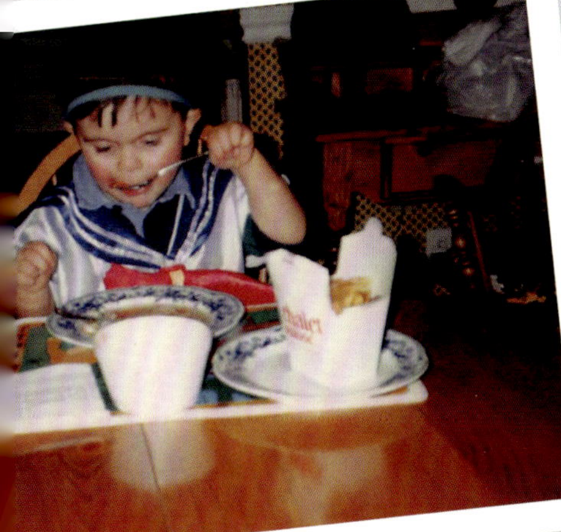

What's a rarer sighting than the Loch Ness monster? A photo of me and my dad.

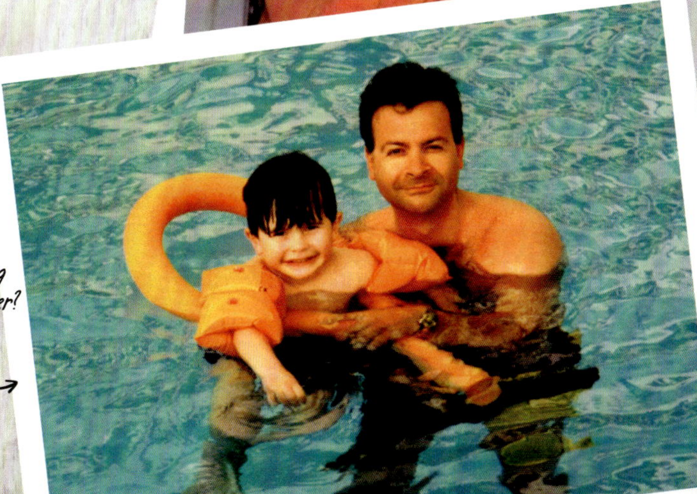

KHICHRI AND AIR-FRIED TOFU

1 (8oz / 225g) block extra-firm tofu
1 tbsp (15ml) soy sauce
½ tbsp (8ml) sesame oil
½ garlic clove, minced
½ cup (100g) dried barley
½ cup (100g) dried red lentils
1½ tsp (4.5g) cumin
1 tsp (3g) turmeric
½ tsp (1.5g) chili powder
2 tsp (10g) fresh grated ginger
1 bay leaf
½ cup (15g) fresh cilantro, chopped
Salt, to taste

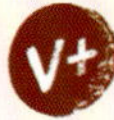

makes 2 servings

NUTRITION (PER SERVING)

445 calories	**10.5g** fat
29.5g protein	**58g** net carbs

While it's not a substitute for "finding yourself" in Bali after your college ex calls you a selfish jerk, this less-than-traditional take on rice and lentils will help you find someone new to spend a night crossing spoons with. Khichri is the ultimate comfort food, great for when you're sick, you need a reset, or you just want something cozy. This version swaps out the usual rice for barley, giving it a nuttier bite and extra fiber, while the blend of cumin, turmeric, and ginger levels up the flavor. The air-fried tofu brings a crispy contrast, because let's be honest—sometimes khichri can look like baby food if left unaccompanied.

1. At least 30 minutes before cooking, remove the tofu from the packaging. Wrap it in a paper towel, place it on a plate or cutting board, and set an object on top of the wrapped tofu to weigh it down (a frying pan works well!) to drain its moisture.
2. If using a conventional oven, preheat it to 400°F (200°C) and line a baking sheet with parchment paper. If using an air fryer, skip this step.
3. In a medium bowl, place the tofu and add the soy sauce, sesame oil, and garlic. Marinate for at least 15 minutes.
4. At the same time, in a large bowl, place the barley and lentils and submerge them in cold water. Set aside to soak for 15 minutes.
5. Place a large pot over medium-high heat and spray it with nonstick cooking spray. Add the cumin, turmeric, chili powder, ginger, and bay leaf and let them toast, stirring often, for 4 to 5 minutes to bring out the aroma.
6. Drain the barley and lentils and add them to the pot with the spices. Sauté for another 4 minutes. Add 5 cups (1.2L) water. Reduce the heat to medium and cover with the lid to let the khichri simmer, stirring occasionally, for 25 minutes.
7. While the khichri is simmering, cut the marinated tofu into 1-inch (2.5cm) blocks. If using a conventional oven, spread the tofu blocks evenly on the prepared baking sheet. If air frying, transfer directly to the air fryer basket.
8. Air fry at 375°F (190°C) for 15 minutes or bake for 20 to 25 minutes, flipping halfway, until the tofu is golden brown and slightly crispy around the edges.
9. Once the khichri is the consistency of a thick soup, add the cilantro and season with salt. Spoon the soup into bowls and top with the air-fried tofu. Enjoy!

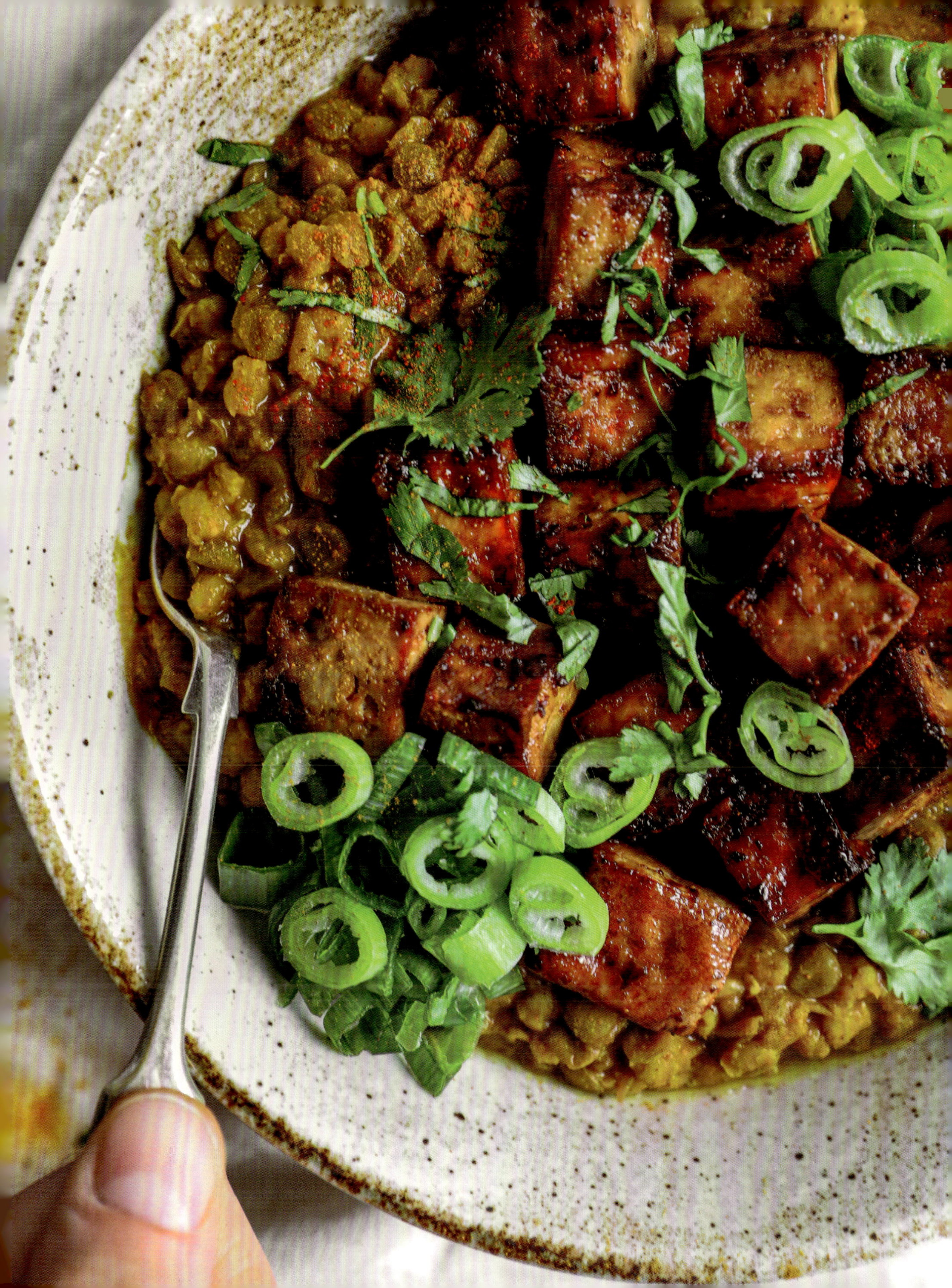

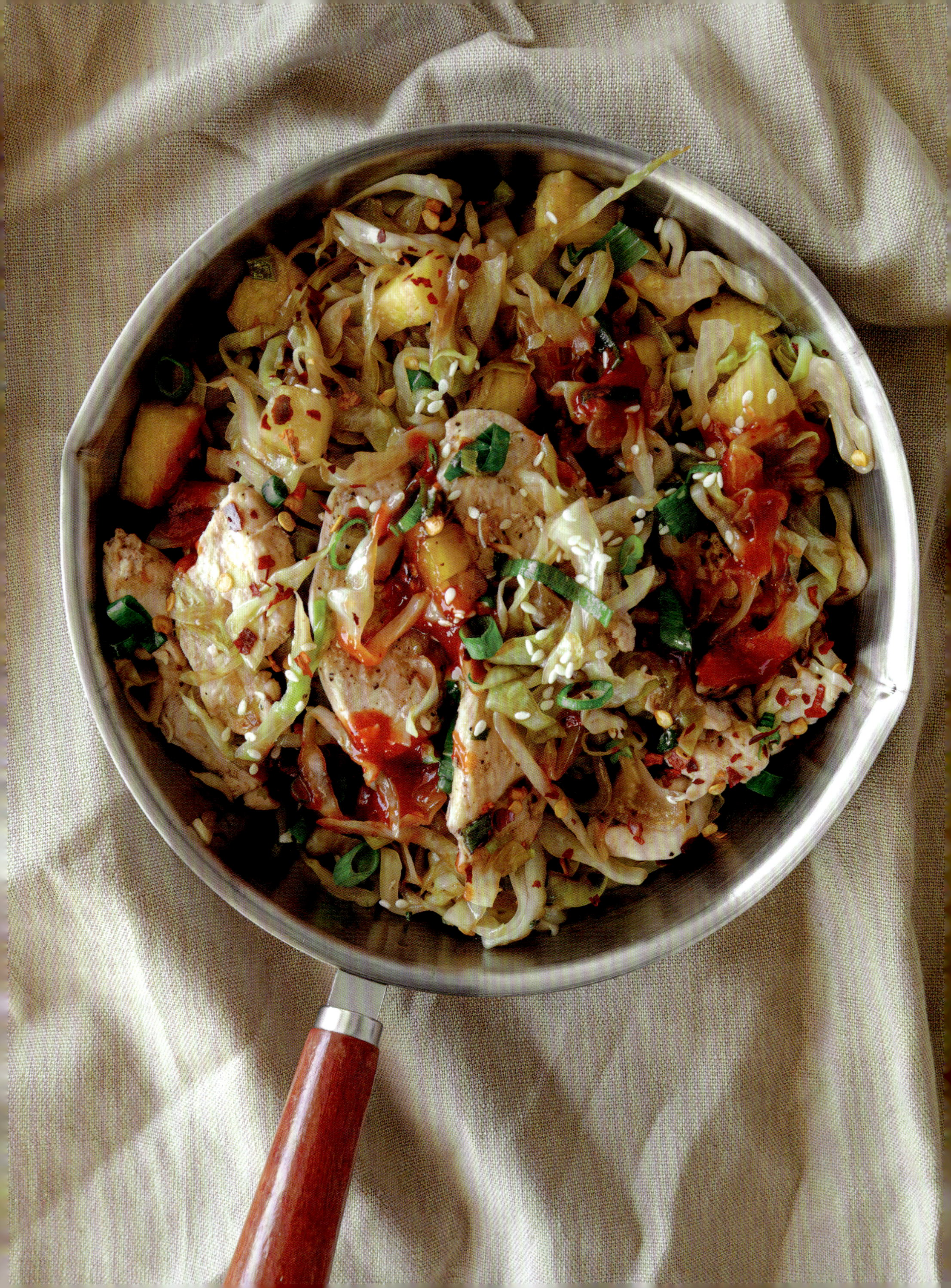

CABBAGE AND CHICKEN STIR FRY

2 stalks of green onion, diced, whites and greens separated
½-inch (1cm) knob of fresh ginger, diced
1 garlic clove, diced
4–6 cups (300–400g) cabbage, thinly sliced
1½ tbsp (23ml) soy sauce
1 chicken breast, about 8oz (225g), sliced into bite-size pieces
Salt and pepper, to taste
½ cup (70g) diced pineapple
½ tsp (1.5g) chili flakes

This dish requires only 15 minutes from start to finish. In my experience, only a baby takes less time to make. Any type of cabbage works here, depending on your preference: Green cabbage gives you a classic crunch (my go-to cabbage), red cabbage adds color and a peppery bite, Napa cabbage softens quickly for a more delicate texture, and Savoy cabbage brings a buttery, tender feel. Pick your poison, and get stir-frying.

1. Preheat a large frying pan over medium heat and spray it with nonstick cooking spray. Add the whites of the green onion, the diced ginger, and garlic, and sauté for 2 to 3 minutes, until softened.
2. Add the cabbage and sauté for another 2 minutes, until the cabbage begins to wilt.
3. To a small bowl, add the soy sauce and 4 tablespoons water and mix.
4. To the pan with the cabbage, pour in the soy-sauce mixture and stir for about 3 minutes, until the cabbage is cooked all the way through.
5. Season the chicken with salt and pepper.
6. Separate the cabbage in the pan to make a well in the middle. Add the chicken to the well and fold the cabbage mixture over top. Let cook for 5 to 7 minutes, stirring occasionally, until the chicken is just about fully cooked.
7. Add the pineapple, chili flakes, and the greens of the green onion, and mix together.
8. Plate up and feel free to add toppings of your choice, such as sesame seeds, sesame oil, or hot sauce.

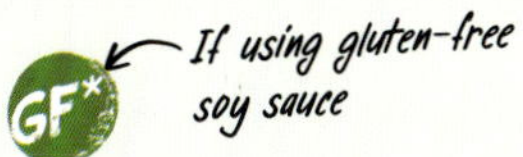

makes 1 serving

NUTRITION (PER SERVING)

427 calories	**2g** fat
57g protein	**43g** net carbs

ONE-POT HEARTY VEGETABLE CHICKEN STEW

- 4¼ cups (450g) butternut squash, peeled and cut into thin fries
- 3½ cups (450g) turnip, peeled and cut into thin fries
- 2⅔ cups (450g) rutabaga, peeled and cut into thin fries
- 2 cups (250g) zucchini, cut into thin fries
- 1 tsp (3g) cumin
- 1 tsp (3g) garlic powder
- 2 tsp (6g) salt, plus more to taste
- Pepper, to taste
- 1 lb (450g) lean ground chicken
- ½ cup (30g) fresh parsley, roughly chopped

A recipe with a built-in workout, all the veggie chopping will create such an appetite, you might try to turn this one-potter into just one meal. If you have some extra calories, top the stew with my tahini dressing: In a small bowl, stir to combine 2 tablespoons (32g) tahini, 2 tablespoons (30ml) water, ¾ teaspoon (3.75ml) lemon juice, 1 teaspoon (3g) cumin, 1 teaspoon (3g) chili powder, and a dash of salt and pepper. And if you're on a cut, this stew will satisfy you all on its own.

1. In a large stock pot, place the butternut squash, turnip, rutabaga, and zucchini. Add the cumin, garlic powder, salt, and pepper and toss to coat.
2. Add 4 to 5 cups (960ml to 1.2L) water, and place the pot over high heat until the water comes to a boil. Once boiling, reduce the heat to medium-low, cover with the lid, and stew for 15 to 20 minutes, until the vegetables soften and become fork tender.
3. When the vegetables have softened, add the ground chicken to the pot, season with additional salt and pepper, and use a spatula or wooden spoon to break up the meat into small morsels. Let cook for 8 to 10 minutes, until the chicken has browned and cooked through.
4. Remove from the heat and toss in the parsley to finish.

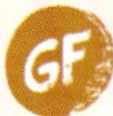

makes 4 servings

NUTRITION (PER SERVING)

260 calories	**6g** fat
28g protein	**22g** net carbs

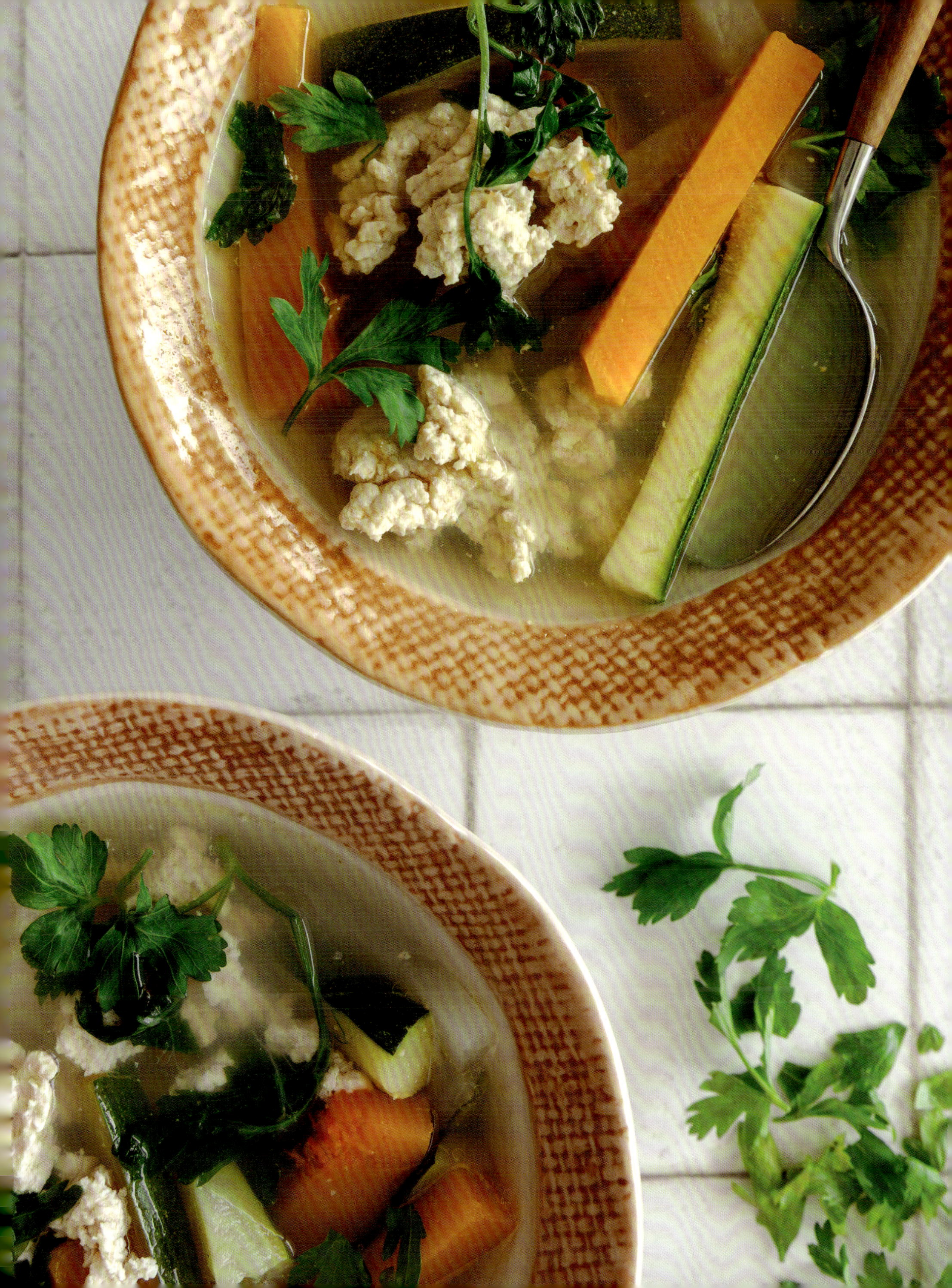

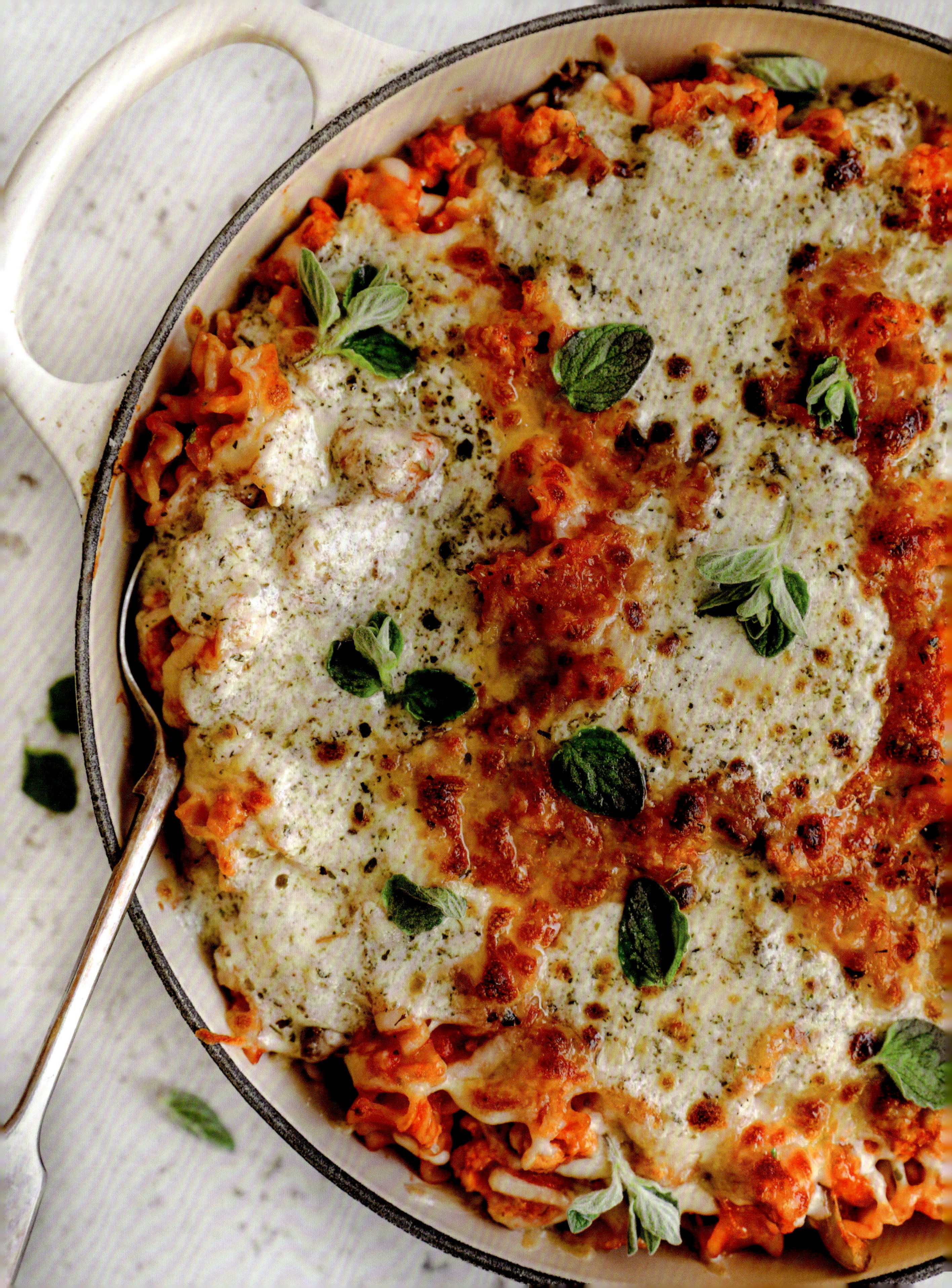

ONE-POT DECONSTRUCTED LASAGNA

1 lb (450g) extra-lean ground turkey
1 large yellow onion, diced
1 green bell pepper, diced
1 cup (240g) sliced white mushrooms
Salt and pepper, to taste
2 garlic cloves, minced
1 (23oz / 652g) jar tomato sauce
8oz (225g) dried pasta of choice
½ cup (124g) low-fat or fat-free ricotta cheese
1 tbsp (7.5g) grated Parmesan cheese
1 tsp (3g) Italian seasoning
⅔ cup (60g) shredded part-skim mozzarella cheese

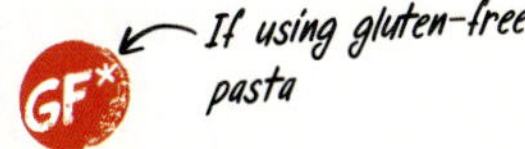

makes 4 servings

NUTRITION (PER SERVING)

575 calories	**13g** fat
41g protein	**73g** net carbs

Like a packed limo on prom night, everyone in this dish is heading to the big dance together before things really heat up and they make their way to the epic afterparty—your mouth. This deconstructed lasagna stays fresh in the fridge for up to 4 days when stored in an airtight container. To prevent the pasta from getting too soft, let it cool completely before sealing it up. If meal prepping, store the ricotta mixture separately, and add it fresh when reheating for the best texture. To reheat, microwave a serving on high for 2 to 3 minutes. Then add the ricotta mixture, and broil for a minute to crisp up the cheese (just make sure you're using an oven-safe container)!

1. Preheat an oven-safe high-sided saucepan or Dutch oven over medium-high heat and spray it with nonstick cooking spray.
2. Add the turkey, onion, bell pepper, and mushrooms. Season with salt and pepper. Sauté, stirring often, for 8 to 10 minutes, or until the turkey is brown and cooked through. Then add the garlic and sauté for an additional 1 to 2 minutes.
3. Add the tomato sauce and 2 cups water. Stir and let simmer for 3 minutes.
4. Add the pasta, cover with the lid, and simmer, stirring occasionally, for 2 to 3 minutes longer than the package instructions, or until al dente.
5. While the pasta is cooking, in a medium bowl, combine the ricotta, Parmesan, and Italian seasoning and stir.
6. Once the pasta is cooked, remove the pan from the heat and top with the ricotta-cheese mixture and mozzarella.
7. Broil in the oven for 1 to 2 minutes, or until the cheese appears golden brown. Voilà!

STUFFED CHICKEN BREAST

WITH SPINACH, SUN-DRIED TOMATO, AND RICOTTA FILLING

1 chicken breast, about 8oz (225g)
¼ cup (62g) ricotta cheese
1 tsp (2.5g) grated Parmesan cheese
¼ cup (62g) frozen spinach, thawed and drained
1¼ tbsp (18g) egg whites
½ tsp (1.5g) garlic powder
Salt and pepper, to taste
1 tbsp (14g) oil-packed sun-dried tomato

We all know chicken breast is the missionary of meats, so I thought I'd add a few kinks that will spice up dinnertime—and your date night. Serve this alongside mashed potatoes, cauliflower mash, or roasted veggies for a balanced meal, or slice it up over a simple arugula salad for a lighter option. Want to jazz it up even more? Drizzle it with a balsamic glaze or serve it with a side of Greek yogurt mixed with lemon and herbs for a fresh, macro-friendly dip.

1. Preheat the oven to 350°F (180°C). Line a baking sheet with parchment paper.
2. Place the chicken breast on a cutting board and cover it with plastic wrap. With a mallet, pound the chicken to flatten to about ½-inch (1cm) thick. Remove the plastic wrap.
3. In a medium bowl, mix the ricotta, Parmesan, spinach, egg whites, and garlic powder and season with salt and pepper.
4. Scoop the spinach-ricotta mixture into the middle of the flattened chicken breast, spreading it evenly. Place the sun-dried tomatoes on top of the spinach ricotta mixture.
5. Fold the chicken breast in half, keeping the stuffing in the center. Season with more salt and pepper.
6. Heat a medium skillet over medium-high heat and spray it with nonstick cooking spray. Sear the chicken for 4 to 5 minutes per side.
7. On the prepared baking sheet, place the seared chicken. Bake for 10 minutes, or until the chicken reaches an internal temperature of 165°F (74°C).

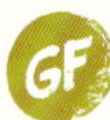

makes 1 stuffed chicken breast / 1 serving

NUTRITION (PER SERVING)

276 calories	**9g** fat
61g protein	**5g** net carbs

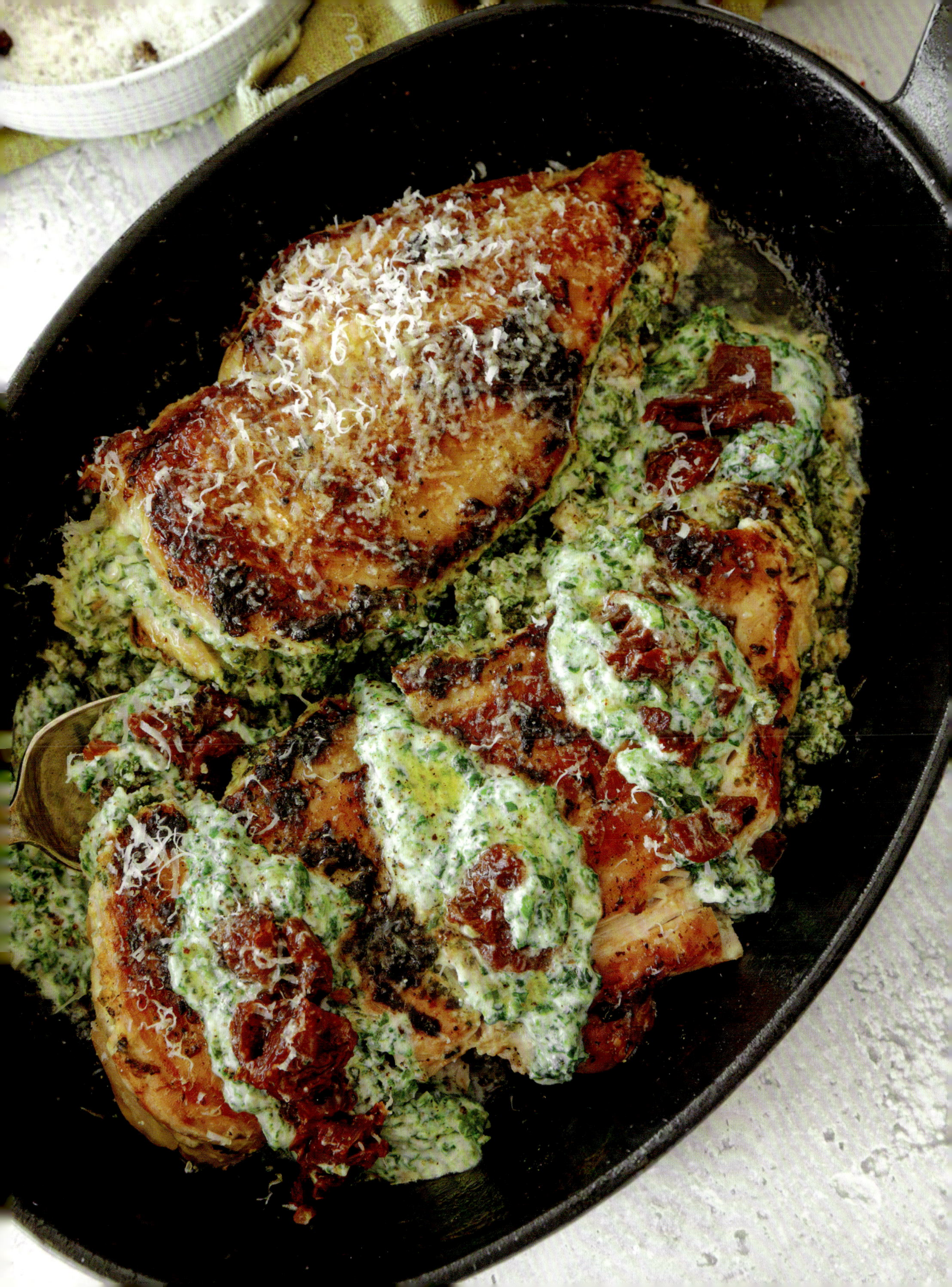

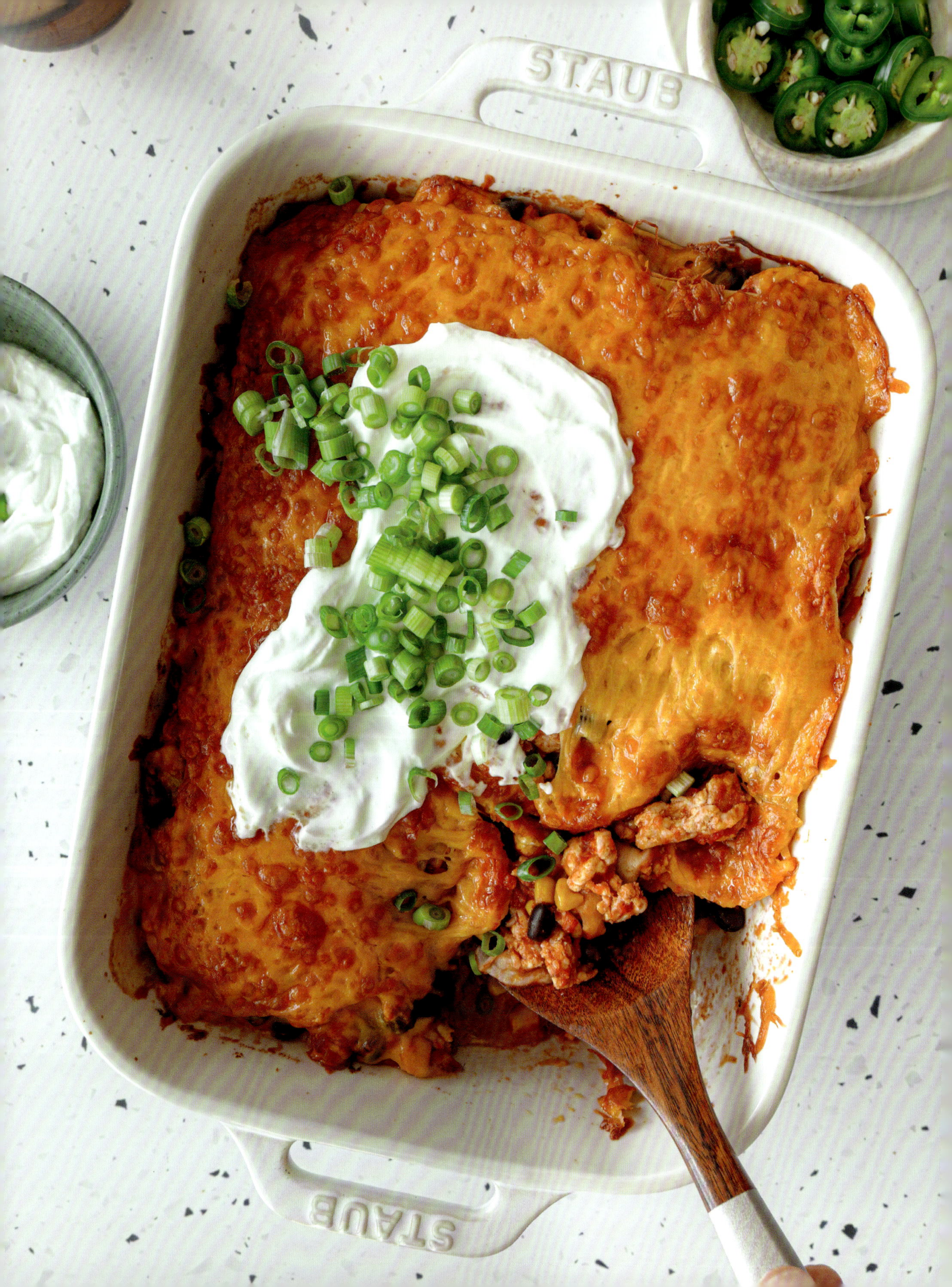
STAUB
STAUB

MEXICAN LASAGNA

2–3 stalks of green onion
½ medium white onion, diced
2lb (900g) ground chicken
Salt and pepper, to taste
2 tsp (6g) cumin
1 tsp (3g) garlic powder
2 tbsp (18g) chili powder
14½oz (411g) can stewed tomatoes
1 cup (135g) frozen corn
1 (15oz / 425g) can black beans, drained
8 flour tortillas, about 2oz (60g) each, cut into quarters
2½ cups (280g) shredded low-fat cheddar cheese
6 tbsp (90g) nonfat Greek yogurt

In honor of my buddy's abuela, this is a recipe *The Great British Bake Off* wished they had in their Mexican week episode. One of my favorite addictive cross-border imports, this can fuel your entire week. Store leftovers in the fridge for up to 4 days, or freeze portions for up to 6 months for an easy, satisfying meal when you're feeling lazy. Want to switch things up? Swap in lean ground beef or turkey, use whole-wheat tortillas for extra fiber, or throw in some bell peppers or jalapeños for a little heat. This dish is hard to mess up—and even harder to stop eating.

1. Preheat the oven to 425°F (220°C).
2. Dice the white and light-green parts of the green onions and set aside. Discard the darker green stalks.
3. Preheat a large frying pan over medium-high heat and spray it with nonstick cooking spray. Add the diced onion and ground chicken, using a spatula or wooden spoon to break apart the chicken. Season with salt and pepper, as well as the cumin, garlic powder, and chili powder. Cook, stirring often, for 8 to 10 minutes, until the chicken is brown.
4. Once the chicken is cooked through, add the stewed tomatoes, corn, and black beans. Stir together and let simmer for 5 minutes.
5. Along the bottom of a large oven-safe casserole dish, place a layer of the ground-chicken mixture, followed by ¼ (70g) of the cheese and a layer of tortilla triangles. Top with more of the chicken mixture, followed by another ¼ (70g) of the cheese, and tortilla triangles, and repeat the layers until the casserole dish is full, finishing with a layer of cheese at the top.
6. Bake for 15 minutes, until the cheese is melted and golden brown.
7. Let rest for 5 to 10 minutes so the lasagna can set, then slice into 6 pieces and top each serving with 1 tablespoon (15g) of the Greek yogurt and the diced green onion.

makes 1 lasagna / 6 servings

NUTRITION (PER SERVING)

655 calories
18g fat
56g protein
56g net carbs

CHICKEN PARMESAN BAKE WITH QUINOA

for the tomato sauce:

3 cups (750ml) strained tomatoes
½ tsp (1.5g) dried oregano
½ tsp (1.5g) dried basil
½ tsp (1g) Parmesan-and-herb seasoning
½ tsp (1.5g) garlic powder
Salt and pepper, to taste

for the chicken parm:

1 cup dry quinoa
1 cup (240ml) low-sodium chicken broth
1 green pepper, diced
1 cup (240g) button mushrooms, chopped
1 yellow onion, chopped
6½ tbsp (100g) egg whites
1 cup (120g) all-purpose flour
¾ cup (80g) shredded Parmesan cheese
½ tsp (1.5g) garlic powder
½ tsp (1g) Parmesan-and-herb seasoning
Salt and pepper, to taste
4 chicken breasts, about 5oz (140g) each

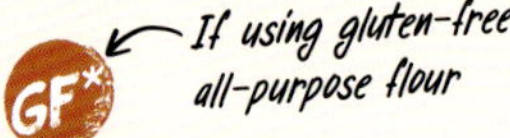

makes 4 servings

NUTRITION (PER SERVING)

480 calories
11g fat
49.5g protein
45.6g net carbs

This recipe will feed the whole family, the homies, or that one guy who's always on a bulk. Taking anabolic Italian food to the next level, even your nonna will approve of this. It's also a solid meal-prep option, though the quinoa will soften as it sits and the chicken won't stay as crispy. To keep the texture on point, store everything in individual containers, and reheat in the oven at 350°F (180°C) for 10 to 12 minutes (covered, then uncovered for crispiness) or in the air fryer at 375°F (190°C) for 5 to 7 minutes. Covering the dish with foil at the start keeps the chicken juicy and ensures the quinoa absorbs all the flavor—just give it a quick broil at the end if you want a little extra crisp.

1. Preheat the oven to 375°F (190°C).
2. **To make the tomato sauce:** To a medium bowl, add the strained tomatoes, oregano, basil, Parmesan-and-herb seasoning, garlic powder, and salt and pepper. Stir to combine.
3. **To make the chicken parm:** Along the bottom of an oven-safe casserole dish, evenly spread the quinoa and top with the tomato sauce, chicken broth, green pepper, mushrooms, and onion. Stir together until the veggies are coated.
4. In a medium bowl, pour the egg whites. In a separate medium bowl, combine the flour, 2 tablespoons (20g) of the Parmesan, the garlic powder, and Parmesan-and-herb seasoning, and season with salt and pepper.
5. One at a time, dip the chicken breasts first in the egg whites, then roll them in the Parmesan coating.
6. On top of the quinoa mixture, place each chicken breast and sprinkle the remaining 60g Parmesan on top. Cover with foil.
7. Bake covered for 40 minutes, then bake uncovered for an additional 20 to 25 minutes.

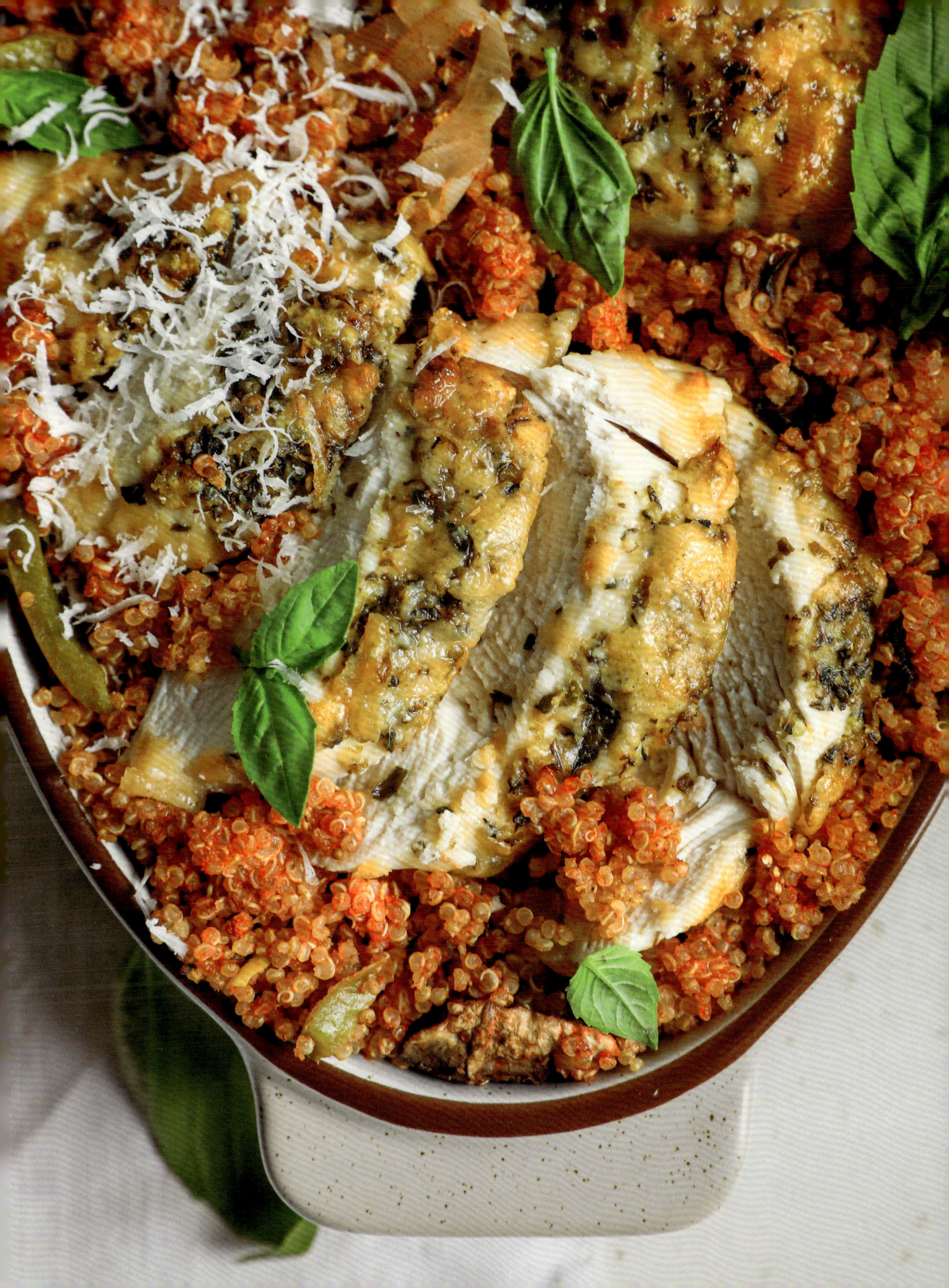

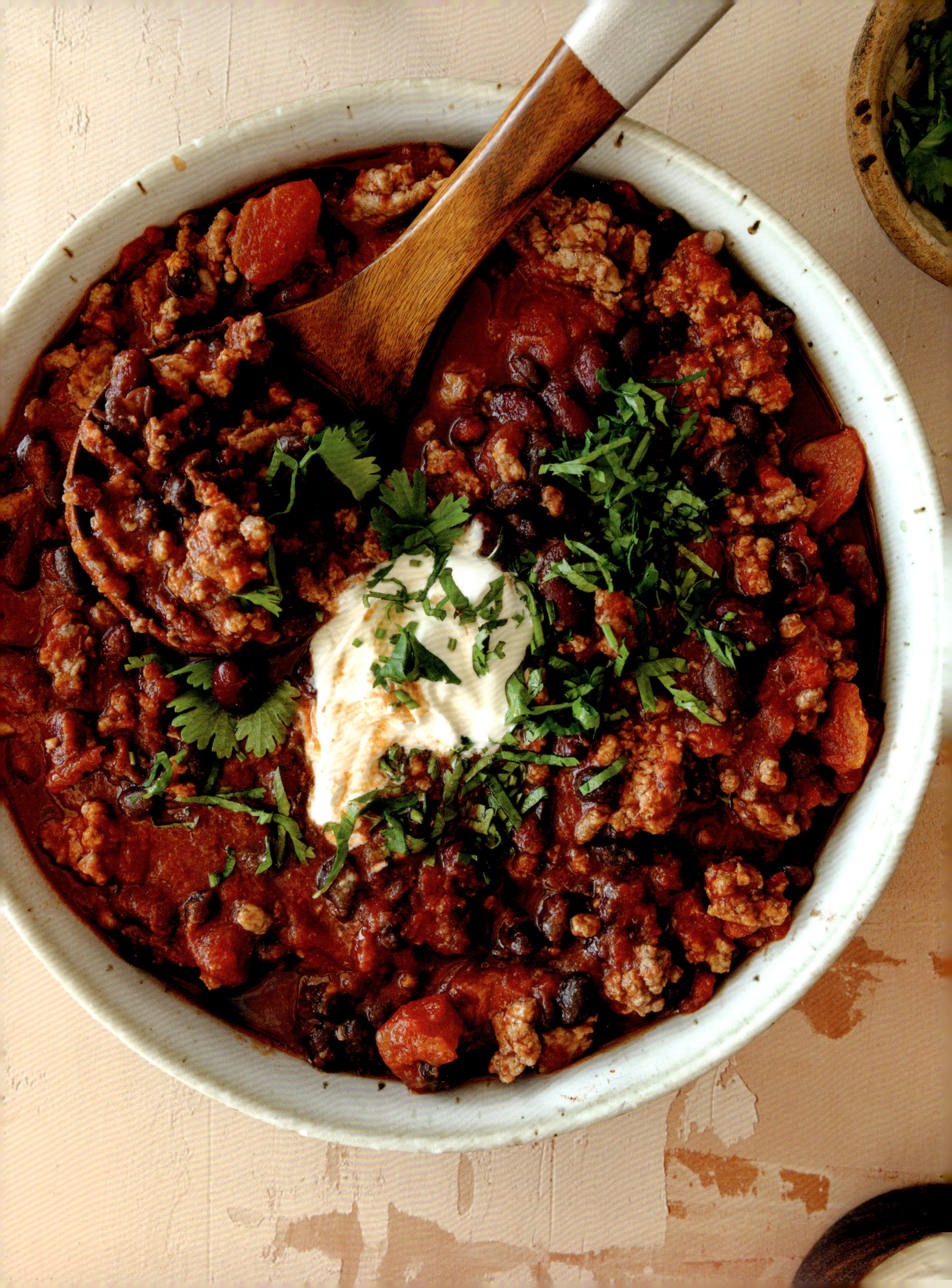

BUDGET-FRIENDLY CHILI

- 2 tbsp (30ml) olive oil
- 1 small yellow onion, chopped
- 2 garlic cloves, minced
- 1 lb (450g) ground beef
- 1 (5½oz / 156ml) can tomato paste
- 1 (28oz / 796ml) can diced tomatoes
- 1 (19oz / 540ml) can red kidney beans, drained and rinsed
- 1 (15oz / 425g) can black beans, drained and rinsed
- 1 tbsp (9g) chili powder
- ½ tbsp (6g) Swerve brown sugar
- 1 tsp (3g) cumin
- ¼ tsp (750mg) cayenne pepper
- ½ tsp (1.5g) garlic powder
- ½ tsp (1.5g) onion powder
- Salt and pepper, to taste

A meal you won't have to wait for pay day to indulge in, this budget-friendly chili will keep both you and your wallet full. It's hard to believe, but the flavors get even better after a day or two in the fridge. Store leftovers in an airtight container for up to 5 days, or freeze portions for up to 3 months for an easy, no-effort meal later on. Serve it on its own or bulk it up with rice, baked potatoes, or toast, and don't forget a dollop of Greek yogurt or sour cream. However you top it, this is one of those recipes that'll have you coming back for seconds—without breaking the bank.

1. Heat a large stock pot over medium heat and add the olive oil. Once hot, add the onion and sauté for 5 to 7 minutes, until the onion is translucent. Then add the garlic and ground beef and sauté for 8 to 10 minutes, until browned.
2. Add the tomato paste and stir into the ground beef. Let cook for 2 minutes.
3. Add the diced tomatoes, kidney beans, black beans, and 1 cup (240ml) water and stir until thoroughly combined. Season with the chili powder, brown sugar, cumin, cayenne pepper, garlic powder, and onion powder and season with salt and pepper. Stir well to combine.
4. Cover with the lid and let simmer for 30 minutes so the flavors can combine and the chili can thicken slightly.

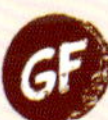

makes 6 servings

NUTRITION (PER SERVING)

415 calories	**18g** fat
27g protein	**38g** net carbs

COCONUT CHICKEN CURRY

4 cups (400g) butternut squash, peeled and cubed
1¾ cup (225g) zucchini, chopped
1¼ cups (150g) eggplant, chopped
½ cup (100g) leeks, sliced
1 chicken breast, about 7oz (200g), grilled and shredded
1½ heaping tbsp (13.5g) curry powder
Salt and pepper, to taste
1¾ cups (400ml) light coconut milk
1¾ cups (400ml) vegetable broth
1 white-flour pita

My grandma grew up in India, and she always made us the most amazing and authentic curry dishes, which still have a special place in my heart. She would be horrified by this recipe, but it's delicious. This dish is also a great way to clean out your fridge, as almost any vegetable works here. Bell peppers, carrots, cauliflower, spinach, and mushrooms all make great additions or swaps, depending on what you have on hand. You can also switch up the protein—shrimp is an easy swap, or skip the meat entirely and keep it vegan. However you customize it, just promise me that my grandma won't find out.

1. Preheat a large stock pot over medium-high heat and spray it with nonstick cooking spray. Add the butternut squash and sauté, stirring occasionally, for 3 minutes. Add the zucchini, eggplant, and leeks and sauté for 8 to 10 minutes, until the vegetables are soft.
2. Add the shredded chicken and stir to combine. Season with the curry powder, and salt and pepper, and mix to evenly coat the vegetables and chicken.
3. Add the coconut milk and vegetable broth and stir. Cover with the lid and let simmer for 10 to 15 minutes, until the curry is bubbling and the squash is easily punctured with a fork.
4. Remove from the heat and enjoy with pita on the side.

makes 2 servings

NUTRITION (PER SERVING)

458 calories | **14g** fat
35g protein | **48g** net carbs

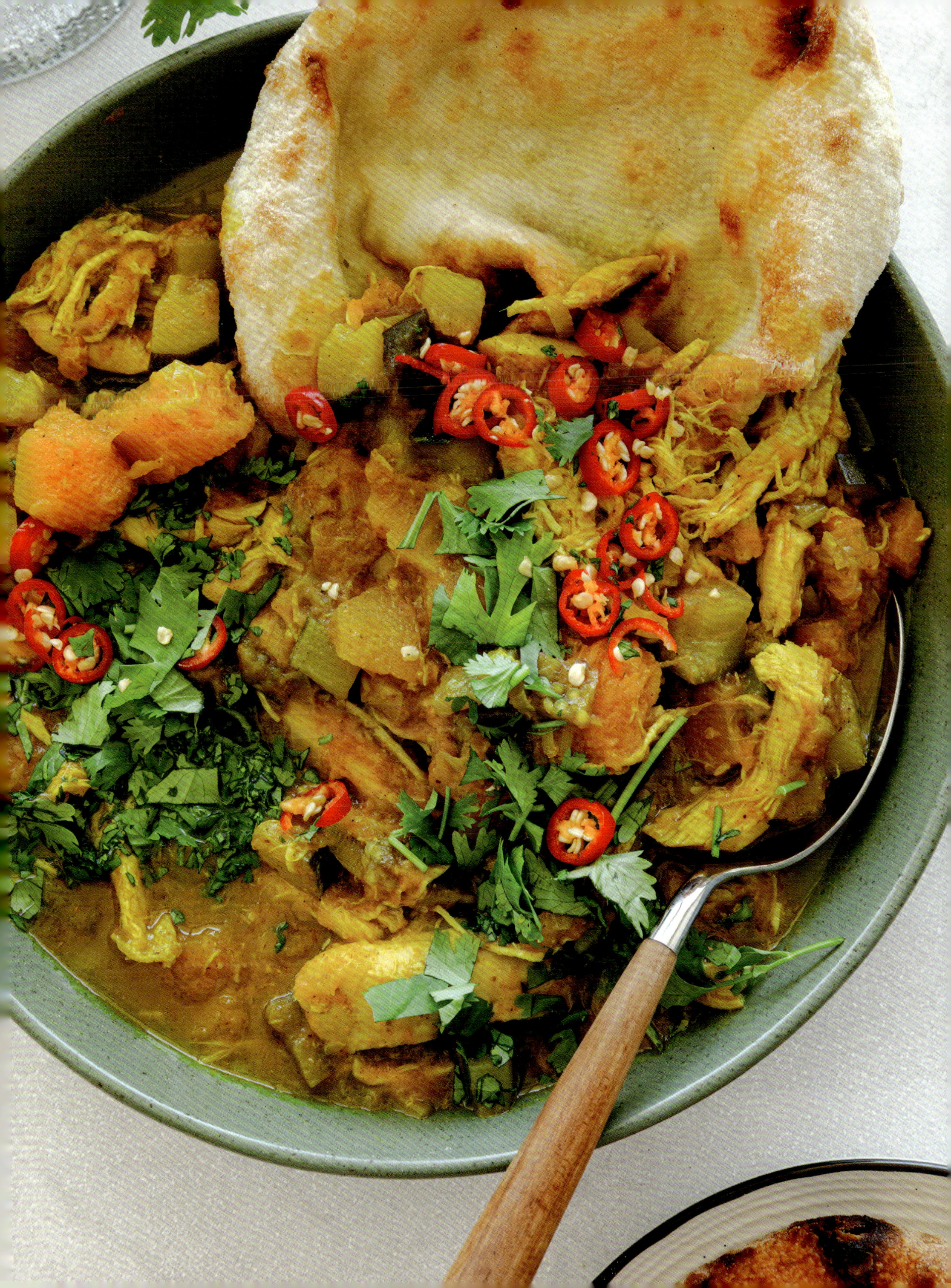

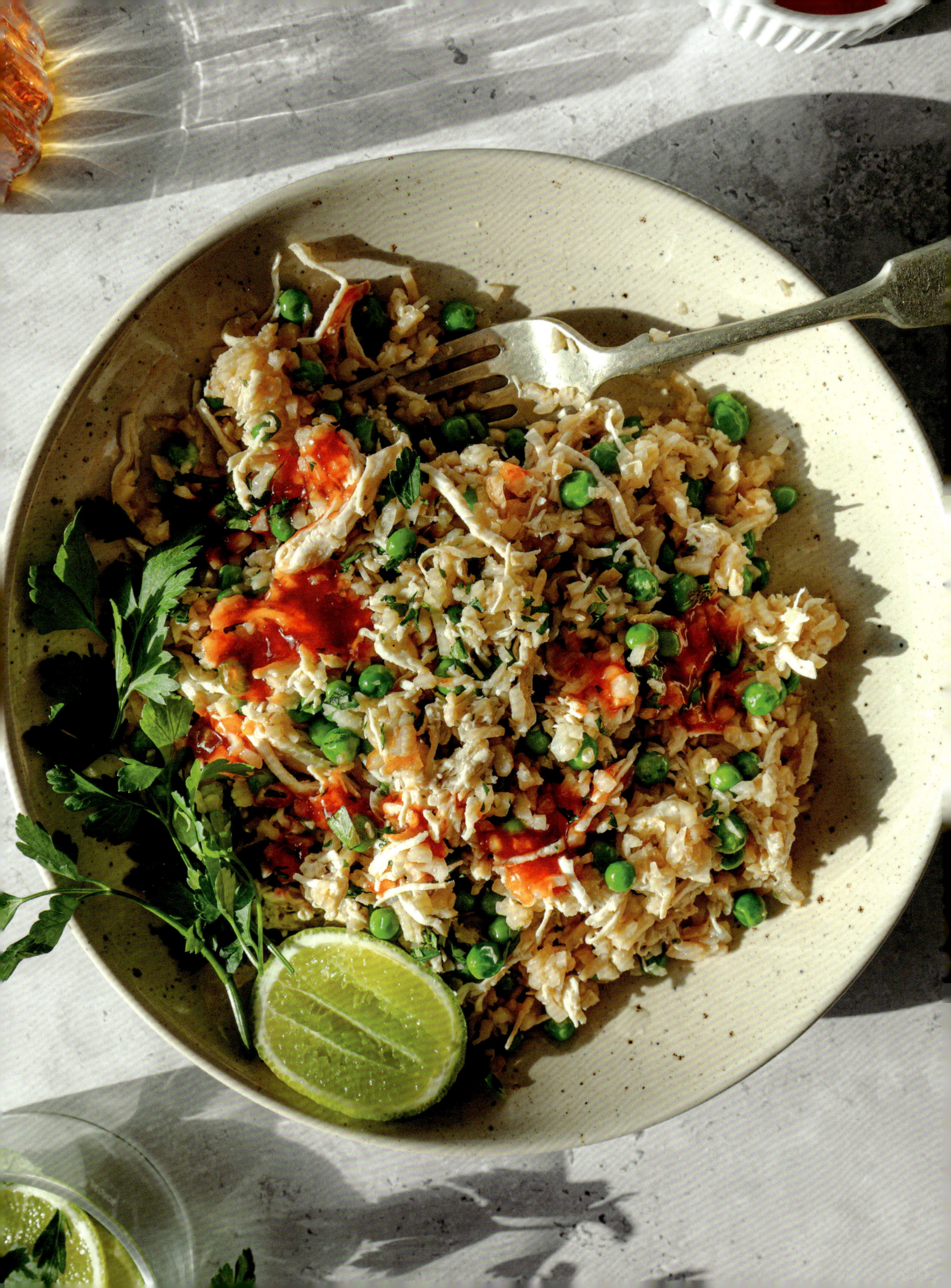

CHICKEN CAULIFLOWER FRIED RICE

1 egg
2 cups (133g) frozen cauliflower rice
½ cup (67g) frozen green peas
1 tbsp (15ml) soy sauce
1 tsp (5ml) sesame oil
3oz (85g) rotisserie chicken, shredded
Sriracha (optional)

Other than my sauce collection, there's nothing I turn to more often than cauliflower rice. Sure, it's not real rice, but unlike zucchini noodles, which are just a wet, crunchy lie, it actually holds up as a solid substitute. It soaks up flavor, gives you that classic tried rice texture, and lets you save your carbs for dessert. Plus, with rotisserie chicken and a quick stir-fry sauce, this dish comes together faster than takeout.

1. Heat a small frying pan over medium-high heat and spray it with nonstick cooking spray. Into the pan, crack the egg and lightly whisk while it cooks to form a scrambled egg patty. Once the egg is cooked, remove from the heat and set aside.
2. Heat a large skillet over medium-high heat and spray it with nonstick cooking spray. Add the cauliflower rice and green peas and allow them to thaw and heat through for 5 minutes.
3. To a small bowl, add the soy sauce and sesame oil and stir to combine.
4. To the hot skillet with the rice and peas, add the soy-sauce mixture, rotisserie chicken, and cooked egg. Mix until the sauce evenly coats the rice, mashing the egg into smaller bite-size pieces as you go.
5. Once the fried rice is heated through, plate and drizzle with the sriracha for some heat (if using).

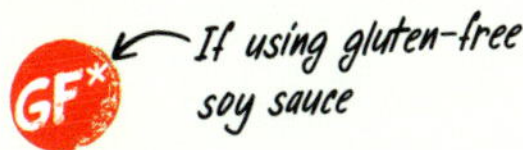

makes 1 serving

NUTRITION (PER SERVING)

350 calories
13g fat
38g protein
16g net carbs

CAULIFLOWER-RICE ARANCINI WITH TURKEY SAUSAGE

- 1 (28oz / 794g) can whole peeled San Marzano tomatoes
- ½ tsp (1.5g) salt, plus more to taste
- ¼ tsp (750mg) chili flakes
- ½ tsp (1.5g) garlic powder
- ¼ tsp (750mg) dried basil
- 1 turkey sausage, about 3⅓oz (94g), casing removed
- 2¼ cups (150g) cauliflower rice
- 1 tsp (1g) Parmesan-and-herb seasoning, plus more to garnish
- Pepper, to taste
- ⅔ cup (50g) shredded part-skim mozzarella
- 1 egg
- 1 cup (110g) bread crumbs
- Fresh basil, to garnish

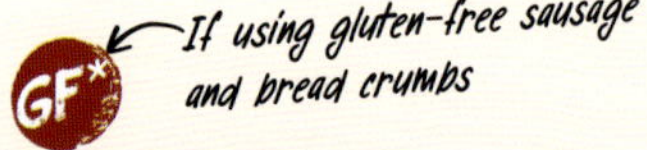

makes 6 arancini / 3 servings

NUTRITION (PER SERVING)

274 calories	**6g** fat
18g protein	**30g** net carbs

Hi, cookbook readers, Mama Tenny here! Have you ever picked up fried rice balls (arancini) from your local Italian bakery? They are sooooo good, but sooooo high in calories and fat. These healthier cauliflower-rice arancini balls will make you feel like you're in Italy, without the jet lag! If you don't have turkey sausage on hand, no problem. Just use ground turkey, and season it with salt, pepper, garlic powder, fennel seeds, and a pinch of red pepper flakes to get that classic sausage flavor. *Buon appetito!*

1. Preheat the oven to 425°F (220°C). If using an air fryer, do not preheat the oven. Line a baking sheet with parchment paper.
2. To a medium saucepan over medium heat, add the tomatoes, salt, chili flakes, garlic powder, and basil. Stir to combine, using a spatula to break the tomatoes apart. Reduce the heat to low and allow the sauce to simmer while preparing the other components of the dish.
3. Preheat a large frying pan over medium-high heat and spray it with nonstick cooking spray. Add the turkey sausage, breaking it apart with a wooden spoon or spatula. Sauté for 5 minutes, or until browned.
4. Add the cauliflower rice and 2 tablespoons (30ml) of the simmering tomato sauce. Season with the Parmesan-and-herb seasoning and salt and pepper. Stir together and sauté for 5 minutes, or until the cauliflower softens.
5. Once the cauliflower is cooked, remove from the heat and add the mozzarella. Fold in the cheese as the cauliflower mixture cools. Set aside to cool more.
6. In a small bowl, whisk the egg. On a large plate, pour the bread crumbs.
7. Once the cauliflower mixture is cooled, form it into 6 balls. Dip the cauliflower balls first into the egg, then roll to coat the balls in the bread crumbs.
8. On the prepared baking sheet, place the arancini. Bake for 25 minutes, or until golden brown. If using an air fryer, air fry at 400°F (200°C) for 17 to 20 minutes.
9. To plate, on the bottom of a wide pasta bowl, spoon a generous scoop of tomato sauce. Place the arancini balls on top of the tomato sauce, and top with basil and a sprinkle of Parmesan-and-herb seasoning.

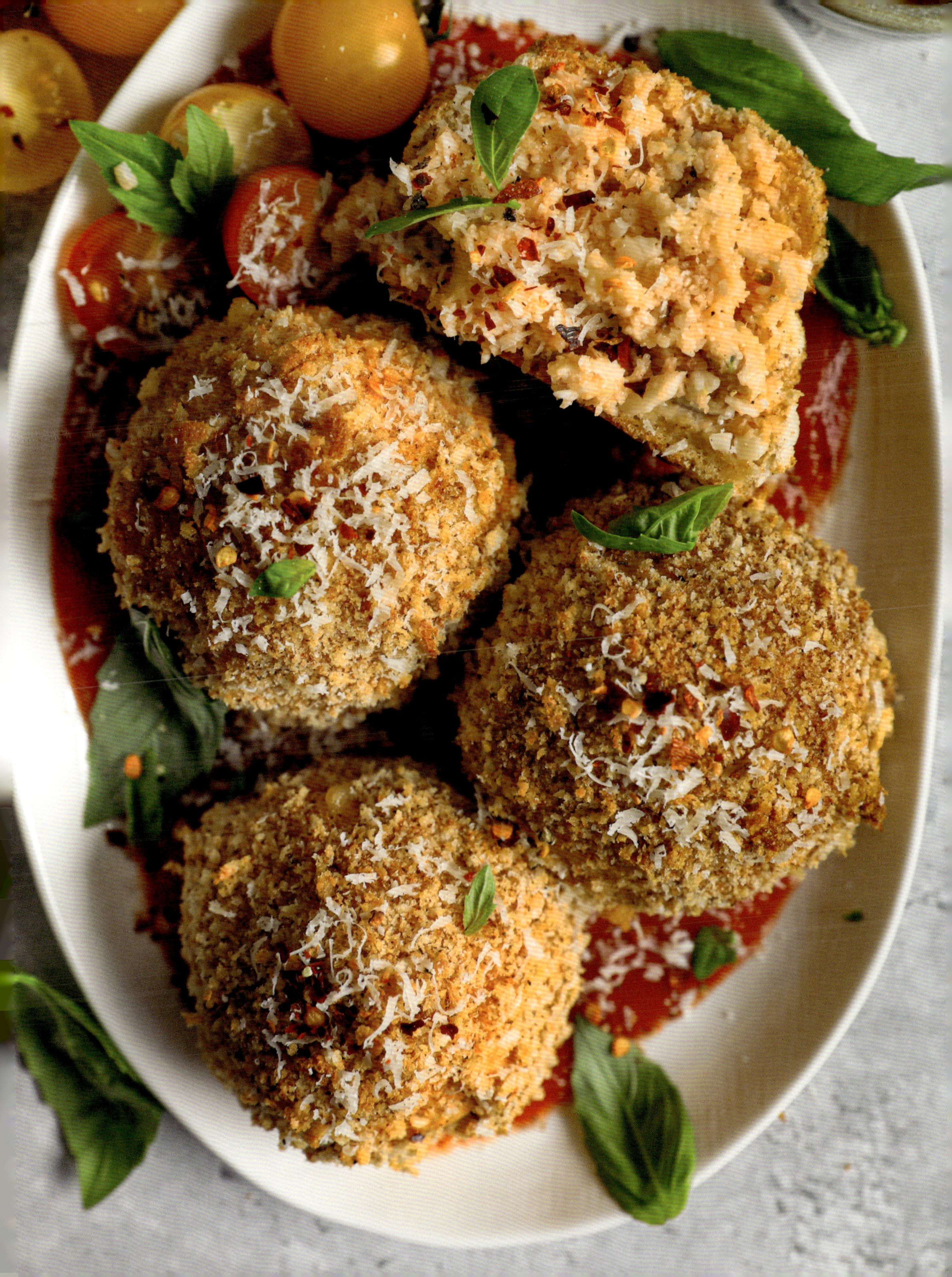

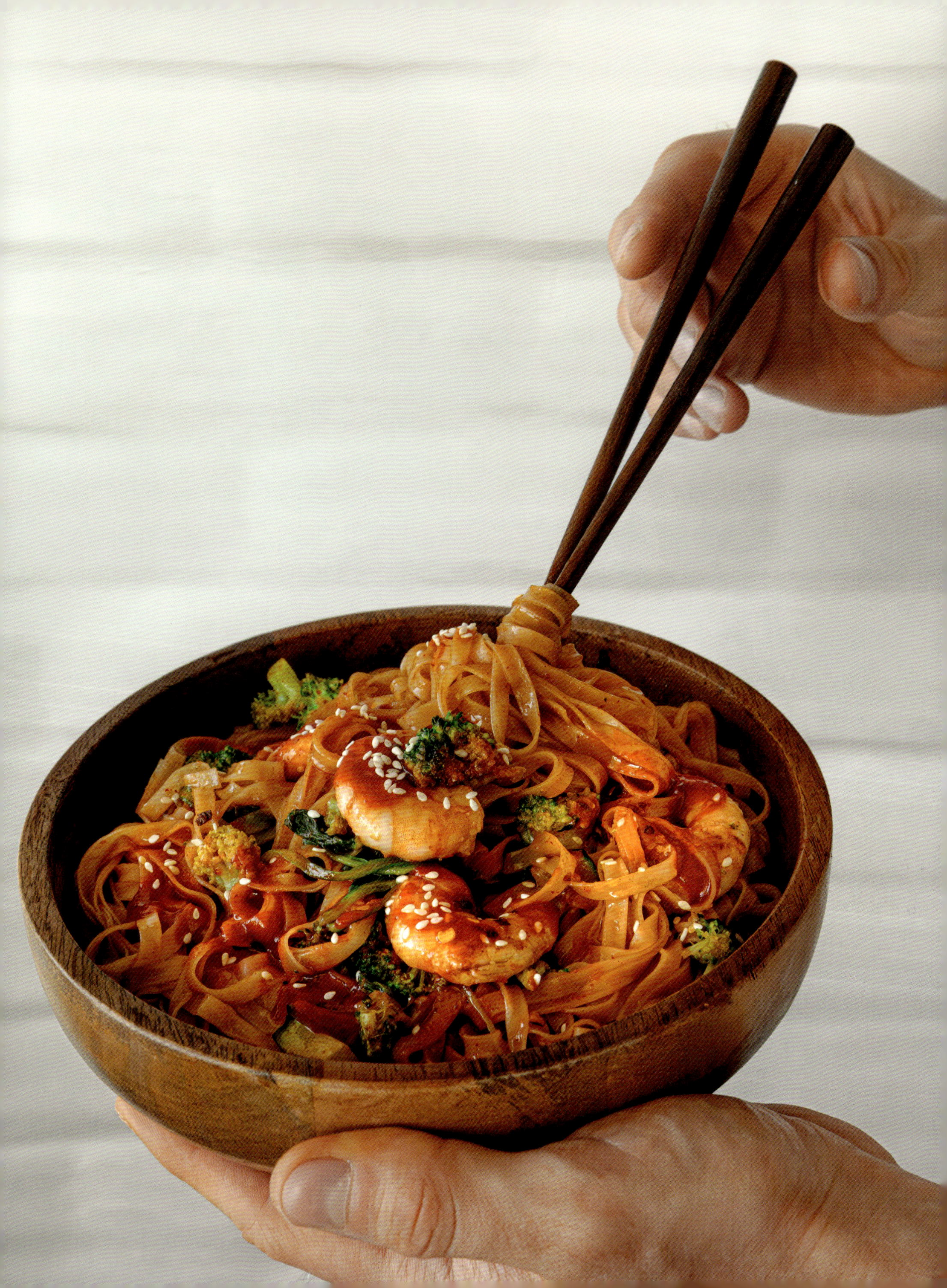

HEALTHY PAD THAI

¼ cup (26g) PB2 Powdered Peanut Butter
2 tsp (10ml) sesame oil
1 tsp (5ml) soy sauce
2 tsp (10ml) sriracha, plus more to garnish, if desired
1 tsp (5ml) rice vinegar
1 garlic clove, finely chopped
1 tsp (5g) finely chopped raw ginger
½ cup (50g) broccoli, chopped
1 medium zucchini, chopped
6 raw jumbo shrimp, thawed and peeled
5½oz (150g) rice noodles
1½ cups (45g) spinach
¼ tsp (750mg) black-and-white sesame seeds

A nod to the other lean sources of protein I discovered while backpacking through Asia, this shrimp pad thai will increase your gains instead of your waistband. For extra freshness, top your pad thai with chopped green onions and thinly sliced chile peppers . . . if you can handle the heat. For added crunch, mix in shredded cabbage or bean sprouts. Not a seafood fan? Questionable, but I'll allow it—just swap the shrimp for chicken, tofu, or beef, and you're good to go.

1. Bring a medium stock pot half full of water to a boil.
2. While waiting for the water to boil, to a small bowl, add the PB2 Powdered Peanut Butter, sesame oil, soy sauce, sriracha, rice vinegar, garlic, ginger, and 2 tablespoons (30ml) water. Mix to combine and set aside.
3. Heat a large skillet over medium-high heat and spray it with nonstick cooking spray. Add the broccoli, zucchini, and shrimp and sauté for 3 to 5 minutes, until the shrimp are pink and the veggies are softened.
4. When the water in the stockpot begins to boil, add the rice noodles and cook until al dente according to the package instructions. Strain and transfer the rice noodles directly to the skillet with the shrimp and veggies.
5. Add the spinach and PB2 mixture and stir to combine. Once the spinach is wilted and the sauce is heated through, remove from the heat.
6. Transfer the pad thai to a large bowl and top with the sesame seeds and more sriracha, if desired.

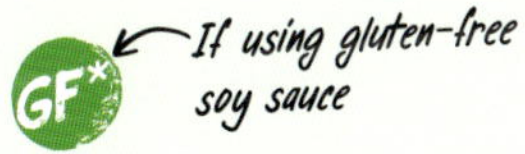

makes 1 serving

NUTRITION (PER SERVING)

568 calories | **20g** fat
33g protein | **55g** net carbs

COTTAGE-CHEESE FETTUCCINI ALFREDO

1 cup (230g) low-fat or fat-free cottage cheese
¼ cup (60ml) 10% cream or half-and-half
¼ cup (30g) grated Parmesan cheese
1 garlic clove
1 tsp (2.5g) cornstarch
¼ cup (60ml) Silk unsweetened cashew milk
1½ tsp (4.5g) salt, plus a pinch of salt
½ tsp (1.5g) black pepper
1 (12oz / 340g) package fettuccini, or pasta of choice
About 10oz (300g) medium frozen raw shrimp, thawed and peeled
¾ tsp (2.25g) garlic powder

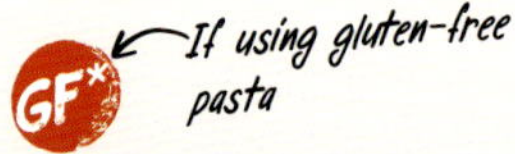

makes 4 servings

NUTRITION (PER SERVING)

442 calories	**5.6g** fat
30.9g protein	**68.1g** net carbs

The only thing heavier than a bowl of fettuccini Alfredo is the nap you take after eating it. This version lightens things up without sacrificing creaminess, thanks to the blended cottage cheese—a high-protein swap that keeps the sauce rich but macro-friendly. The shrimp adds a lean protein, but if seafood isn't your thing, swap it for grilled chicken, tofu, or even sautéed mushrooms for a vegetarian option. To keep the sauce smooth, it's important to reserve the pasta water—the starch helps bind everything together for that classic consistency. Top with fresh parsley, basil, or a squeeze of lemon juice to brighten the flavors, and suddenly this "healthier" Alfredo feels just as indulgent as the original, without the food coma.

1. Fill a large pot halfway with water and bring it to a boil over high heat.
2. While waiting for the water to boil, in a blender, combine the cottage cheese, cream, Parmesan, garlic, cornstarch, cashew milk, 1 teaspoon (3g) of the salt, and the black pepper. Blend until the mixture becomes a smooth and creamy Alfredo sauce. Set aside.
3. Once the water in the pot is boiling, add a pinch of salt and the pasta and cook according to the package instructions. Strain the pasta, reserving ½ cup (120ml) of the pasta water in a heatproof measuring cup or mug with a handle. Set the pasta water aside.
4. Return the pasta to the pot. Pour the Alfredo sauce over the pasta. Place the pot over medium-low heat and stir the pasta and sauce together until the sauce is warmed through.
5. Gradually add the reserved pasta water, stirring constantly, until the sauce reaches your desired consistency. You may not need to use the entire ½ cup (120ml) pasta water. Set aside.
6. In a medium bowl, season the shrimp with the garlic powder and remaining ½ teaspoon (1.5g) salt, coating both sides evenly.
7. Heat a small frying pan over medium-high heat and spray it with nonstick cooking spray. Add the shrimp and sauté for 3 to 5 minutes, until the shrimp are pink.
8. Plate the pasta, top with the shrimp, and *buon appetito*!

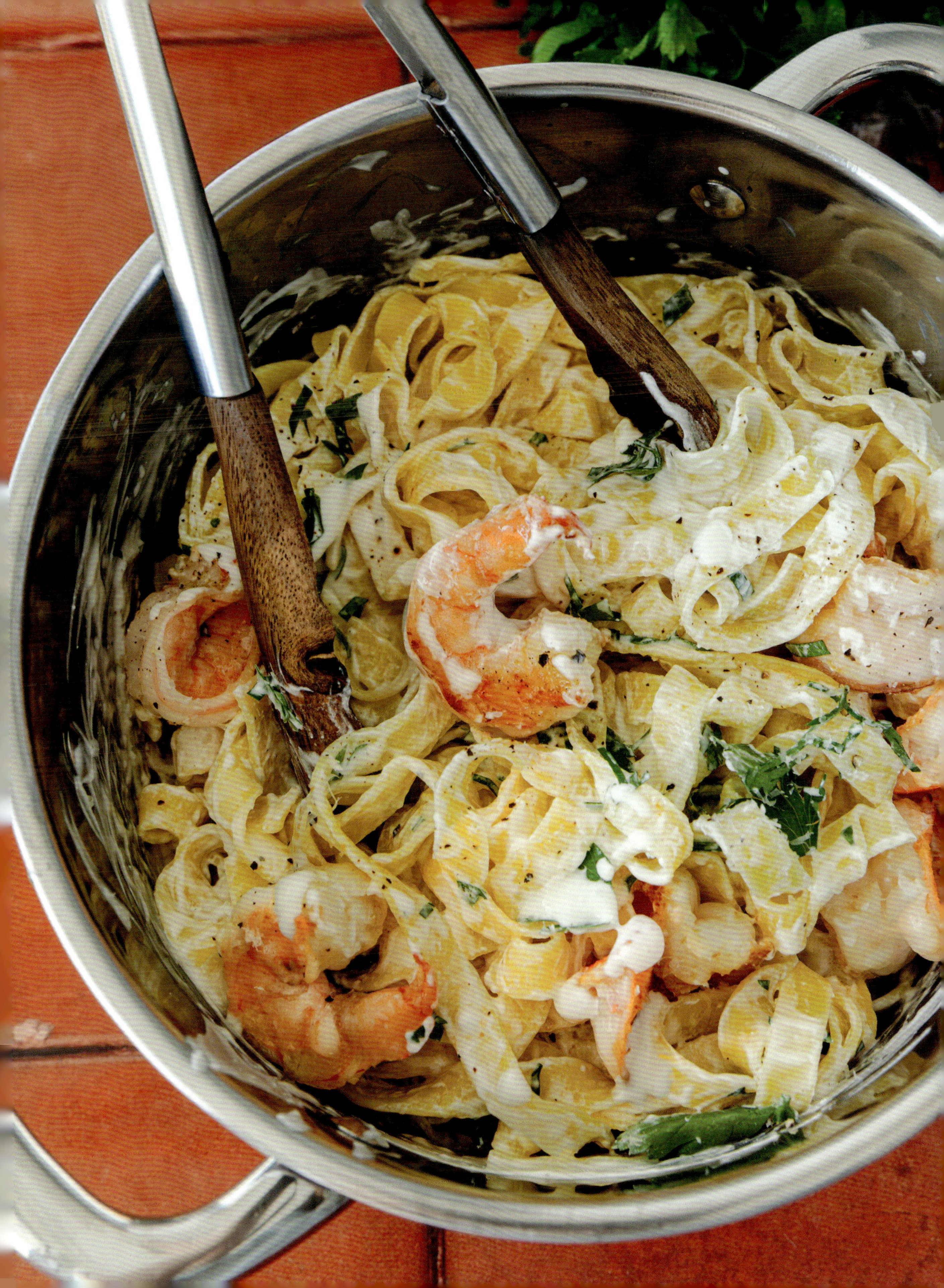

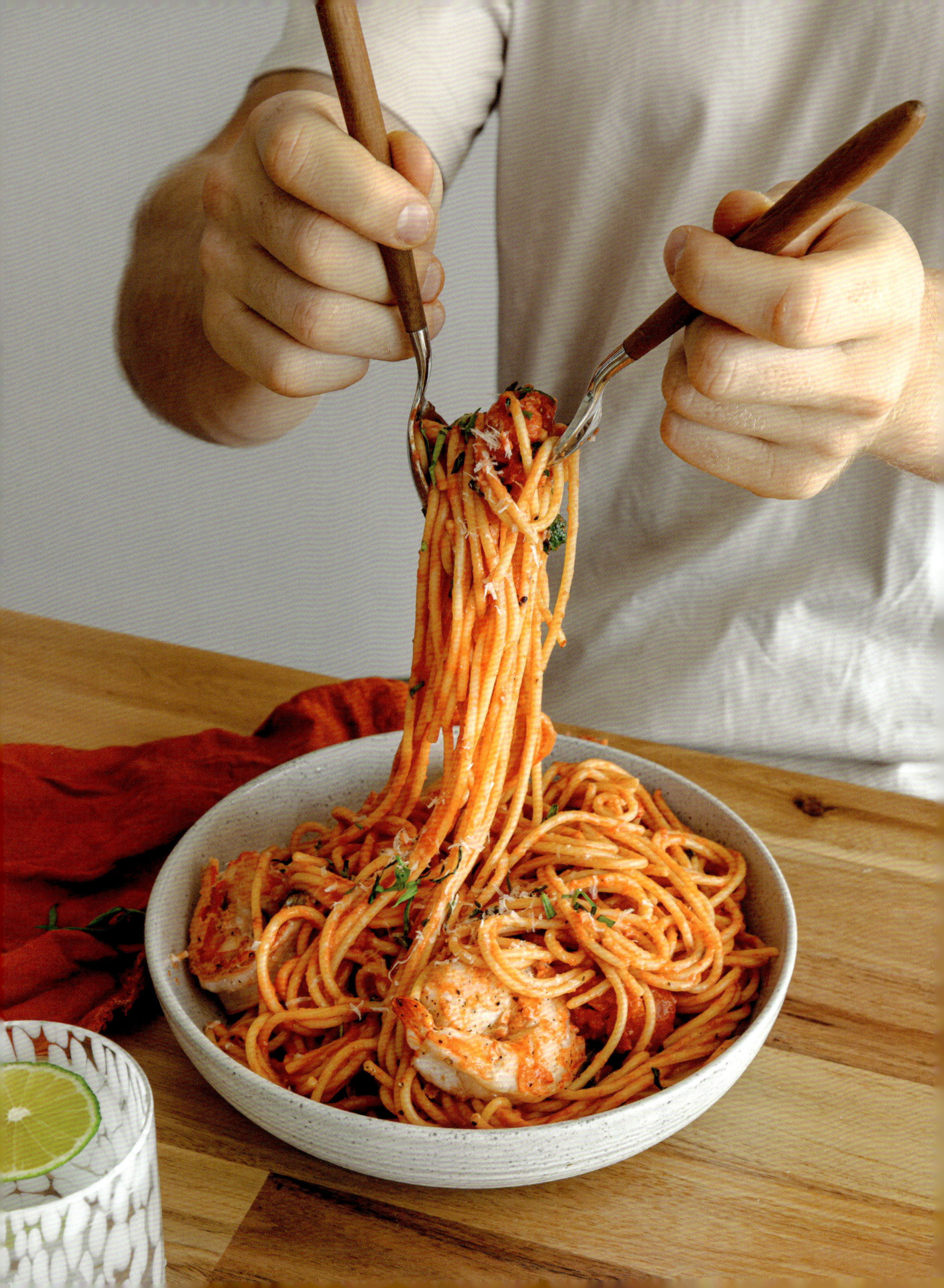

CREAMY TARRAGON SHRIMP PASTA

1 cup (100g) white onion, diced
½ cup (75g) red bell pepper, diced
2 garlic cloves, diced
13oz (375g) canned whole peeled San Marzano tomatoes
2½ cups (75g) fresh spinach
¼ cup (7g) fresh tarragon, chopped
2 tsp (6g) salt
6oz (170g) spaghetti
About 10oz (300g) medium frozen raw shrimp, thawed and peeled
1½ tsp (4.5g) garlic powder
3 tbsp (45ml) 10% cream or half-and-half
¼ cup (30g) grated Parmesan cheese

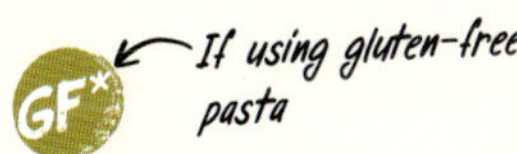

makes 2 servings

NUTRITION (PER SERVING)

578 calories	**8.5g** fat
49.5g protein	**76g** net carbs

Tarragon, but not forgotten—this underrated herb gives shrimp pasta a sneaky upgrade. It adds a hint of fancy flavor (kind of like mild licorice, but trust me, it works) and makes the creamy tomato sauce taste next level. Parmesan and 10% cream keep things rich but still macro-friendly, and the spinach lets you feel slightly more responsible while inhaling carbs. Cook the pasta just al dente so it holds up, and smash those canned tomatoes like they wronged you. Toss everything together, and look at that—gourmet pasta, low effort, high protein. What more do you need?

1. Fill a medium pot halfway with hot water and bring it to a boil over high heat.
2. While waiting for the water to boil, heat a large saucepan over medium-high heat and spray it with nonstick cooking spray. Add the onion and bell pepper and sauté for 6 to 8 minutes, or until the onions are brown and translucent. Add the garlic and sauté for 1 additional minute, or until fragrant.
3. Add the tomatoes and, using a wooden spoon or spatula, break them apart to form a thick sauce.
4. Stir in the spinach, tarragon, and 1 teaspoon (3g) of the salt. Mix well and cook while preparing the pasta and the shrimp, until the sauce begins to bubble and the spinach wilts. Reduce the heat to low.
5. Once the water in the pot begins to boil, add the spaghetti and cook until al dente according to the package instructions. Strain the pasta and set aside.
6. In a medium bowl, season the shrimp with the garlic powder and the remaining 1 teaspoon (3g) salt, coating both sides evenly.
7. Gently place the shrimp in the sauce, ensuring they are fully covered. Cover with the lid and let the mixture simmer for 6 to 8 minutes, or until the shrimp turn pink.
8. Remove the pan from the heat and stir in the cream and Parmesan until the sauce is smooth and creamy.
9. To the saucepan, add the cooked spaghetti and toss until the pasta is evenly coated in the sauce. Plate the spaghetti and serve immediately. Enjoy!

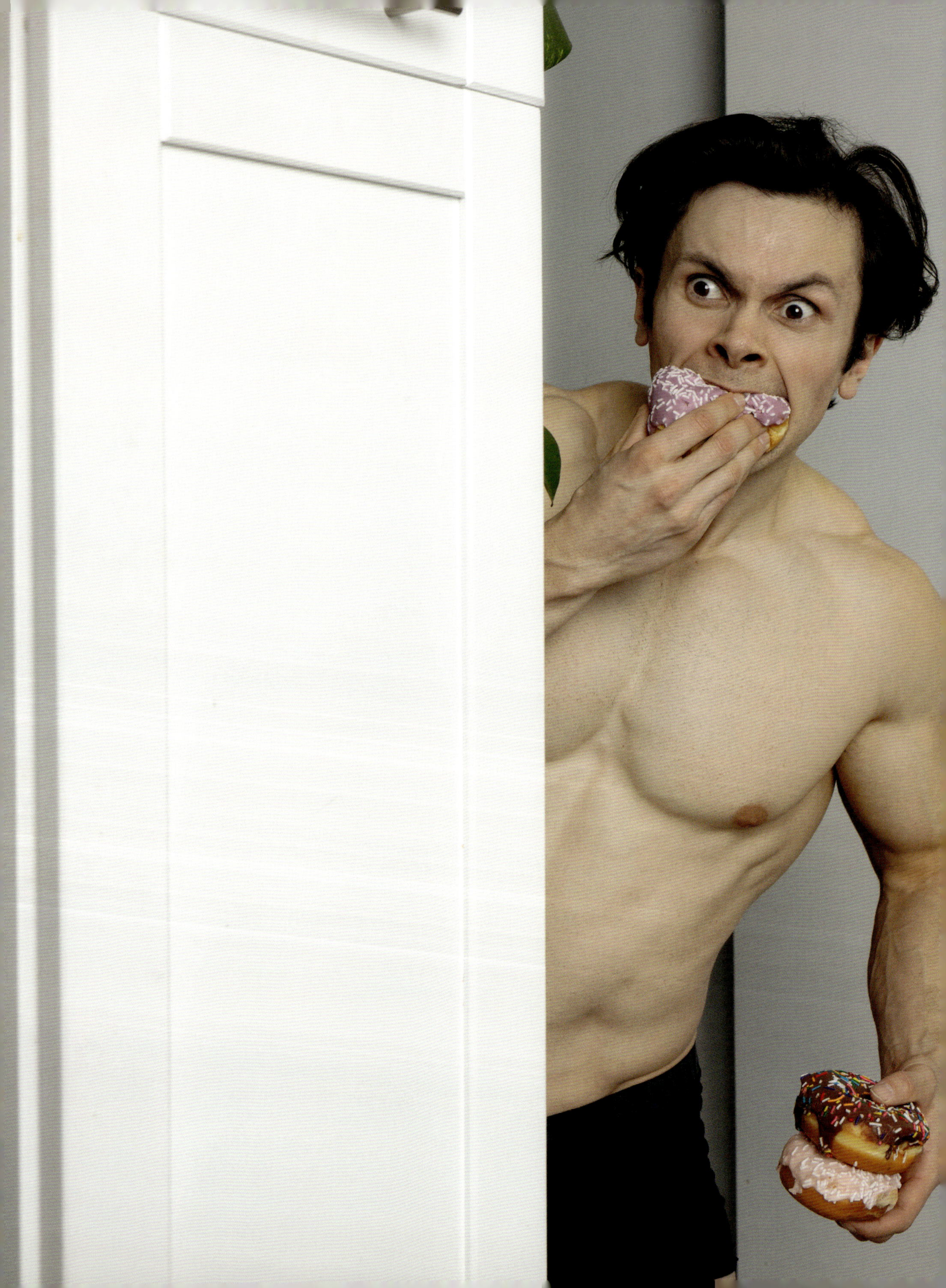

—CHAPTER 6—

CHEAT CODES

FAKE THE TAKEOUT

OLLIE "THE GOAT" TENNYSON

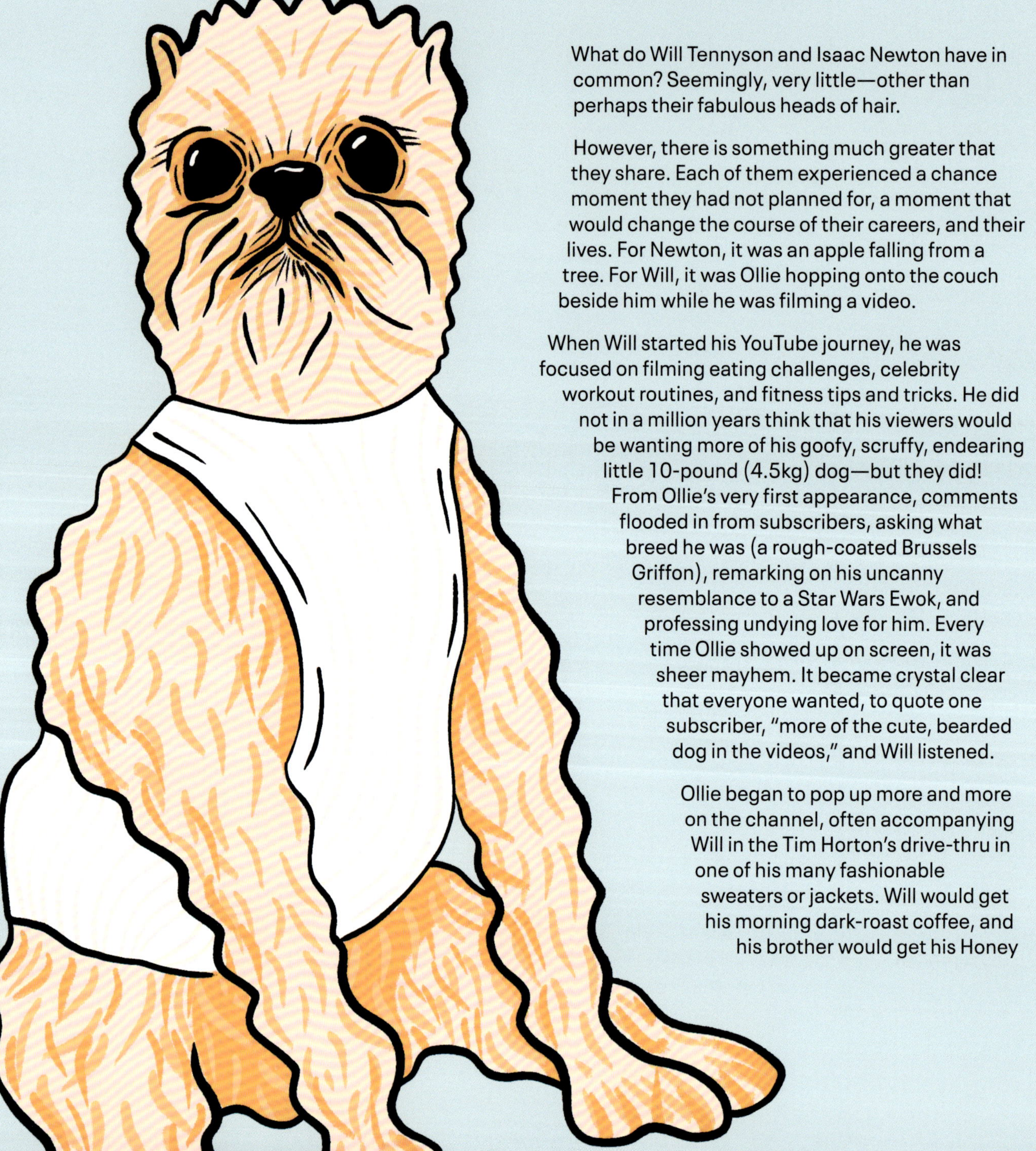

What do Will Tennyson and Isaac Newton have in common? Seemingly, very little—other than perhaps their fabulous heads of hair.

However, there is something much greater that they share. Each of them experienced a chance moment they had not planned for, a moment that would change the course of their careers, and their lives. For Newton, it was an apple falling from a tree. For Will, it was Ollie hopping onto the couch beside him while he was filming a video.

When Will started his YouTube journey, he was focused on filming eating challenges, celebrity workout routines, and fitness tips and tricks. He did not in a million years think that his viewers would be wanting more of his goofy, scruffy, endearing little 10-pound (4.5kg) dog—but they did! From Ollie's very first appearance, comments flooded in from subscribers, asking what breed he was (a rough-coated Brussels Griffon), remarking on his uncanny resemblance to a Star Wars Ewok, and professing undying love for him. Every time Ollie showed up on screen, it was sheer mayhem. It became crystal clear that everyone wanted, to quote one subscriber, "more of the cute, bearded dog in the videos," and Will listened.

Ollie began to pop up more and more on the channel, often accompanying Will in the Tim Horton's drive-thru in one of his many fashionable sweaters or jackets. Will would get his morning dark-roast coffee, and his brother would get his Honey

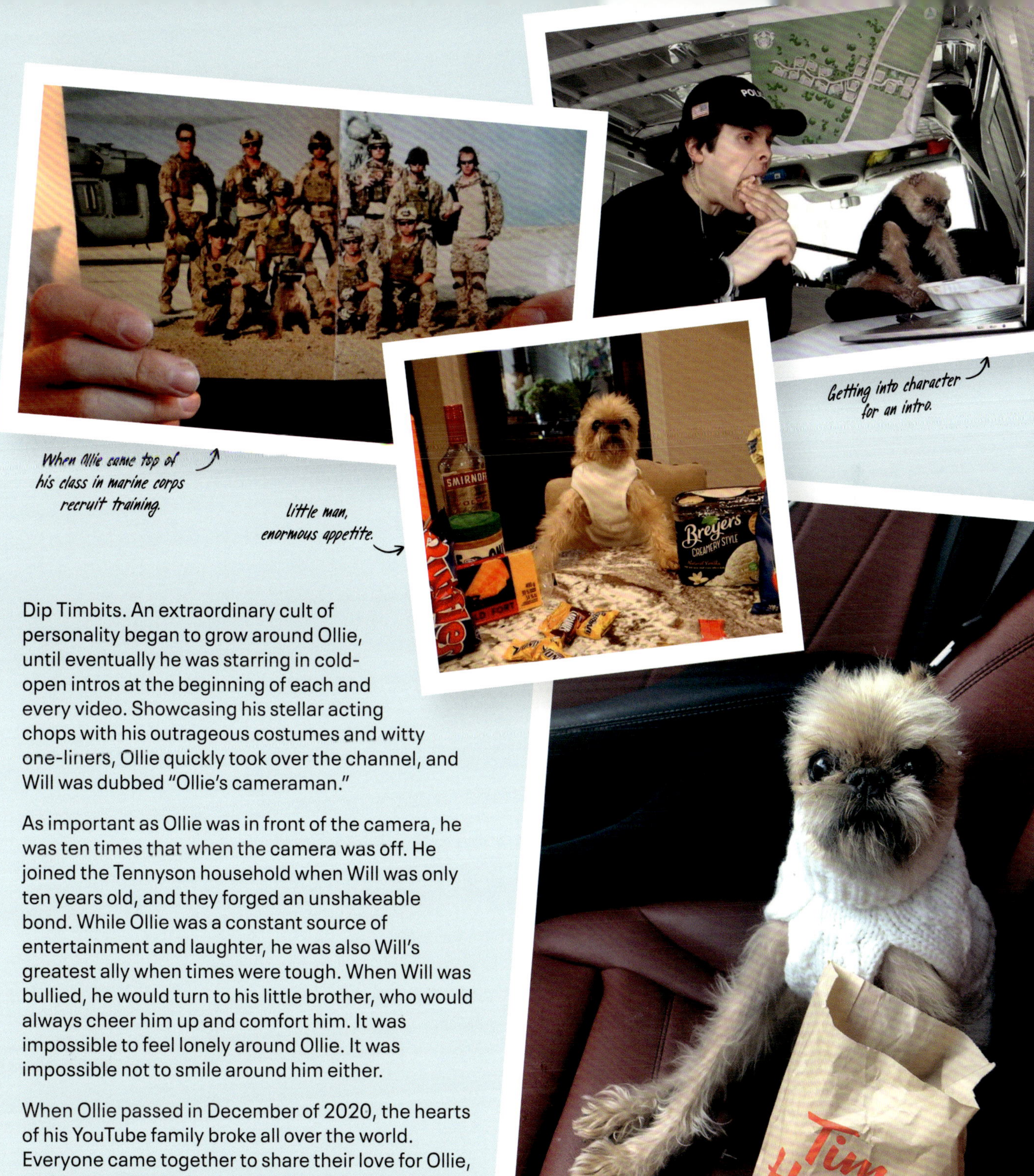

When Ollie came top of his class in marine corps recruit training.

Getting into character for an intro.

little man, enormous appetite.

Posing with his snack of choice, the Honey Dip Timbits.

Dip Timbits. An extraordinary cult of personality began to grow around Ollie, until eventually he was starring in cold-open intros at the beginning of each and every video. Showcasing his stellar acting chops with his outrageous costumes and witty one-liners, Ollie quickly took over the channel, and Will was dubbed "Ollie's cameraman."

As important as Ollie was in front of the camera, he was ten times that when the camera was off. He joined the Tennyson household when Will was only ten years old, and they forged an unshakeable bond. While Ollie was a constant source of entertainment and laughter, he was also Will's greatest ally when times were tough. When Will was bullied, he would turn to his little brother, who would always cheer him up and comfort him. It was impossible to feel lonely around Ollie. It was impossible not to smile around him either.

When Ollie passed in December of 2020, the hearts of his YouTube family broke all over the world. Everyone came together to share their love for Ollie, and to give thanks for the positive impact he had on so many people. And to think this all started by accident! While he is now gone from this world, his legacy has been immortalized—something that his brother, sisters, and parents are eternally grateful for. To this day, it is still his channel, and Will is just the cameraman.

—XX Victoria

ANABOLIC PIZZA

for the dough:

1 cup (230g) nonfat Greek yogurt
1½ cups (180g) self-rising flour
1 tsp (3g) salt

for the pizza sauce:

½ cup (120ml) strained tomatoes
½ tsp (1.5g) garlic powder
1½ tsp (0.75g) fresh or ½ tsp (0.3g) dried basil
¼ tsp (750mg) salt
¼ tsp (750mg) crushed red chili flakes (optional)

for the pizza:

⅔ cup (60g) shredded part-skim mozzarella cheese
⅔ cup (100g) banana peppers, sliced
3½ oz (25g) turkey pepperoni
½ cup (130g) tomato, sliced
¾ oz (20g) canned pineapple

With great pizza comes great responsibility. While I won't judge you for your toppings, you'll be sending a pretty clear message to your partner if this pizza's presented with no pineapple in sight. If you don't have self-rising flour on hand, you can use all-purpose flour instead, but just know the dough won't rise quite the same way. To make up for it, add 2¼ teaspoons (12g) baking powder and ⅓ teaspoon (1g) salt to your 1½ cups (180g) all-purpose flour to mimic self-rising flour. Without that extra lift, your crust will be a bit denser, but still delicious!

1. **To make the dough:** Preheat the oven to 450°F (230°C). Line a baking sheet with parchment paper.
2. To a large bowl, add the Greek yogurt, flour, and salt. With a spoon, mix until it begins to resemble a lumpy, well-mixed dough.
3. Using your hands, knead the dough until smooth and roll it into a ball. In a bowl, place the dough ball and cover it with plastic wrap. Let it sit for 15 minutes to rest.
4. Once the dough has rested, on the prepared baking sheet, spread the dough out. To prevent sticking, dip your fingers in water as you push the dough.
5. **To make the pizza sauce:** To a small bowl, add the strained tomatoes, garlic powder, basil, salt, and chili flakes (if using) and stir to combine.
6. **To make the pizza:** With a spoon, spread the pizza sauce onto the dough, leaving roughly 1 inch (2.5cm) all the way around for the crust.
7. Sprinkle the mozzarella over the surface of the pizza and top with the banana peppers, turkey pepperoni, tomato, and pineapple.
8. Bake on the middle rack for 20 to 25 minutes.
9. Remove the pizza from the oven, let sit for 2 minutes, slice, and dig in!

makes 1 personal pizza / 1 serving

NUTRITION (PER SERVING)	
1084 calories	**16g** fat
66g protein	**165g** net carbs

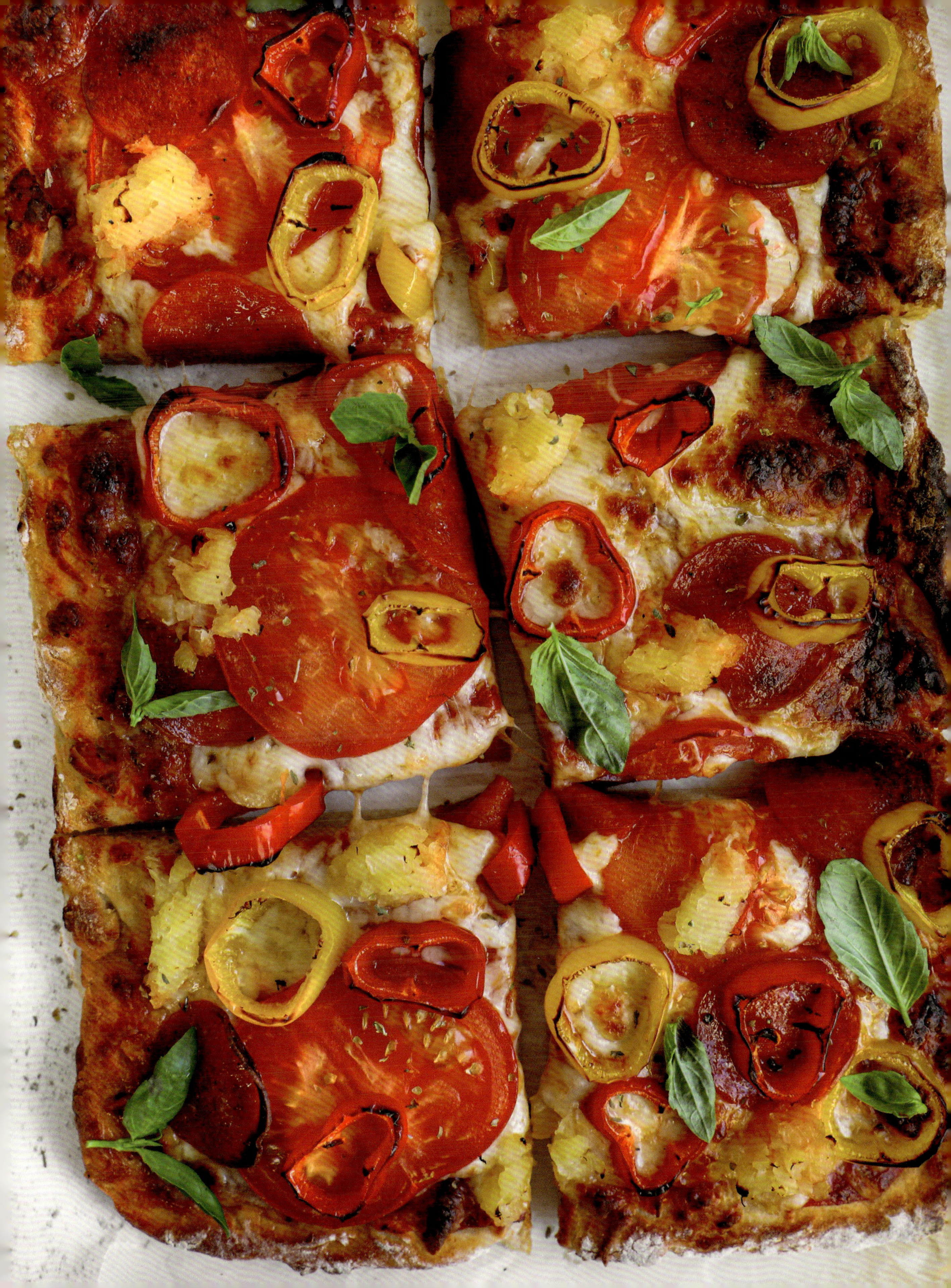

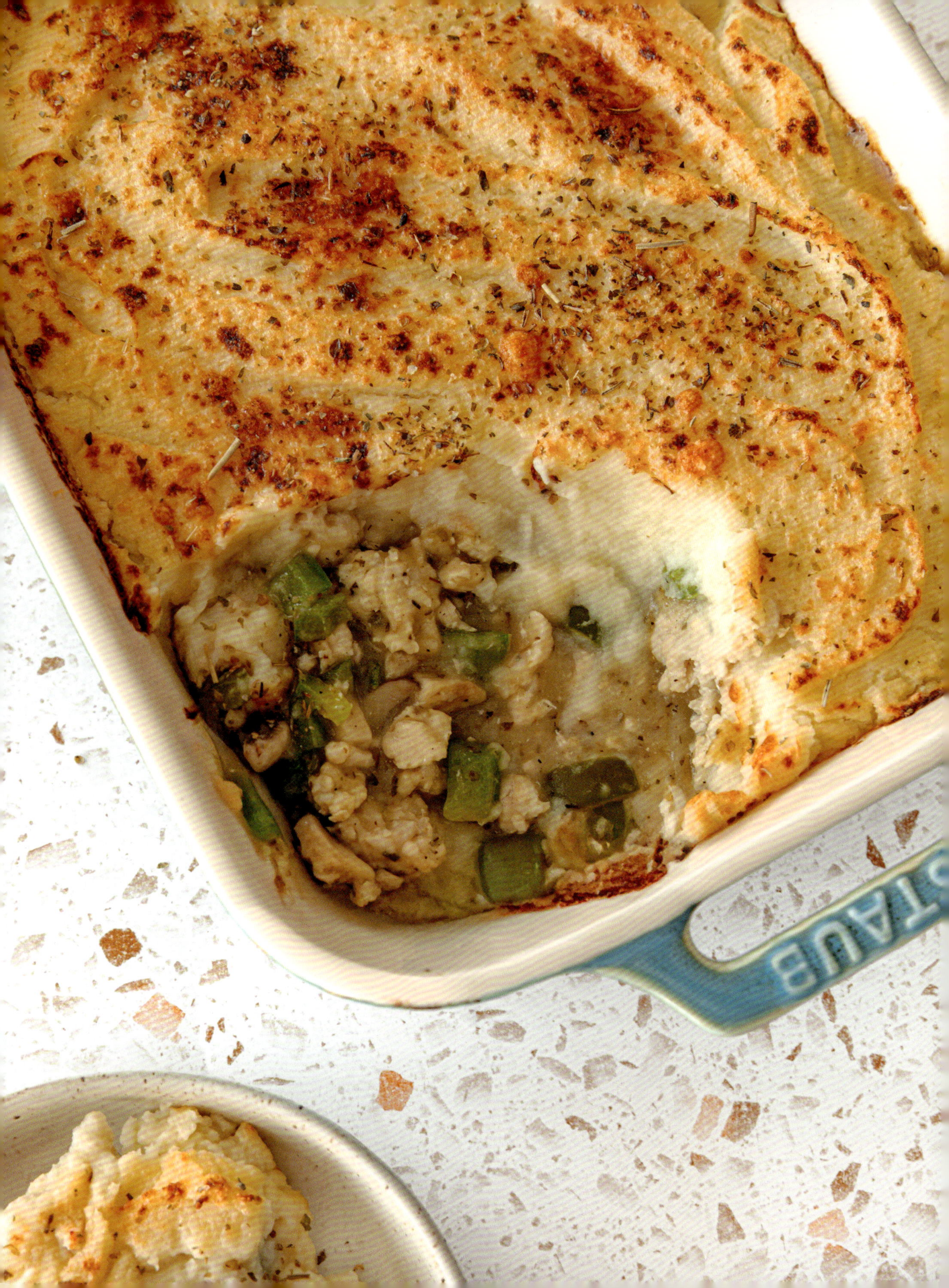
STAUB

ANABOLIC SHEPHERD'S PIE

9½ cups (800g) cauliflower florets
2–4 garlic cloves, or to taste
1 lb (450g) ground chicken
½ medium zucchini, chopped
½ yellow onion, chopped
1 cup (240g) button mushrooms, chopped
1 tbsp (6g) fresh rosemary, finely chopped
⅔ cup (160ml) chicken stock
1 tbsp (7.5g) all-purpose flour
1 tbsp (15g) nonfat Greek yogurt
Salt and pepper, to taste
2 tbsp (12g) Parmesan-and-herb seasoning

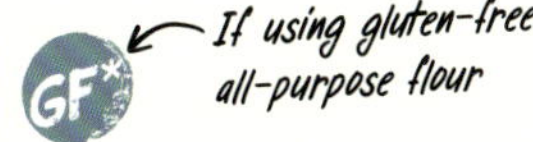

makes 4 servings

NUTRITION (PER SERVING)

229 calories	**6g** fat
29g protein	**18g** net carbs

You'll definitely think you're getting lucky when you try this pie—a healthy, high-protein, high-volume take on a warm, down-to-earth comfort classic. Boiling the cauliflower until it's supersoft makes it blend into a smoother, more convincing mash. For the crispy, golden-brown finish, a sprinkle of Parmesan-and-herb seasoning does the trick. If it's not on hand, a quick mix of grated Parmesan, dried oregano, basil, garlic powder, onion powder, and black pepper creates the same savory topping. This dish stores well for up to 4 days in the fridge or 6 months in the freezer. Reheat in the microwave for 2 to 3 minutes or in the oven at 350°F (180°C) for 15 to 20 minutes, and it's just as good as fresh.

1. Bring a large pot of water to a boil over high heat. Add the cauliflower and garlic and boil for 15 to 20 minutes, or until very soft. Strain from the water and set aside.
2. Heat a large skillet over medium to medium-high heat and spray it with nonstick cooking spray. Add the ground chicken and sauté for 8 to 10 minutes.
3. Once the chicken is cooked through, remove it from the skillet, keeping the stove on, and set aside. To the same hot skillet over medium to medium-high heat, add the zucchini, onion, mushrooms, and rosemary and sauté for 6 to 8 minutes, until the vegetables are softened.
4. Return the cooked chicken to the skillet and stir to combine. Add the chicken stock and evenly dust the flour over top, stirring to incorporate. Let simmer over medium heat for 5 minutes.
5. Meanwhile, to a blender, add the boiled cauliflower and garlic cloves and the Greek yogurt, seasoning with salt and pepper. Blend until smooth.
6. Preheat the oven to 400°F (200°C) convection bake or 425°F (220°C) regular bake.
7. Into a 9 x 9-inch (23 x 23cm) baking dish, pour the ground chicken filling and top with the blended cauliflower purée. For a crispy top, sprinkle with the Parmesan-and-herb seasoning.
8. Bake for 20 to 30 minutes, or until the top is thoroughly browned.
9. Let the pie cool for 10 minutes before serving.

CHEESEBURGER SPRING ROLLS

WITH THOUSAND ISLAND DIP

for the spring rolls:

1 large onion, diced
1 lb (450g) extra-lean ground beef
1 tbsp (15ml) Worcestershire sauce
1 tsp (3g) salt
½ tsp (1.5g) black pepper
2 garlic cloves, diced
1 cup (120g) shredded low-fat cheddar cheese
10 spring roll pastry sheets, about ¼oz (8g) each

for the Thousand Island dip:

¼ cup (60g) nonfat Greek yogurt
¼ cup (60ml) low-fat mayonnaise
¼ cup (60ml) sugar-free ketchup
¼ cup (60g) relish
2 tbsp (30ml) mustard
½ tsp (1.5g) onion powder
½ tsp (1.5g) garlic power
½ tsp (1.5g) smoked paprika

makes 10 rolls / 5 servings

NUTRITION (PER SERVING)

348 calories	**14g** fat
30g protein	**25.6g** net carbs

A burger and a crispy wonton walked into a bar—this is what happened next. This cheeseburger spring roll takes everything you love about a classic burger—savory beef, melty cheese, and tangy sauce—and wraps it in a golden, flaky shell. The real star? Thousand Island dressing, which is basically the OG special sauce. While most people just think of it as a burger condiment, it was actually invented in the Thousand Islands region between Ontario and New York—which, as someone from Ontario, makes me feel like I have a rightful claim to it. Call it patriotic, call it delicious, just don't forget to dunk.

1. **To make the spring rolls:** Preheat the oven to 425°F (220°C). Line a large baking sheet with parchment paper.
2. Heat a medium frying pan over medium heat and spray it with nonstick cooking spray. Add the onion and cook for 4 to 5 minutes, stirring often, until it becomes translucent.
3. Add the ground beef, Worcestershire sauce, salt, and pepper. Stir the seasoning into the meat and increase the heat to medium-high. Sauté for 6 to 8 minutes, or until the beef begins to brown. Add the garlic and sauté for 1 to 2 minutes, or until the garlic is fragrant.
4. Remove the beef filling from the heat and fold in the cheese. Set the mixture aside to cool for at least 10 minutes.
5. On a flat surface, place a spring roll pastry sheet with one corner facing you, like a diamond. Add some of the filling, leaving 1 to 2 inches (2.5 to 5cm) on each side. Fold the bottom corner over the filling, then fold in the sides, and roll tightly toward the top. Moisten the top corner with water to seal the roll securely. Repeat with the remaining pastry sheets and filling.
6. On the prepared baking sheet, evenly arrange the spring rolls and lightly spray them with nonstick cooking spray.
7. Bake on the middle rack for 15 minutes. Flip each spring roll and bake for an additional 10 minutes, or until the pastry is golden brown and crispy. Remove the sheet from the oven and let cool for at least 5 minutes.
8. **To make the Thousand Island dip:** In a medium bowl, combine the Greek yogurt, mayonnaise, ketchup, relish, mustard, onion powder, garlic powder, and smoked paprika. Stir until well combined. Serve the spring rolls warm with the Thousand Island dip on the side.

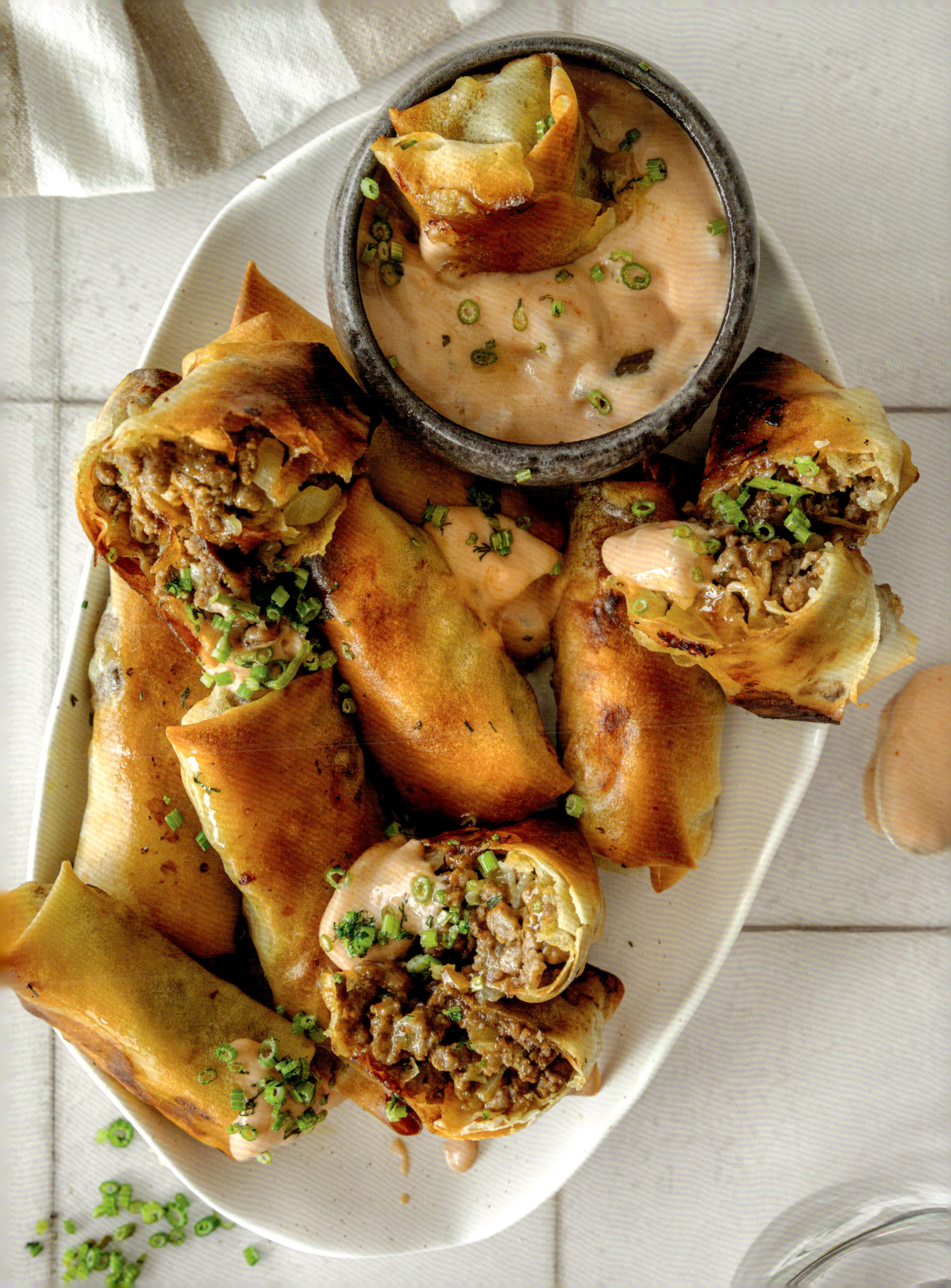

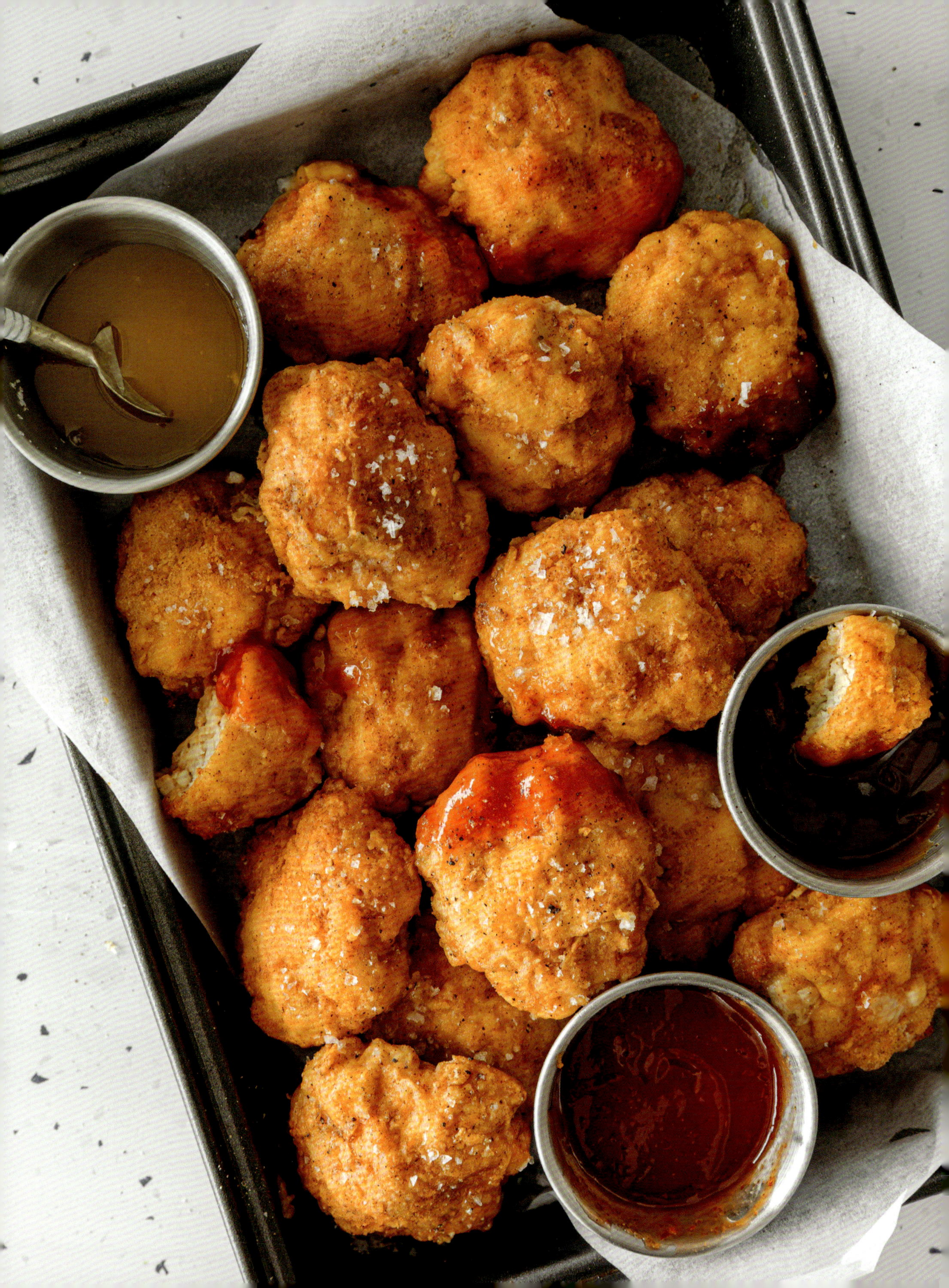

CHICKEN NUGGIES

- 1 lb (450g) lean ground chicken
- 1 egg
- ¼ cup (30g) grated Parmesan cheese
- 1 tsp (3g) chili powder
- 2 tsp (6g) garlic powder
- 2 tsp (6g) onion powder
- 2 tsp (6g) salt
- 6¾ tbsp (50g) all-purpose flour
- 1 tsp (5g) baking powder
- ½ tsp (1.5g) cayenne pepper
- 4½ tbsp (70g) egg whites

Like every kid, I used to beg for fast-food nuggets, only to hear the classic, "We have food at home." Spoiler: "Food at home" was never nuggets. So, I finally made a version that actually hits. The air fryer is the move for that fast-food crunch, but the oven still gets the job done if that's what you've got. Dipping is mandatory, and I switch between plum sauce, honey mustard, and sriracha, depending on my mood (or how daring I'm feeling with spice that day). However you sauce them up, these nuggies are proof that sometimes, food at home is actually the better option.

1. If using an oven, preheat it to 425°F (220°C). Line a large baking sheet with parchment paper. If using an air fryer, skip this step.
2. In a medium mixing bowl, combine the ground chicken, egg, Parmesan, chili powder, and 1 teaspoon (3g) each of the garlic powder, onion powder, and salt. Mix until well combined, ensuring the chicken is fully coated in the seasoning.
3. Shape the chicken mixture into 15 equal nugget pieces about 35g each and place them on the prepared baking sheet.
4. Place the baking sheet in the freezer for 25 minutes to allow the chicken nuggets to firm up.
5. Meanwhile, in a medium bowl, mix the flour, baking powder, and the remaining 1 teaspoon (3g) each of the garlic powder, onion powder, and salt, and the cayenne pepper to create the nugget coating.
6. Fill a small bowl with the egg whites.
7. Remove the nuggets from the freezer. Dip each nugget first into the egg whites, ensuring it is fully coated, then roll in the flour-coating mixture. Place the coated nuggets either back on the prepared baking sheet or in the air fryer basket.
8. Bake for 25 minutes or air fry at 400°F (200°C) for 16 minutes, or until the nuggets are crispy and golden brown.
9. Remove the nuggets from the heat and let cool for a few minutes. Serve with your favorite dipping sauce and enjoy!

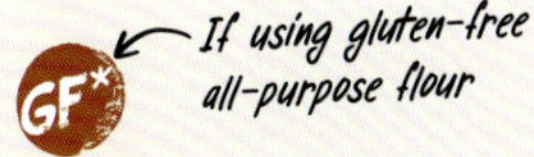

makes 15 nuggets / 3 servings

NUTRITION (PER SERVING)

300 calories	**14g** fat
36.5g protein	**7.5g** net carbs

ANIMAL-STYLE FRIES

for the fries:

4 tsp (12g) salt

1¼lb (550g) russet potatoes, cut lengthwise into ¼in-thick sticks

1 tsp (3g) garlic powder

1 tsp (3g) onion powder

½ tsp (1.5g) paprika

1¼ cups (150g) shredded low-fat cheddar cheese

for the caramelized onions:

3 cups (300g) diced white onion

½ tsp (1.5g) salt

for the sauce:

1¾ tbsp (25g) low-fat mayonnaise

5 tsp (25g) nonfat Greek yogurt

1 tbsp (15ml) sugar-free ketchup

1 tbsp (13g) pickle relish

¼ tsp (1.25ml) hot sauce

¼ tsp (750mg) onion powder

¼ tsp (750mg) garlic powder

¼ tsp (750mg) paprika

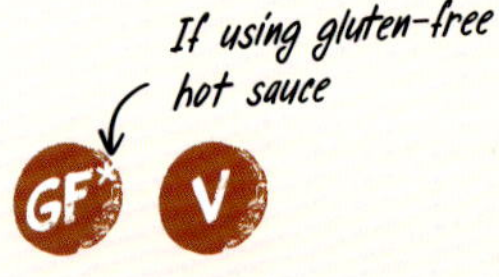

makes 2 servings

NUTRITION (PER SERVING)

423 calories	**9g** fat
16.5g protein	**69g** net carbs

You know that song about doing it "like they do on the Discovery Channel"? Pretty sure they were talking about making this recipe. In-N-Out's animal-style fries have earned their cult status for a reason—golden fries piled high with rich caramelized onions, gooey cheese, and a bold, savory sauce. This version delivers all the same flavors while ditching the deep fryer, making it easier to enjoy without needing a postmeal siesta. Soaking the potatoes before baking helps them crisp up beautifully, giving you that perfect bite every time. Stick to the classic toppings, or throw in some ground meat to make it a full meal—because when it comes to loaded fries, more is always better.

1. Preheat the oven to 425°F (220°C). Line a large rectangular baking sheet with parchment paper.
2. **To prepare the fries:** Fill a large bowl two-thirds with cold water and add 3 teaspoons (9g) of the salt. Place the fries into the saltwater, ensuring they are fully submerged. Soak for 30 minutes to help remove excess starch.
3. Strain the fries. With a paper towel, pat them dry thoroughly. Return the fries to the bowl and add the remaining 1 teaspoon (3g) salt and the garlic powder, onion powder, and paprika. Spray the fries with nonstick cooking spray and toss until evenly coated with the spices.
4. On the prepared baking sheet, evenly spread the fries. Bake for 20 minutes. For extra crispiness, if you have a convection setting, flip the fries halfway and switch to convection bake. Once the fries are browned and crisp, remove them from the oven and set aside, leaving the oven on.
5. **To make the caramelized onions:** Heat a medium frying pan over medium-low heat and spray it with nonstick cooking spray. Add the onions and salt. Sauté for about 30 minutes, stirring often, until the onions are caramelized. If the onions begin to dry out or shrivel, add 2 tablespoons (30ml) water and repeat as needed until golden and soft. Be patient. This can take up to 1 additional cup (240ml) of water.
6. **To make the sauce:** In a small bowl, combine the mayonnaise, Greek yogurt, ketchup, relish, hot sauce, onion powder, garlic powder, and paprika. Stir until smooth and well combined.
7. Over the fries, sprinkle the caramelized onions evenly and top with the cheese. Bake for 5 minutes, or until the cheese is melted and bubbly.
8. Remove the fries from the oven and let sit for 5 minutes before serving.
9. To serve, over the fries, spoon dollops of the sauce. Enjoy immediately!

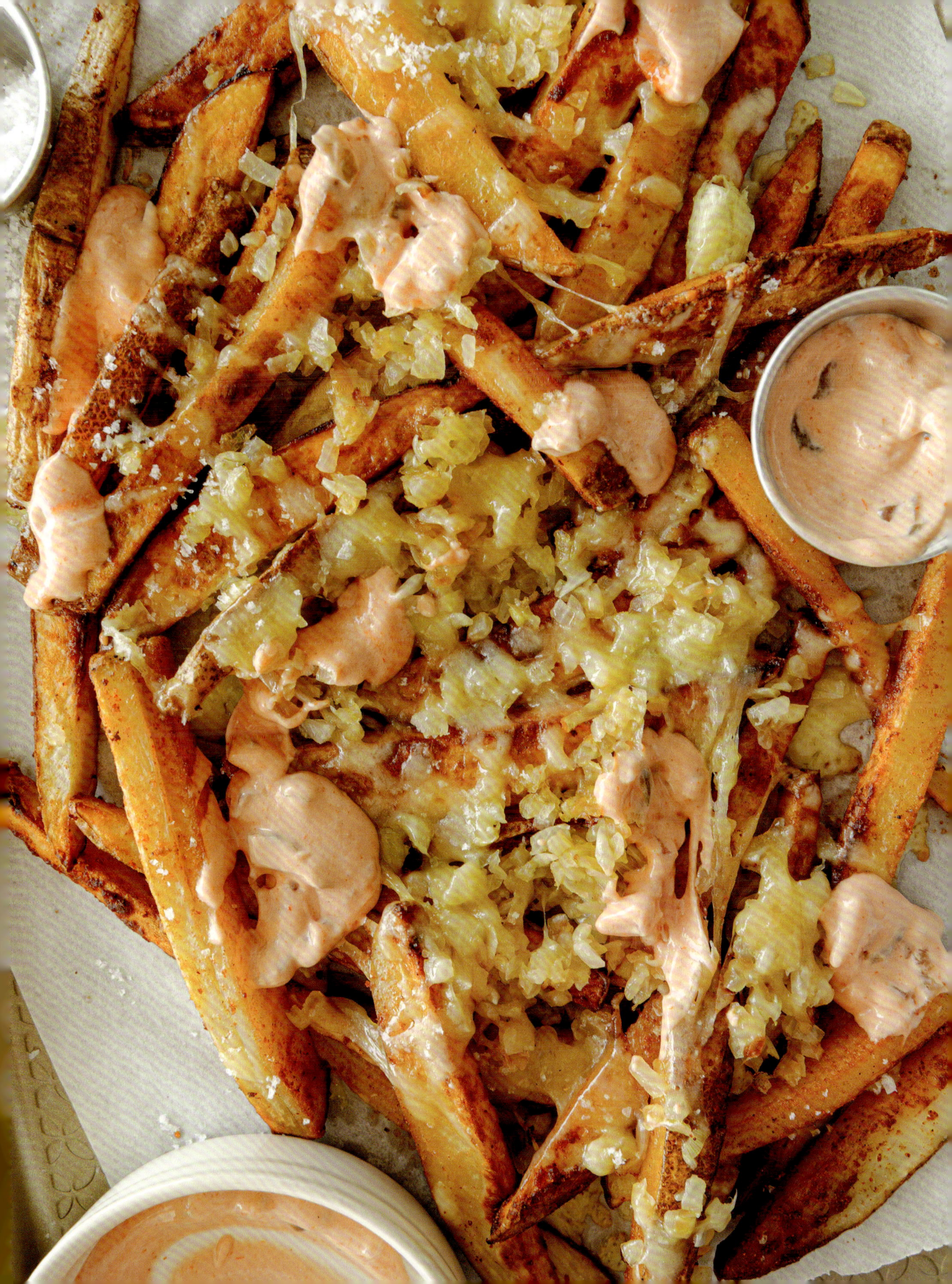

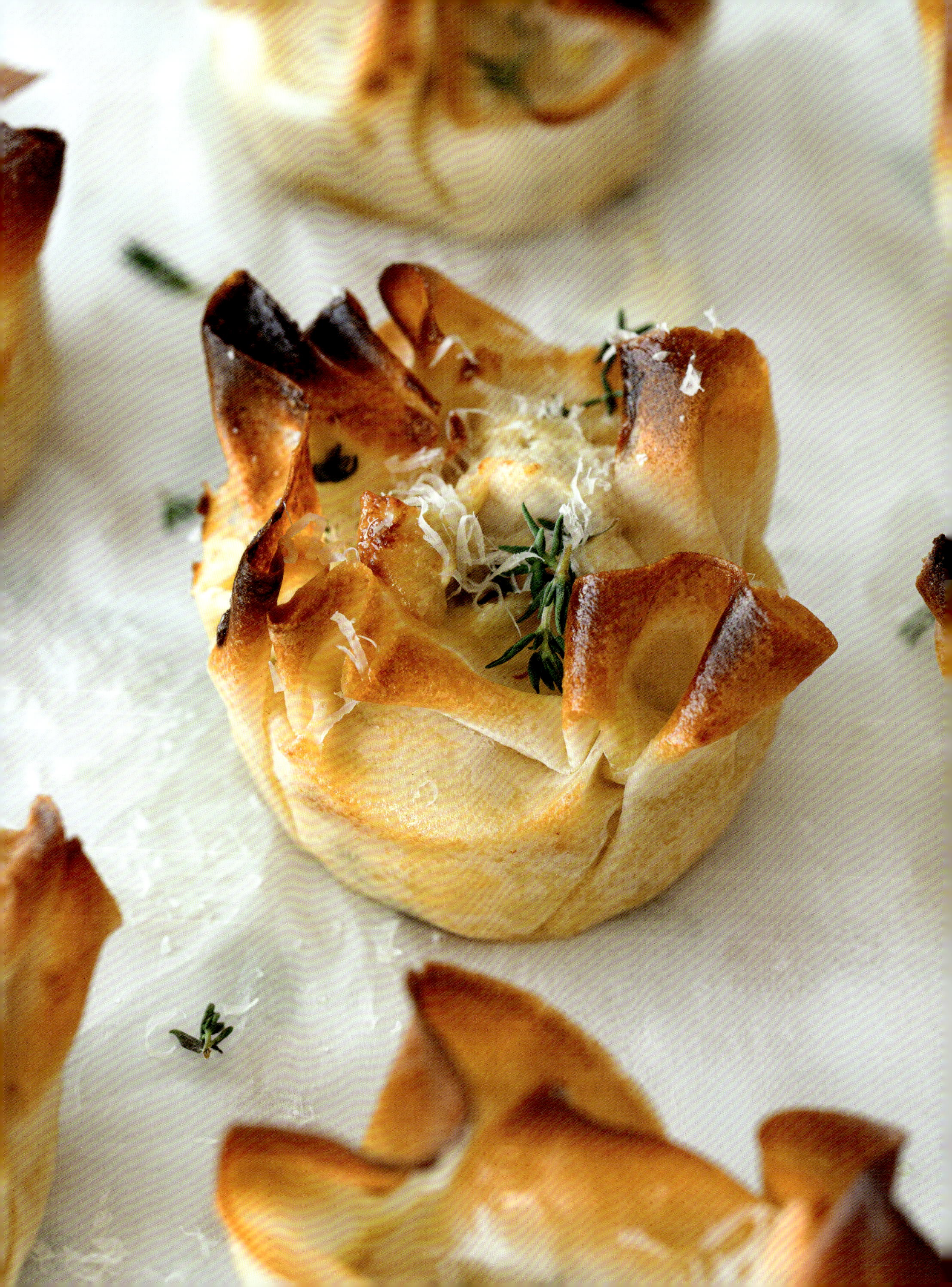

CRISPY CHEESE CHICKEN CUPS

- 1 cup (100g) onion, finely diced
- 2 garlic cloves, finely diced
- 1 cup (250g) light cream cheese, room temperature
- 10oz (283g) can chicken breast, drained
- 1 tsp (1g) fresh thyme leaves
- 2 tbsp (15g) grated Parmesan
- 1 egg
- 12 spring roll pastry sheets

makes 12 cups / 12 servings

NUTRITION (PER SERVING)	
102 calories	**5.2g** fat
7.2g protein	**6.5g** net carbs

Finding the perfect cup size is a struggle—but thankfully, these ones always fit. Inspired by crab rangoon, these crispy, cheesy cups swap out the seafood for a rich, savory chicken filling, while keeping all the crunch and creaminess that makes the original so addictive. Spring-roll pastry sheets bake up thinner and crispier than traditional wonton wrappers, giving you that perfect bite without feeling too heavy. And let's talk about canned chicken—it's underrated, convenient, and blends seamlessly into the filling like it was born to be there. Whether you're making these for a crowd or just meal prepping snacks for the week, they never last long. Store leftovers in an airtight container for up to 4 days or freeze them for up to 3 months. Reheat in the oven at 375°F (190°C) for 8 to 10 minutes from the fridge, or 15 to 18 minutes from the freezer—no thawing needed.

1. Preheat the oven to 425°F (220°C). Lightly spray a 12-cup muffin tin with nonstick cooking spray.
2. Heat a small frying pan over medium heat and lightly spray it with nonstick cooking spray. Add the onion and cook for about 5 minutes, or until it becomes translucent.
3. Add the garlic and cook for 1 minute, or until fragrant. Remove the pan from the heat and allow the mixture to cool.
4. In a large mixing bowl, combine the cooled onion and garlic mixture, cream cheese, chicken, thyme, Parmesan, and egg. Mix until the ingredients are evenly combined.
5. Into each muffin mold, place one spring roll pastry sheet, pressing gently to fit.
6. Among the 12 muffin cups, evenly distribute the cheese and chicken mixture, about 3 tablespoons per muffin.
7. Fold the excess spring roll pastry over the top of the filling, covering it completely. Lightly spray the tops of the wrapped cups with nonstick cooking spray.
8. Bake on the middle rack for 20 minutes, or until the wrappers are golden brown and crispy.
9. Remove from the oven and let the cups cool for a few minutes before serving. Enjoy!

HEALTHIER BAKED MAC AND CHEESE

- 1 small head of cauliflower, roughly chopped into bite-size chunks
- 1 cup (125g) uncooked macaroni pasta
- 2 cups (480ml) Silk unsweetened cashew milk
- 3 tbsp (22.5g) all-purpose flour
- Salt and pepper, to taste
- 2 cups (240g) shredded low-fat cheddar cheese
- ¼ cup (27.5g) bread crumbs

In Canada, we don't just eat mac and cheese—we eat Kraft Dinner (or KD, if you're really in the know). It's practically a food group here, but this version takes things up a notch with a rich cheese sauce, a crispy baked topping, and a sneaky helping of cauliflower to cut the carbs and lighten things up. The cashew milk keeps it smooth, and the cheese sauce still delivers all the comfort-food feels. It's the best of both worlds—nostalgic, satisfying, and a little more balanced. Just don't tell any KD purists what's in it. For meal prep, store in a sealed container for up to 4 days in the fridge. Reheat in the oven at 375°F (190°C) for 15 to 20 minutes (covering with foil to keep it from drying out), or microwave in 30-second bursts with a splash of cashew milk to bring the sauce back to life.

1. Preheat the oven to 400°F (200°C).
2. Fill a medium saucepan halfway with water and bring it to a boil over high heat. Once boiling, add the cauliflower and pasta to the saucepan. Cook for 2 minutes less than the package instructions. Strain and set aside.
3. To a medium saucepan over medium heat, add the cashew milk and flour. Stir together until combined, then bring to a boil and reduce the heat to low. Let simmer for 3 to 4 minutes, until it becomes thick and creamy. Season with salt and pepper.
4. Add the cheese and stir for 1 to 2 minutes, until the cheese melts entirely and creates a cheesy sauce.
5. Pour the pasta and cauliflower into the cheese sauce and stir to coat.
6. In a large baking dish, pour the mixture and dust the top with the bread crumbs.
7. Bake for 25 minutes, until the bread crumbs become golden brown and the cheese sauce bubbles!

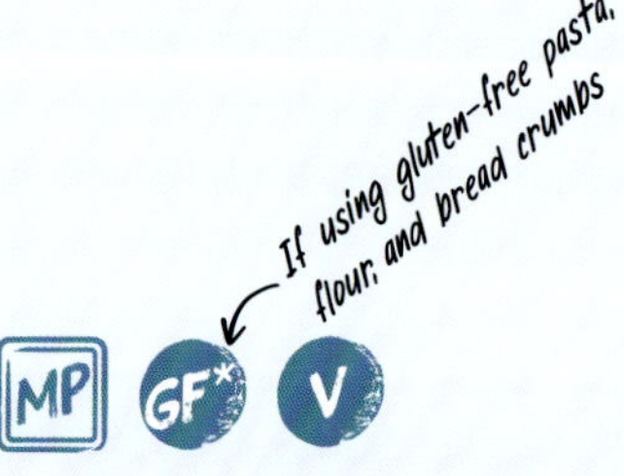

makes 2 servings

NUTRITION (PER SERVING)

541 calories	**12g** fat
42g protein	**61g** net carbs

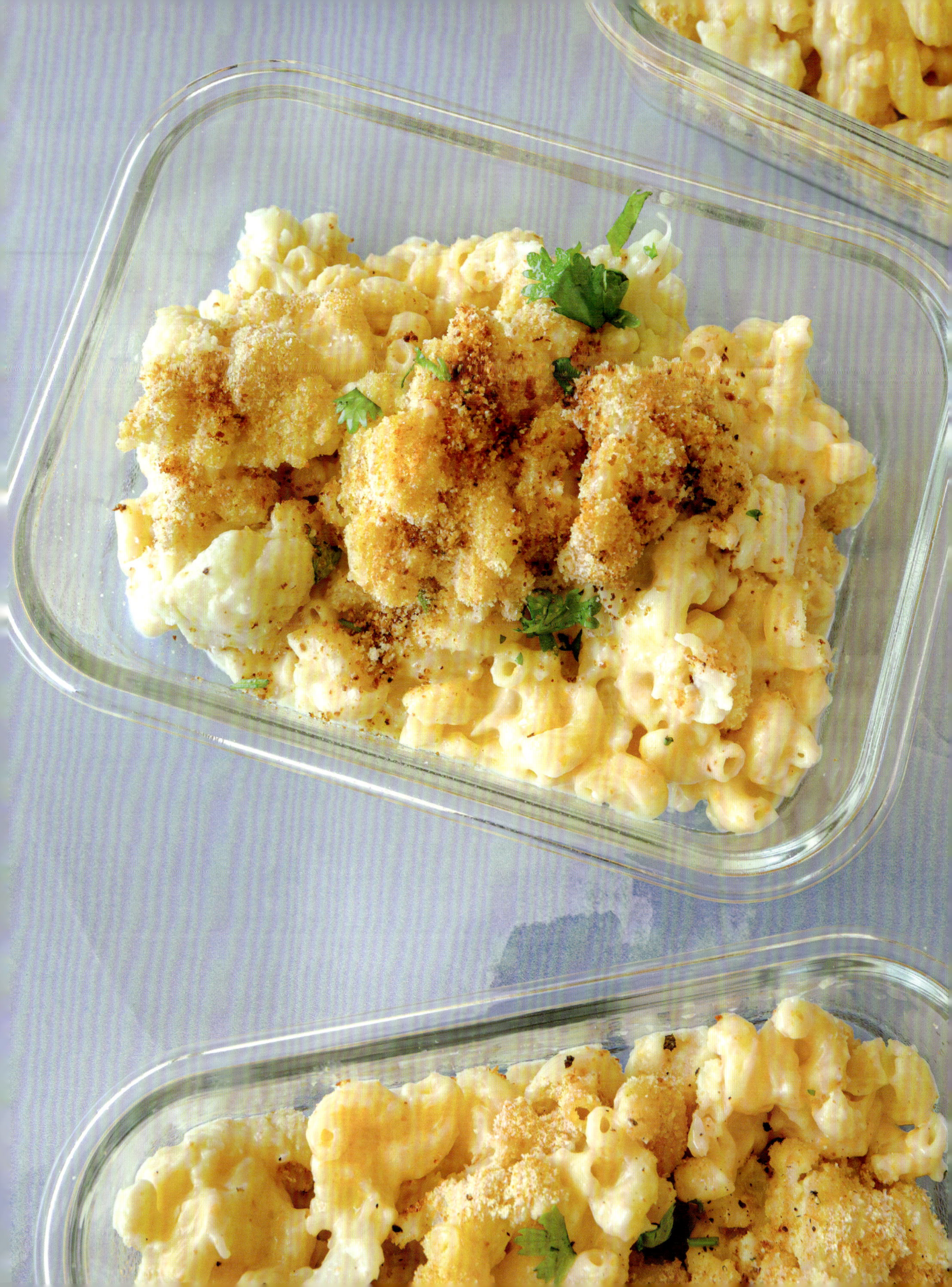

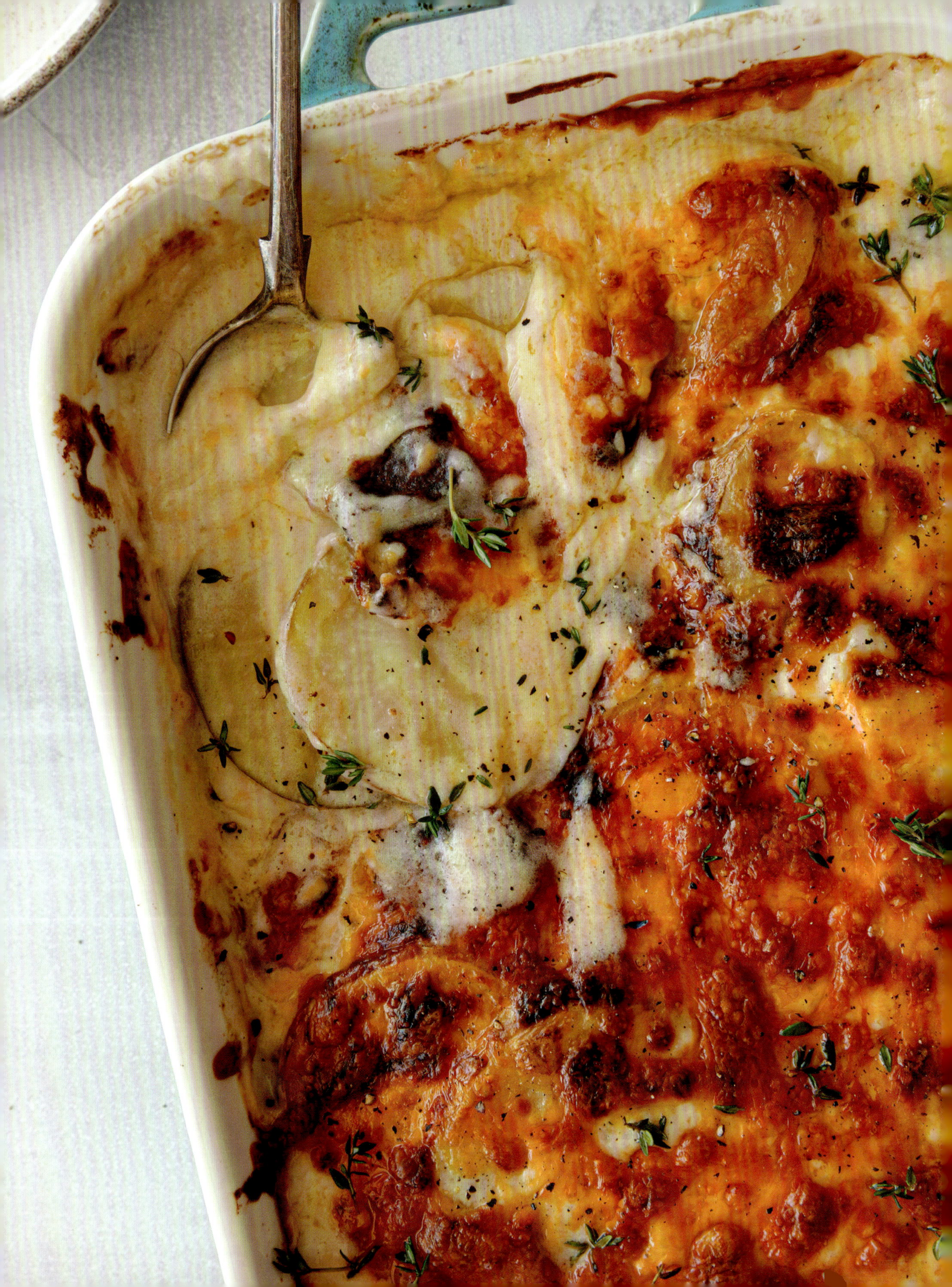

PROTEIN SCALLOPED POTATOES

2 cups (480ml) skim milk, warmed
½ cup (115g) low-fat cottage cheese
½ cup (115g) nonfat Greek yogurt
3 tbsp (14g) butter
3 tbsp (22.5g) all-purpose flour
2 garlic cloves, minced
2 tsp (6g) salt
½ tsp (1.5g) black pepper
2 tbsp (6g) fresh thyme, minced
2½ lb (1.1kg) russet potatoes, peeled and sliced into ⅛-inch (⅓cm) rounds
2 cups (224g) shredded part-skim marble cheese

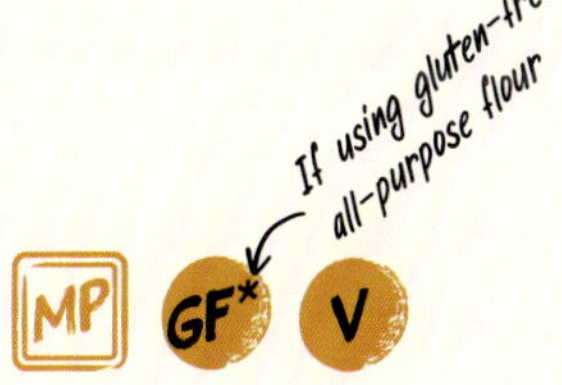

makes 10 servings

NUTRITION (PER SERVING)

228.5 calories
8.5g fat
13.2g protein
24.8g net carbs

Unlike the scallops I accidentally left in my trunk for two months and tried to erase from my memory, these scalloped potatoes will entice you with their delicious aroma. They have a reputation for being indulgent, but this version delivers on comfort while sneaking in extra protein. A mix of Greek yogurt, cottage cheese, and skim milk keeps the sauce thick and velvety without relying on heavy cream. To get the best results, slice the potatoes evenly (if you have a mandoline, this would be the time to use it) so they cook through at the same time, and preboiling them prevents any undercooked layers. Leftovers store well in an airtight container for up to 4 days. When reheating, bake at 375°F (190°C) for 15 to 20 minutes.

1. Preheat the oven to 400°F (200°C). Spray a large, rectangular, oven-safe casserole dish with nonstick cooking spray.
2. In a blender, combine the milk, cottage cheese, and Greek yogurt. Blend on medium speed until smooth.
3. Heat a medium saucepan over medium-low heat and add the butter. Once melted, add the flour and whisk continuously until the mixture bubbles and begins to turn light brown.
4. Add the garlic and sauté for 2 minutes, or until fragrant.
5. While stirring, gradually pour the blended mixture into the saucepan. Increase the heat to medium and cook for 5 minutes, stirring occasionally, until the sauce begins to thicken.
6. Once the sauce is thick enough to coat the back of a spoon, remove from the heat and stir in the salt, black pepper, and thyme.
7. To assemble the scalloped potatoes, layer ⅓ (about 1¼ lb / 367g) of the potato slices on the bottom of the prepared casserole dish. Top with ⅓ of the sauce and ⅓ (about ⅔ cup / 75g) of the cheese. Repeat this process two more times, finishing with a layer of cheese on top.
8. Cover the casserole dish with foil and bake for 30 minutes covered, then for an additional 20 minutes uncovered, or until the top is golden brown and the cheese is bubbly.
9. Remove the casserole from the oven and let rest for 10 to 15 minutes before serving. Enjoy!

FRIED ZUCCHINI CHIPS
WITH MARINARA DIP

for the zucchini chips:

2 medium zucchinis, sliced into round chips ¼-inch (5mm) thick
1 egg
½ cup (55g) bread crumbs
1½ tbsp (12g) powdered Parmesan cheese
1 tsp (3g) garlic powder

for the marinara dipping sauce:

½ cup (120ml) strained tomatoes
1 tsp (3g) dried basil
1 tsp (3g) garlic powder
Salt and pepper, to taste

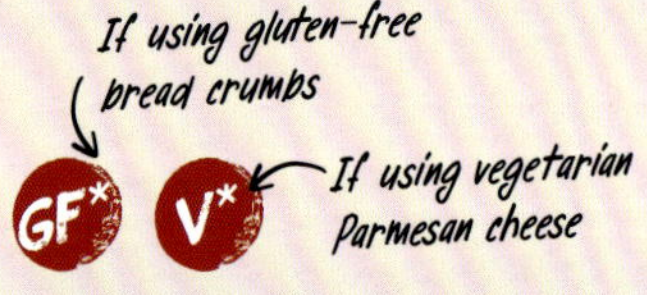

makes 2 servings

NUTRITION (PER SERVING)	
211 calories	**4.5g** fat
10.5g protein	**36.2g** net carbs

While I'm a firm believer that zucchini can be enjoyed raw, it scratches a different itch in chip form. It's mild enough to let the crispy, garlicky coating shine, and once it's golden and dunked in marinara, it's impossible to stop eating. To keep them from turning soggy, lightly salt the zucchini slices and let them sit for 10 minutes before patting them dry—this draws out excess moisture so they crisp up instead of steaming. Baking or air frying in a single layer also helps lock in that crunch. These chips are easy to make, easy to eat, and proof that sometimes, the underdog ingredient steals the show.

1. **To make the zucchini chips:** If using an oven, preheat it to 400°F (200°C) and line a baking sheet with parchment paper. If using an air fryer, skip this step.
2. Into a small bowl, crack the egg and whisk until the yolk and whites are fully combined.
3. In a separate small bowl, mix the bread crumbs, Parmesan, and garlic powder until evenly combined.
4. Dip a zucchini slice first into the whisked egg, ensuring both sides are coated, then into the bread-crumb mixture, pressing gently to adhere the coating to both sides. Repeat with all zucchini slices.
5. If using an air fryer, arrange the coated zucchini chips in a single layer in the air fryer basket and spray them with nonstick cooking spray. Cook at 375°F (190°C) for 12 minutes, flip the zucchini chips, and cook for an additional 5 minutes, or until golden brown and crisp. If using an oven, place the coated zucchini chips in a single layer on the prepared baking sheet. Bake for 20 to 25 minutes, flipping halfway through, until golden brown and crisp.
6. Once the zucchini chips are cooked, remove them from the oven or air fryer and let them rest for 5 minutes.
7. **To make the marinara dipping sauce:** In a small bowl, combine the tomatoes, basil, and garlic powder and season with salt and pepper. Mix thoroughly, then heat in the microwave on high for 1 minute. Serve the sauce alongside the zucchini chips.

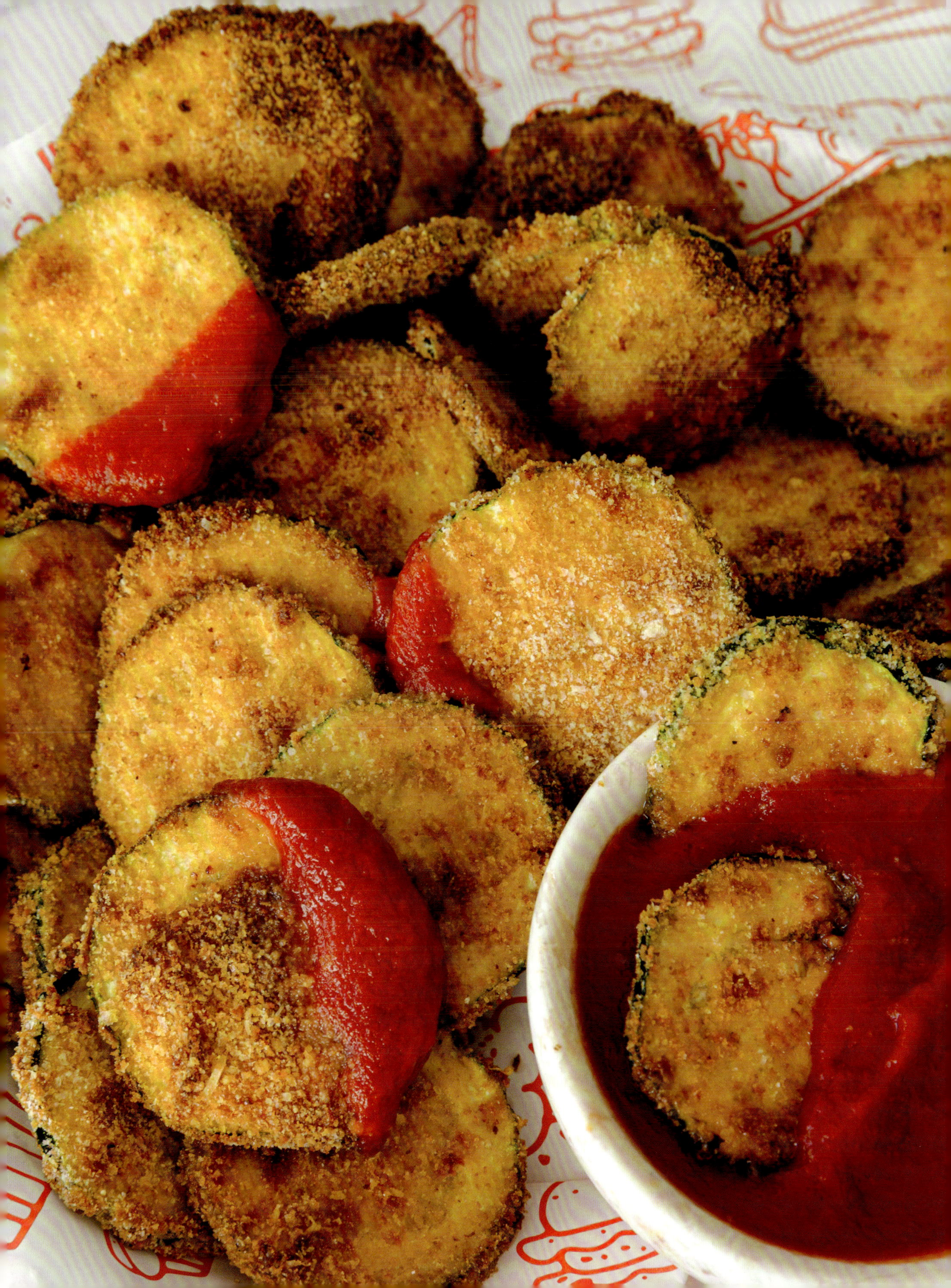

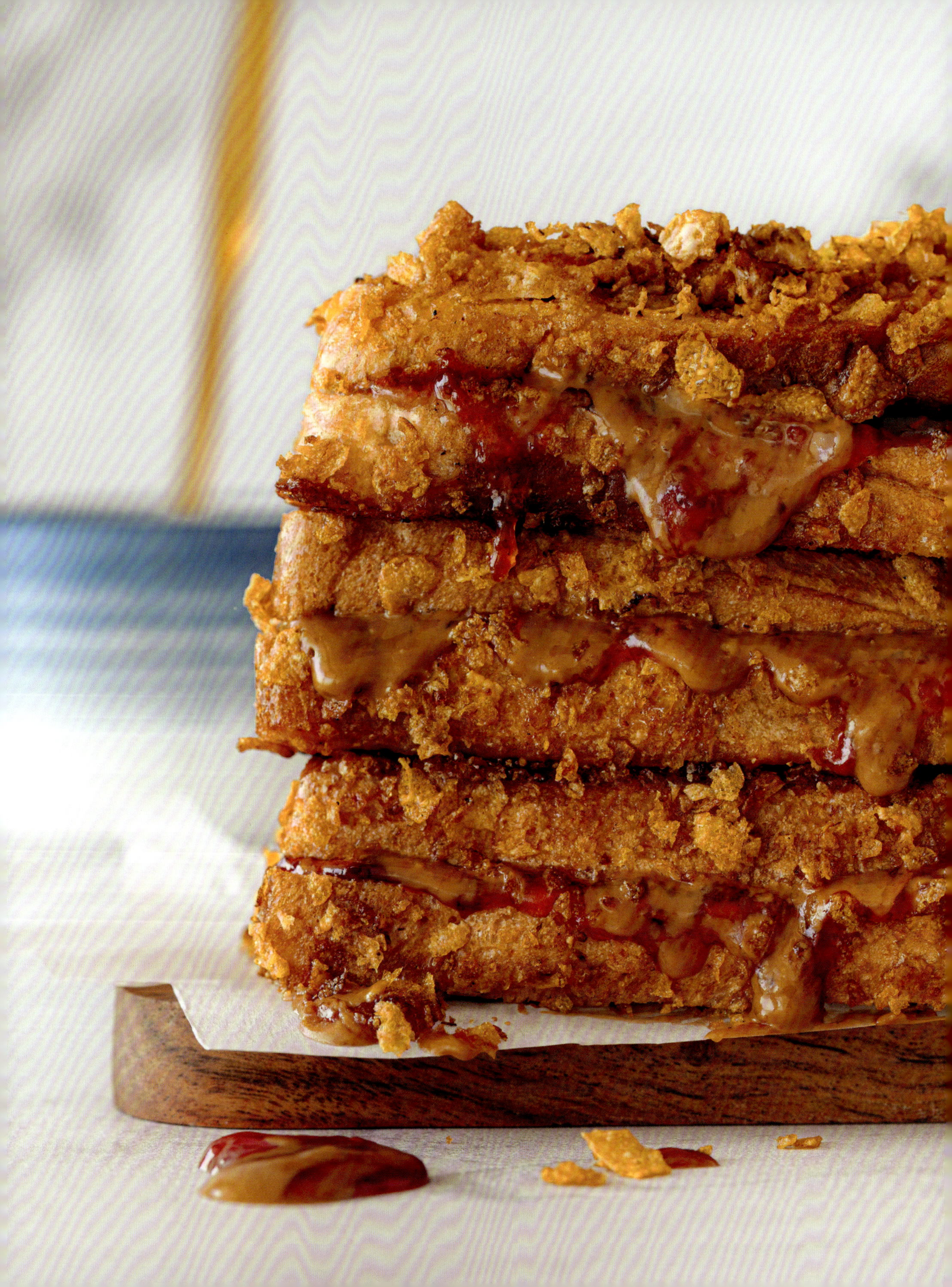

CRISPY FRIED PB&J SANDWICH

- 7 tsp (15g) PB2 Powdered Peanut Butter
- 2 slices of low-calorie white bread
- 1½ tbsp (30g) sugar-free strawberry jam
- ⅔ cup (20g) corn flakes cereal
- 1½ tsp (6g) erythritol
- 4½ tbsp (70g) egg whites
- ½ tsp (2.5ml) vanilla extract
- 1 tsp (5ml) coconut oil

If you've ever been *elevated* to a state where a PB&J sounded like the greatest meal of your life, this one's for you. Crispy on the outside, warm and gooey on the inside, it's like your favorite childhood sandwich went through a rebellious phase, hit the gym, and came out absolutely shredded—perfect for when you're deep in the munchies zone. It cooks fast, though, so don't get too distracted—all stoves are different, and this can go from golden brown to burned in seconds. The crushed cornflakes crust adds the crunch you never knew was missing, and trust me, it's impossible to eat this without moaning. Just try not to burn your mouth in your excitement.

1. In a small bowl, combine the PB2 Powdered Peanut Butter with 1½ tablespoons (23ml) water. Stir slowly until the mixture is smooth and creamy, ensuring there is no dry powder remaining.
2. On one slice of bread, spread the PB2 mixture. On the other slice of bread, spread the strawberry jam, and then sandwich the slices together.
3. In a medium bowl, place the cereal and erythritol. Use a wooden spoon or potato masher to crush the cereal into small chunks, being careful not to turn it into a powder.
4. In a separate medium bowl, whisk the egg whites and vanilla extract until fully combined.
5. Heat a medium frying pan over medium-high heat and add the coconut oil.
6. Dip the sandwich into the egg-white mixture, ensuring both sides absorb the mixture thoroughly. Next, use your hands to coat the sandwich with the cereal mixture, pressing the crushed cereal onto both sides to form an even crust.
7. In the heated pan, place the crusted sandwich and cook for 3 to 5 minutes on each side, or until golden brown and crispy.
8. Remove from the heat, plate, and devour!

If using gluten-free bread and corn flakes

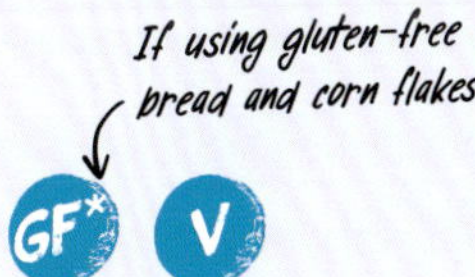

makes 1 serving

NUTRITION (PER SERVING)

346 calories	**10g** fat
21g protein	**43g** net carbs

PIZZA CASSEROLE

- 4–5 cups (450g) short pasta of choice
- 1⅓ cup (150g) chopped white onion
- 6½ tbsp (100g) chopped mushrooms
- 6½ tbsp (100g) chopped green pepper
- 1 lb (450g) extra-lean ground turkey
- 2 garlic cloves, minced
- 1 tsp (3g) salt
- 1 tsp (3g) dried oregano
- 3 cups (700ml) tomato sauce
- 1 cup plus 2 tbsp (250g) low-fat cottage cheese
- 1 cup plus 3 tbsp (100g) part-skim shredded mozzarella
- 16 slices of turkey pepperoni

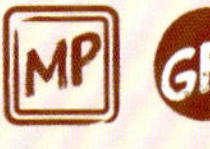

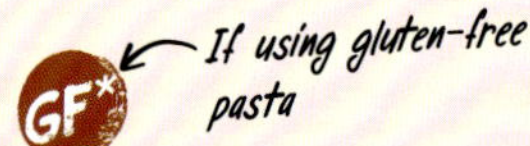

makes 1 casserole / 8 servings

NUTRITION (PER SERVING)

404 calories	**9g** fat
29g protein	**52g** net carbs

Casseroles have a reputation for being the dish your aunt brings to a potluck that nobody actually wants, but this one flips the script. All the cheesy, saucy goodness of a classic pizza, packed into a high-protein, meal-prep-friendly dish that actually delivers. Feel free to mix up the toppings—black olives, jalapeños, banana peppers, or even cooked turkey bacon all work great. I recommend using a tomato sauce that's around 40 to 50 calories per ½ cup (120ml) to keep things light without sacrificing flavor. Make a batch at the start of the week, and store portions in airtight containers in the fridge for up to 4 days. When it's time to eat, reheat in the oven at 375°F (190°C) for 10 to 15 minutes and enjoy!

1. Preheat the oven to 400°F (200°C).
2. Fill a medium pot halfway with water and bring it to a boil. Add the pasta and cook until al dente according to the package instructions. Strain the pasta and set aside.
3. Place a large saucepan over medium-high heat and spray it with nonstick cooking spray. Add the onions, mushrooms, and green peppers. Sauté for 5 to 6 minutes, or until the onions are slightly browned and translucent.
4. Add the ground turkey, garlic, salt, and oregano and mix to combine. Sauté for 5 to 7 minutes, or until the turkey begins to brown and most of the moisture has evaporated.
5. Remove the saucepan from the heat and stir in the tomato sauce and cottage cheese. Mix until a creamy pink sauce forms.
6. Add the cooked pasta to the saucepan and stir until the pasta is fully coated with the sauce.
7. Transfer the pasta mixture to a large oven-safe casserole dish. Spread evenly and top with the shredded cheese and turkey pepperoni.
8. Bake on the center rack for 25 to 30 minutes, or until the cheese begins to brown and the sauce is bubbling.
9. Remove the casserole from the oven and let cool for 10 minutes before serving. Enjoy!

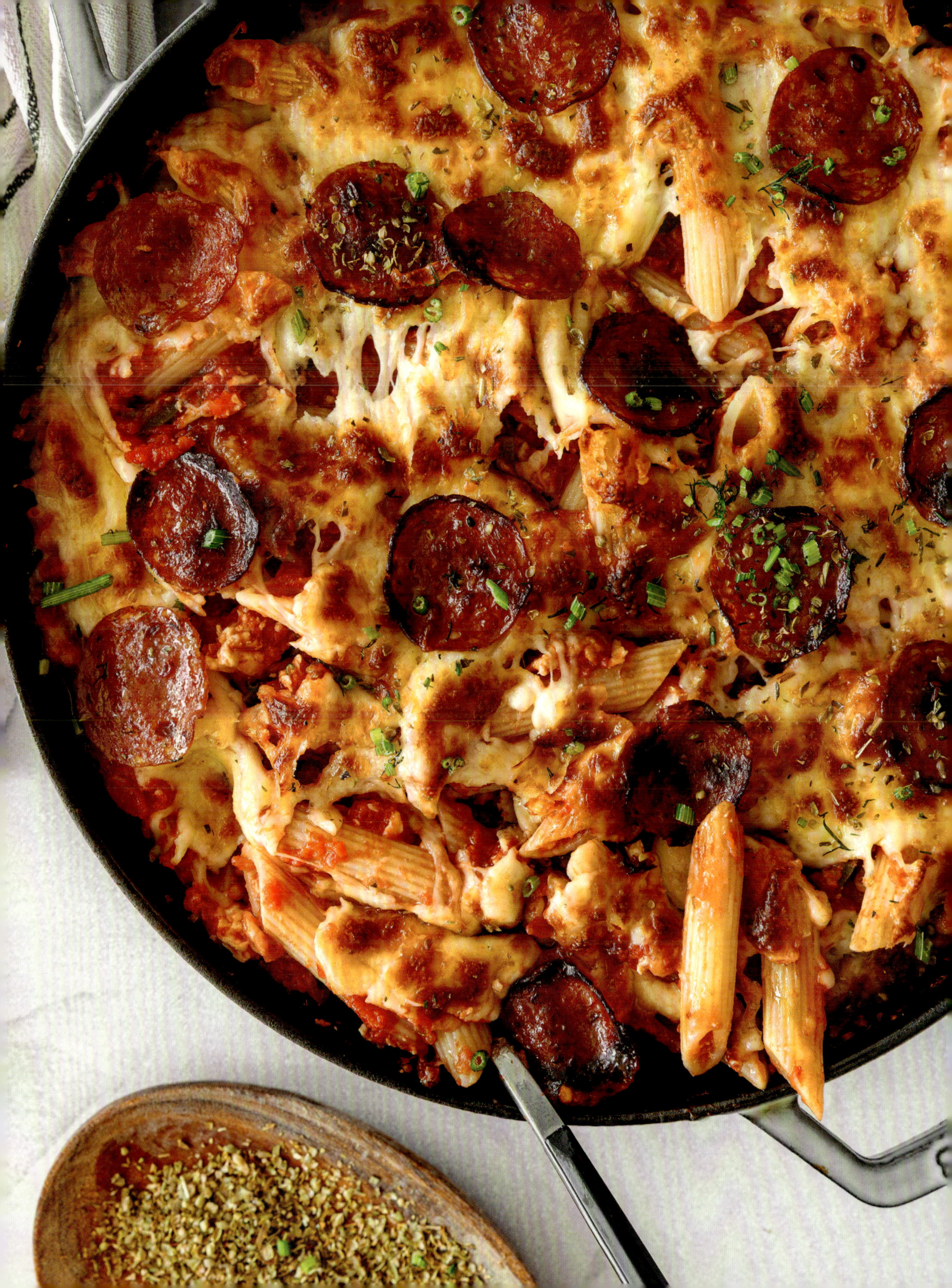

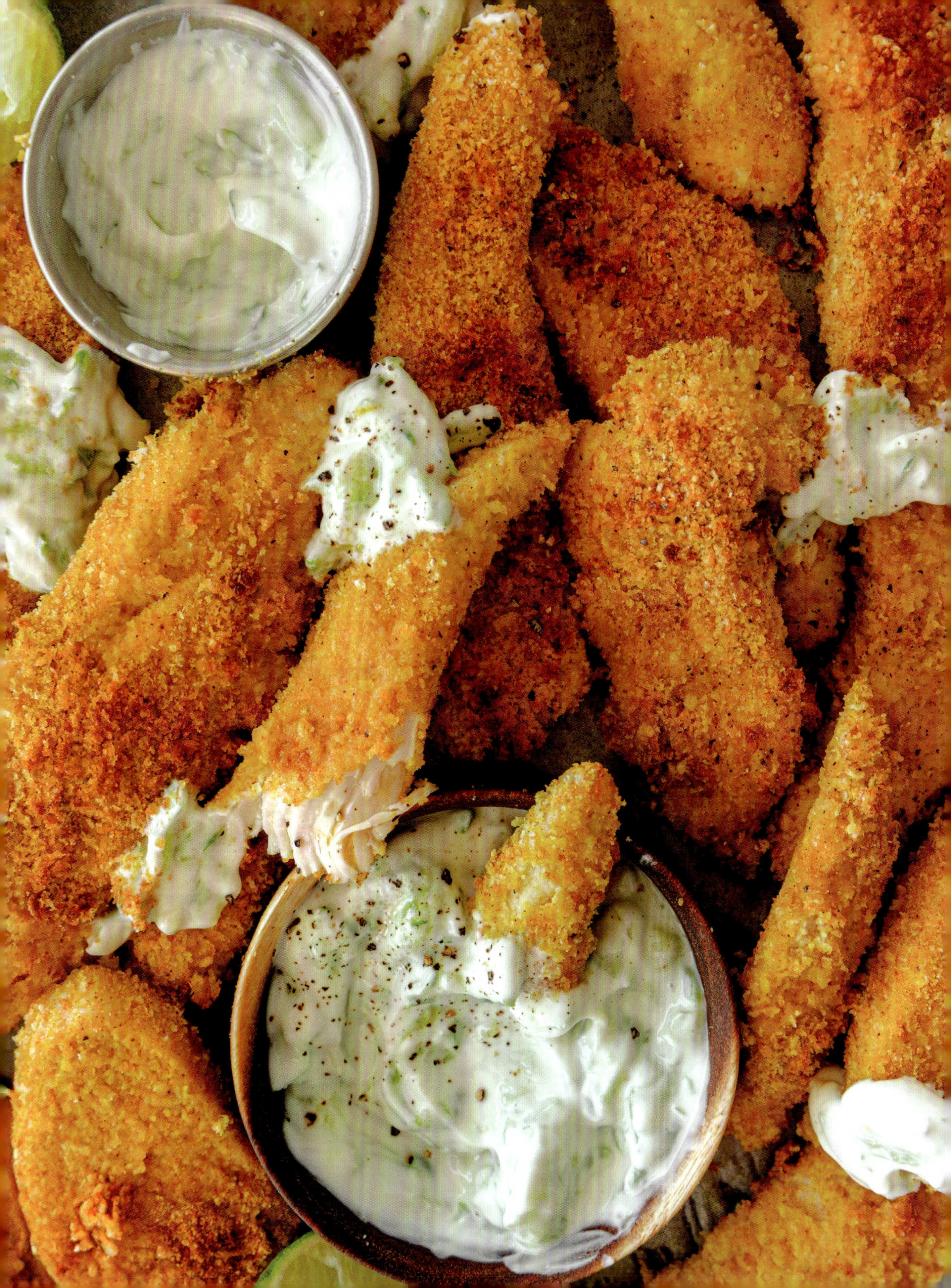

CURRY CHICKEN TENDERS

WITH GREEK-YOGURT DIP

for the chicken tenders:

2 small end pieces from a loaf of sourdough bread, lightly toasted
1 tsp (3g) curry powder
Salt and pepper, to taste
1 egg
1 large chicken breast (350g), sliced lengthwise into long strips

for the dipping sauce:

2 heaping tbsp (45g) nonfat Greek yogurt
Juice of ½ lime
½ tbsp (6g) grated cucumber
¼ tsp (750mg) cumin
¼ tsp (250mg) dried chives
Salt and pepper, to taste

I like my chicken like I like my lovers—tender and spicy. If you don't want to toast and blend your own bread crumbs, store-bought works just fine. Just go for plain bread crumbs so you can season them yourself. Feel free to experiment with the breading mixture—garlic powder, smoked paprika, or even a little cayenne for extra heat can all take this to the next level. If you want a little extra crunch, try using panko instead of traditional bread crumbs. And don't sleep on the dipping sauce—it's creamy, refreshing, and works with the curry like a well-matched Tinder swipe.

1. **To make the chicken tenders:** Preheat the oven to 425°F (220°C). Line a baking sheet with parchment paper.
2. In a blender or food processor, place the bread and pulse until it forms fine bread crumbs. Add the curry powder, season with salt and pepper, and pulse briefly to combine. Transfer the bread crumbs to a medium bowl and set aside.
3. Into another medium bowl, crack the egg. Add 2 tablespoons (30ml) lukewarm water and whisk together until frothy.
4. Dip each chicken strip, one at a time, into the egg wash, ensuring it is fully coated. Then dip the strip into the bread crumbs, pressing gently to adhere the coating to all sides. On the prepared baking sheet, place the coated chicken strips.
5. Lightly spray the coated chicken strips with nonstick cooking spray. Bake for 15 to 18 minutes, flipping the strips halfway through cooking. The tenders are done when they are browned and crisp on the outside and have reached an internal temperature of 165°F (74°C). Remove the chicken strips from the oven and let them cool on the baking sheet for 5 minutes.
6. **To make the dipping sauce:** In a small bowl, combine the Greek yogurt, lime juice, cucumber, cumin, and chives and season with salt and pepper. Stir until well mixed. Serve the dipping sauce on the side of the chicken tenders. Dip and enjoy!

makes 1 serving

NUTRITION (PER SERVING)

470 calories **10.6g** fat
54g protein **35g** net carbs

BLENDED CREAMY VANILLA-PROTEIN ICED COFFEE

9fl oz (250ml) brewed coffee, cooled in the fridge
2½ cups (620ml) Silk unsweetened cashew milk
2½ tbsp (37.5g) 10% cream or half-and-half
1 scoop (31g) vanilla protein powder
2 tsp (8g) erythritol
10oz (285g) ice

We're all broke because we keep buying overpriced coffee, so here's a solution that won't require you to check your bank balance before ordering. For the days when you need caffeine and protein but don't have the energy to make both, this drink does the heavy lifting for you. It's cold, creamy, and suspiciously close to a vanilla Frappuccino, but with actual nutritional value. Serve it as is, or take it up a notch with coconut whipped cream, sugar-free chocolate sauce, or even a cherry on top, if you're feeling bougie. Best enjoyed before a workout, after a workout, or whenever life demands both gains and caffeine.

1. To a blender, add the coffee, cashew milk, cream, protein powder, and erythritol. Blend on low or pulse until the ingredients are fully combined and smooth.
2. Add the ice to the blender and blend on high until the ice is completely crushed and the mixture is thick, smooth, and frothy, resembling a milkshake.
3. Pour the blended iced coffee into 2 glasses. Enjoy immediately!

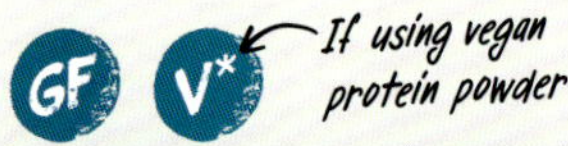

makes 2 drinks / 2 servings

NUTRITION (PER SERVING)

100 calories	**4g** fat
13.5g protein	**2.5g** net carbs

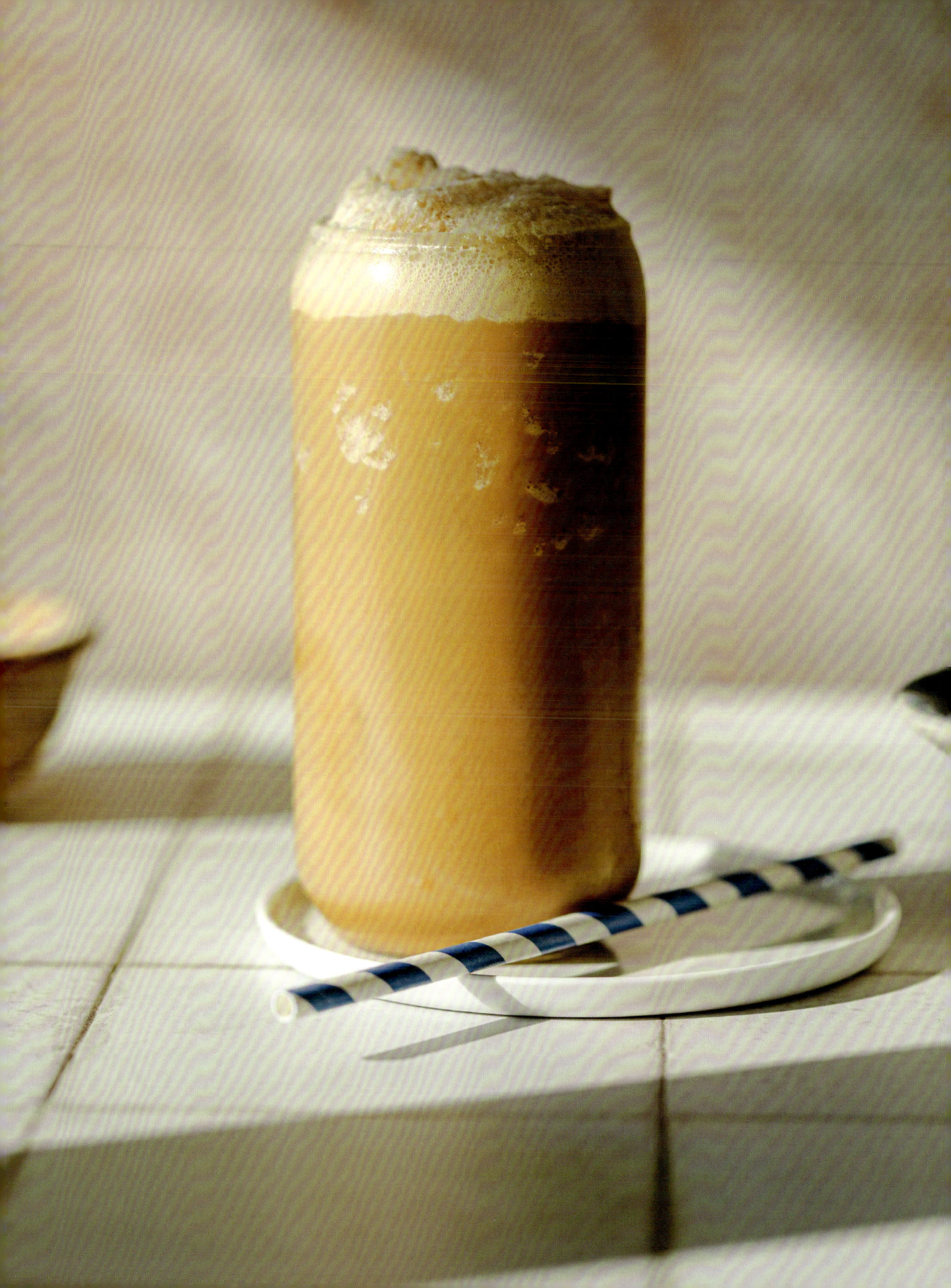

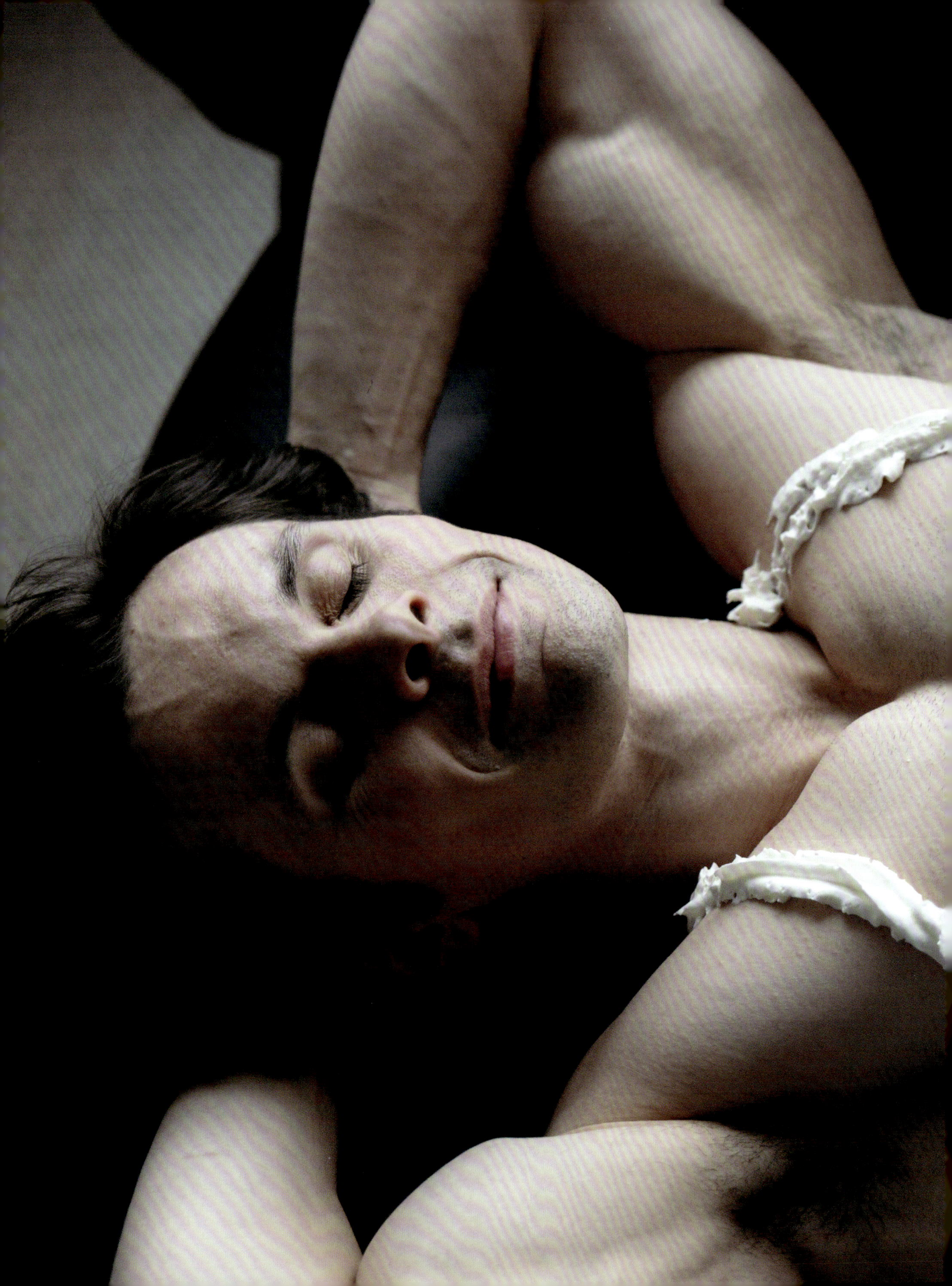

-CHAPTER 7-

HAPPY ENDINGS

DELECTABLE DESSERTS

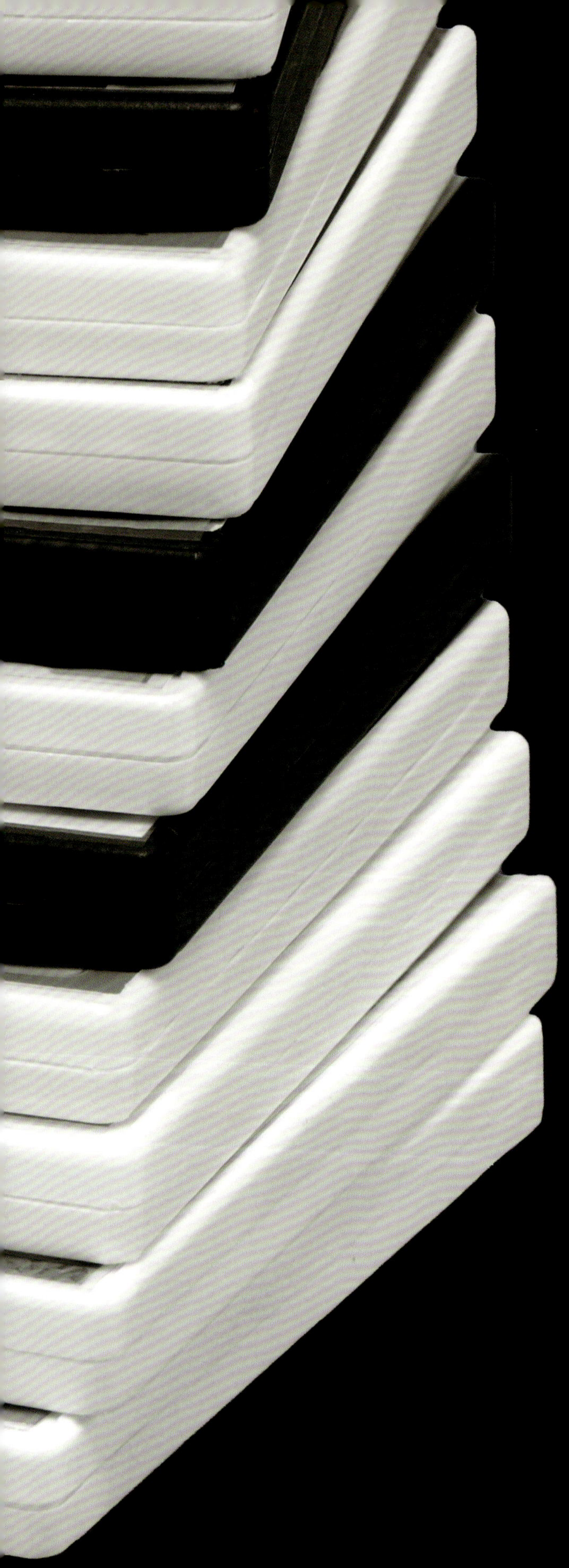

WILL'S FAVORITE MOVIES

We used to eat late-night sweets in the dark with just our shame to keep us company, but the ones in this chapter pair much better with one of my favorite movies:

Oceans 11
(2001)

21 Jump Street
(2012)

Nocturnal Animals
(2016)

Nightcrawler
(2014)

The Dark Knight
(2008)

Shawshank Redemption
(1994)

The Perks of Being a Wallflower
(2012)

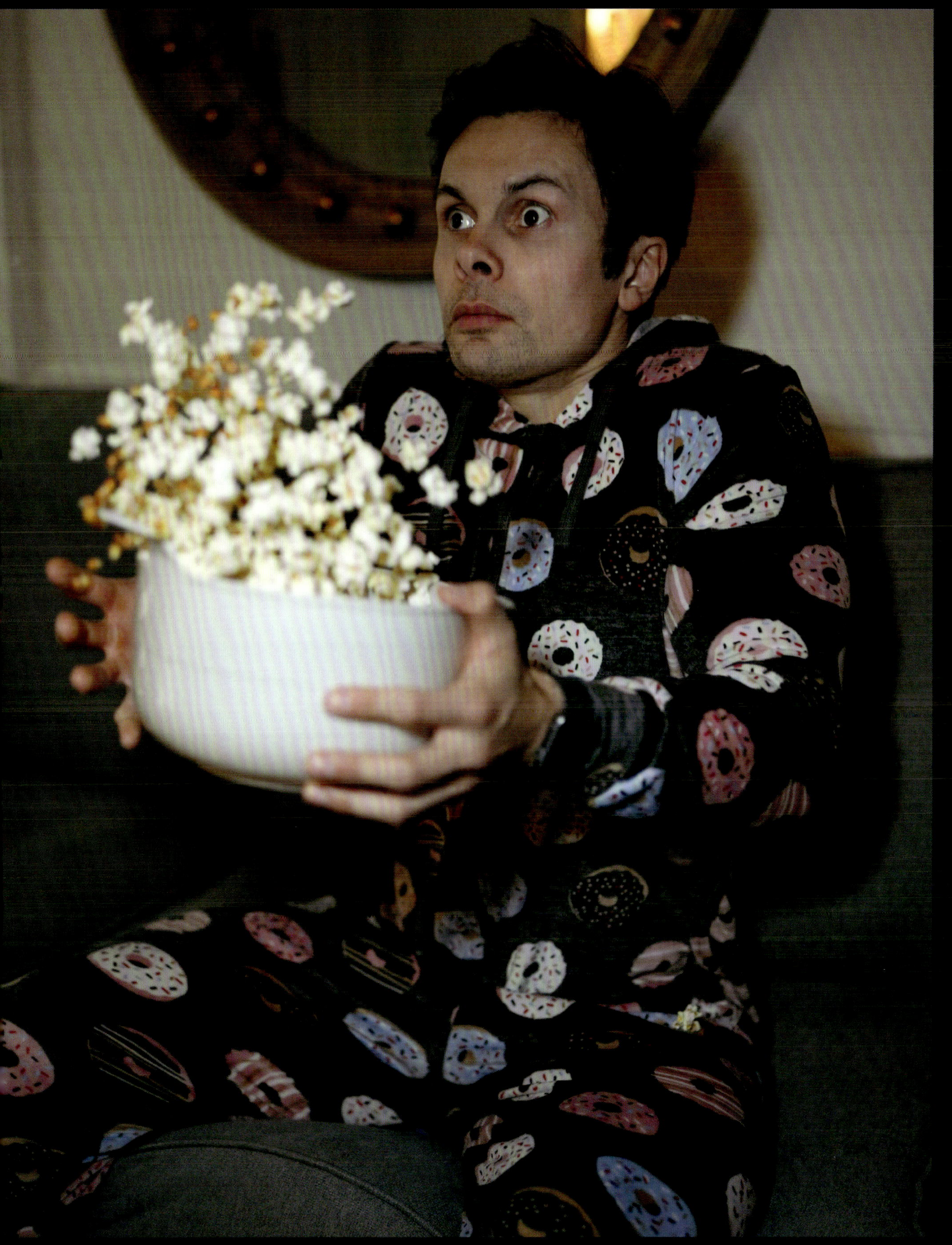

GREEK YOGURT ICE POPS

½ cup (70g) frozen blueberries
½ cup (88g) frozen mango
1 cup (230g) nonfat Greek yogurt
1 scoop (31g) protein powder of choice
2 tsp (14g) honey

It's time to create a sweet treat you see a bit of yourself in. You pick the fruits; you pick the shape. Be proud of your delicious creation regardless of its length, girth, or curvature. No ice-pop mold? No problem. Pour the mixture into an ice-cube tray for bite-size frozen treats, or use small paper cups with ice-pop sticks for a DIY solution. Mango and blueberry are a winning combo, but don't be afraid to mix it up—strawberries, raspberries, peaches, or pineapple all work. However you freeze it, this is the kind of snack that'll cool you down while keeping your macros in check.

1. In a small bowl, place the blueberries; in a second small bowl, add the mango. Microwave the fruit for 60 to 90 seconds until fully thawed.
2. In each bowl of thawed fruit, evenly divide the Greek yogurt, protein powder, and honey and stir to combine well.
3. Pour both mixtures into ice-pop molds that hold at least 2.5 oz (70g) and freeze for at least 2 hours before serving.

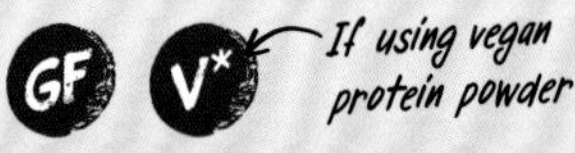

makes 4 ice pops / 4 servings

NUTRITION (PER SERVING)

95 calories	**0.5** g fat
13.5g protein	**9.5g** net carbs

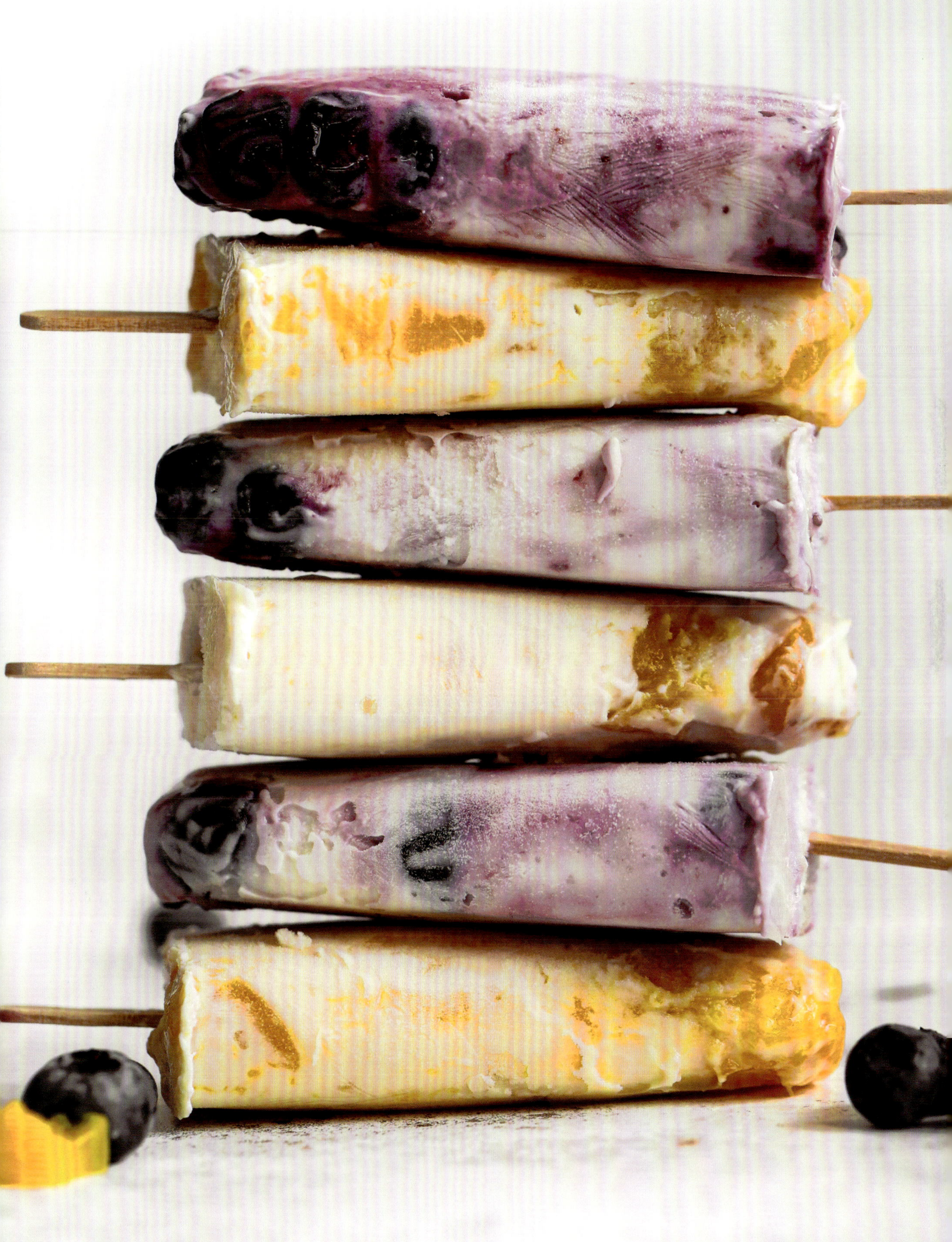

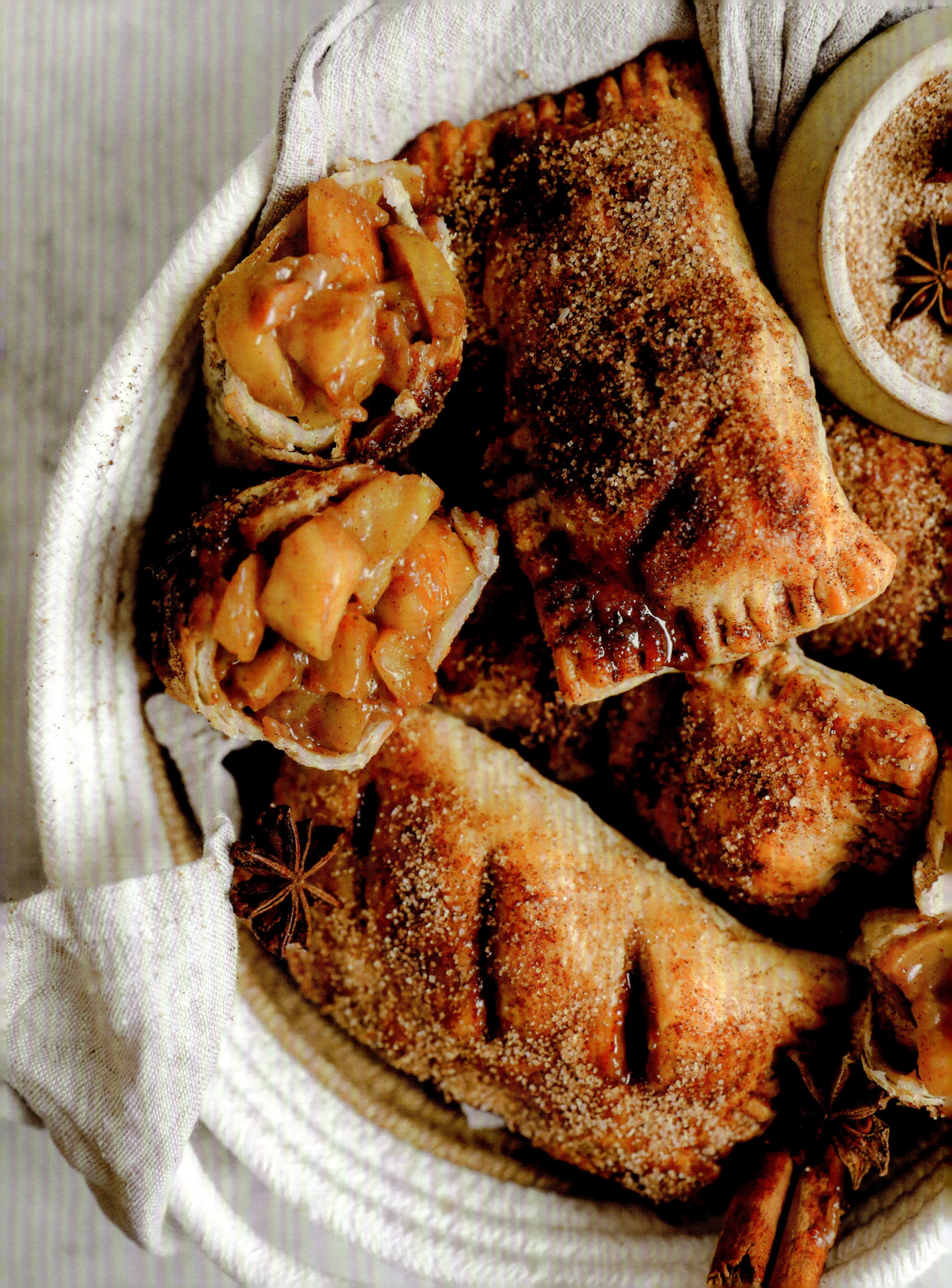

HANDHELD APPLE PIES

- 4 small apples, peeled, cored, and diced
- ¼ cup (56g) unsalted butter
- Juice of 1 large lemon
- ½ tsp (1.5g) salt
- 5 tsp (15g) cinnamon
- 9½ tbsp (115g) Swerve brown sugar
- ¼ tsp (750mg) ground nutmeg
- 3 tsp (7.5g) cornstarch
- 8oz (225g) store-bought puff-pastry dough, thawed
- 2½ tbsp (36g) egg whites
- 1 tbsp (12g) Stevia sweetener

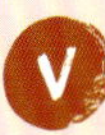

makes 6 pies / 6 servings

NUTRITION (PER SERVING)

287 calories	**15g** fat
4g protein	**50g** net carbs

Say "bye-bye, Miss American Pie" and "Hello" to a take on the McDonald's apple pie that won't supersize your waistband. For the best results, make sure your puff pastry is fully thawed but still cold—this keeps it easy to work with while ensuring a flaky texture. When sealing the edges, press firmly with a fork to avoid leaks during baking. Let the apple filling cool completely before assembling, or the pastry can become too soft and difficult to handle. Cutting small slits on top is key to releasing steam and preventing a soggy crust. If you want an even crispier finish, bake the pies on a wire rack set over a baking sheet to allow hot air to circulate underneath. Enjoy them warm, but be careful—just like the ones from the drive-thru, these can be molten inside! Store these in an airtight container in the fridge for up to 4 days. To reheat, pop them in the oven or air fryer at 350°F (180°C) for 5 to 7 minutes.

1. In a large saucepan, add the apples, butter, lemon juice, salt, 2 teaspoons (6g) of the cinnamon, and the brown sugar. Place the saucepan over medium heat and cook for about 10 minutes, stirring the mixture often, until the apples soften. While stirring, add the ground nutmeg.
2. While the apple filling is softening, in a small bowl, combine the cornstarch and 3 teaspoons (45ml) water. Slowly add the cornstarch mixture to the softened apples and cook for an additional 2 minutes, until the filling thickens.
3. Remove the pot from the heat and let it sit until cool. Transferring to a separate bowl will speed up the cooling time.
4. Preheat the oven to 425°F (220°C). Line a baking sheet with parchment paper.
5. Onto a floured flat surface, roll out the thawed puff pastry to roughly ⅛-inch (3mm) thick and cut it into 6 evenly sized squares. On the prepared baking sheet, place the pastry squares.
6. Scoop 2 heaping tablespoons (about 30g) of the cooled apple-filling mixture into the center of each of the puff pastry squares. Carefully fold the pastry dough over the apple filling and press the edges down with a fork to close the pastry and seal in the apple mixture.
7. Brush each pie lightly with the egg whites to assist with browning in the oven. Cut 3 even slits on the top of each pie. This will help vent the filling and ensure the pie doesn't get soggy.
8. In a small bowl, combine the Stevia and remaining 3 teaspoons (9g) cinnamon to create a cinnamon sugar. Sprinkle over each pastry.
9. Bake for 25 minutes.

MICROWAVE APPLE PIE

1½ tbsp (21g) light margarine
4 tbsp (48g) Swerve brown sugar
2 tsp (6g) cinnamon
½ tsp (1.5g) plus ⅛ tsp (0.25g) nutmeg
2 tbsp (15g) almond flour
2 tbsp (10g) oats
Pinch of salt (optional)
1 apple, cored and diced into ½-inch (1cm) cubes
1 tsp (4g) Stevia sweetener
1 tsp (2.5g) cornstarch

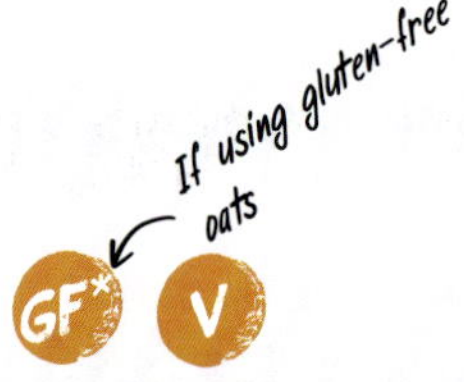

makes 1 pie / 1 serving

NUTRITION (PER SERVING)

266 calories **17g** fat
5g protein **83g** net carbs

Let's pray that Eugene Levy's not around to see me mistreat this beloved American classic. My microwave apple pie may be untraditional, but I've never been one to play it safe. My advice to you is to dice the apples small so they soften quickly. And keep an eye on it while microwaving, as every microwave heats differently, and you don't want to end up with applesauce. Top with Greek yogurt for a breakfast-worthy version, or go all in with ice cream for a late-night dessert that takes less time than a drive-thru run.

1. In a medium bowl, add 1 tablespoon (14g) of the light margarine, 2 tablespoons (24g) of the brown sugar, 1 teaspoon (3g) of the cinnamon, ½ teaspoon (1.5g) of the nutmeg, the almond flour, oats, and a pinch of salt (if using). Mix to create a crumble topping resembling wet sand. Set aside.
2. In a microwave-safe bowl, add the apple and remaining ½ tablespoon (7g) margarine and microwave on high for 1 minute, or until the apples are softened.
3. Once the apples are soft, add the remaining 2 tablespoons (24g) brown sugar, the remaining 1 teaspoon (3g) cinnamon, the remaining ⅛ teaspoon (0.25g) nutmeg, the Stevia, and cornstarch and combine to create the apple-pie filling.
4. Pour the crumble topping evenly over the apple-pie filling. Microwave on high for 2 to 2½ minutes, until the filling is bubbling and the top is melted. Let cool for 5 minutes before eating.

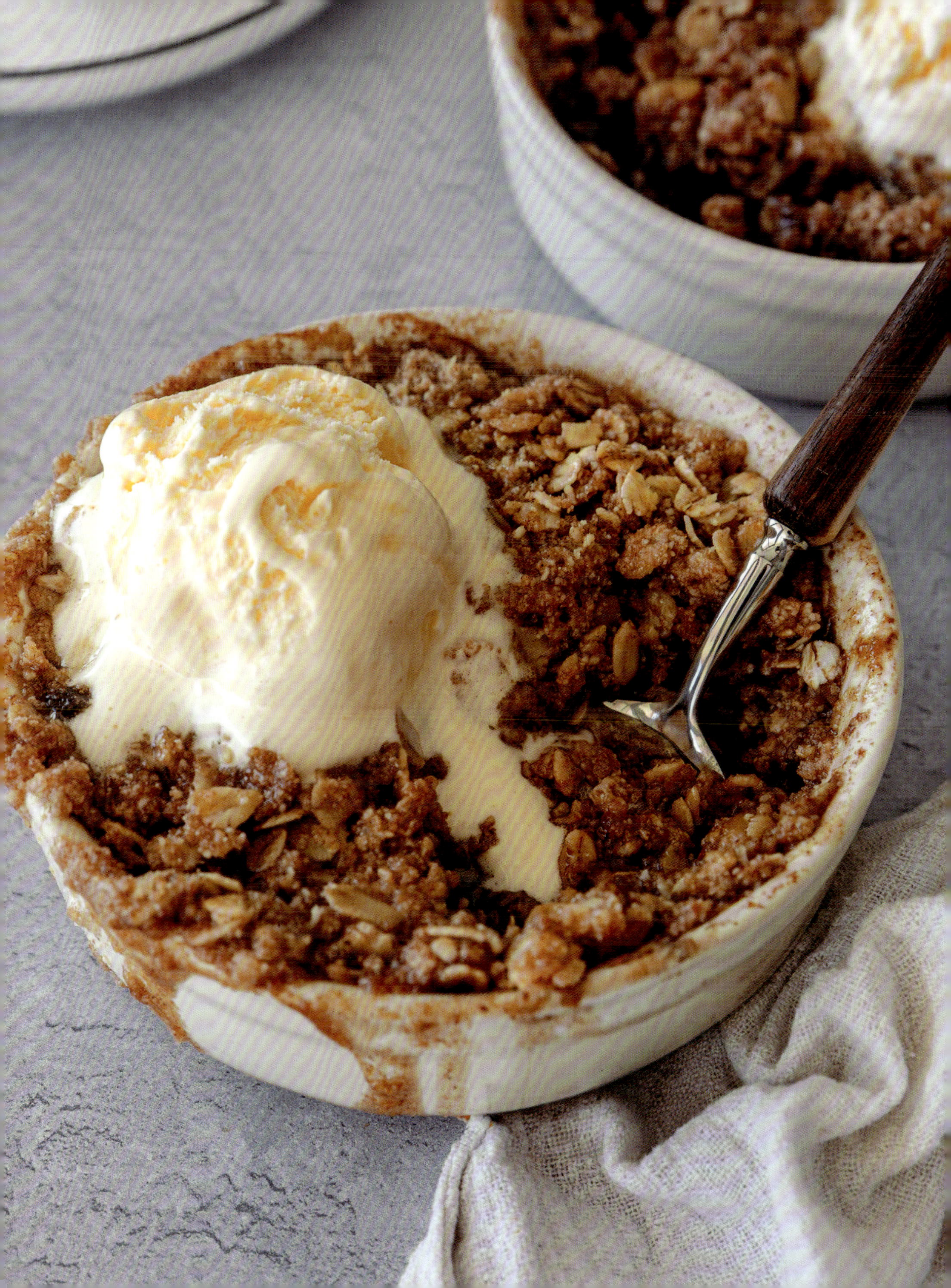

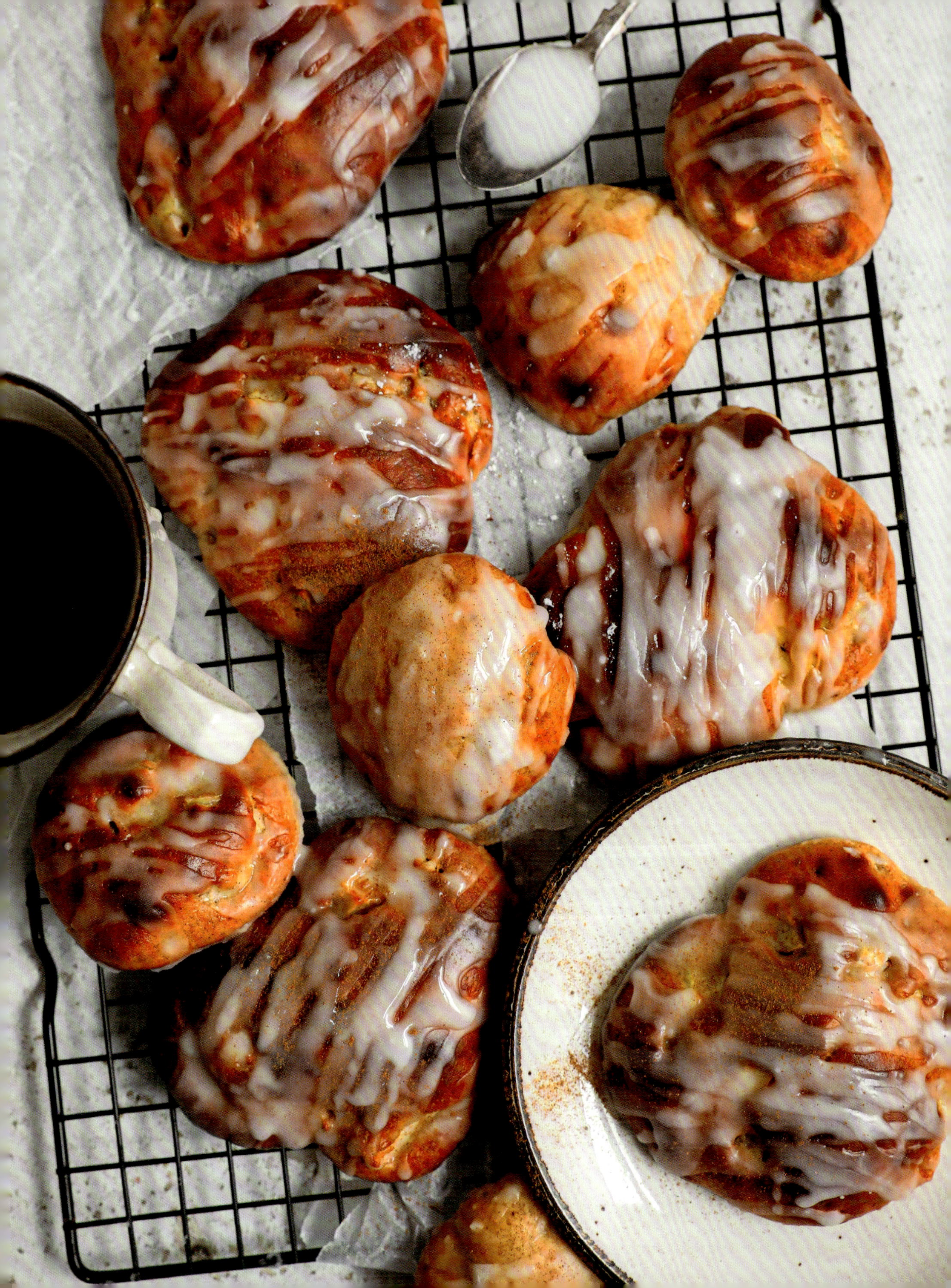

PROTEIN APPLE FRITTERS

- ¼ cup (30g) all-purpose flour
- 1 scoop (31g) protein powder of choice (I used apple pie flavor)
- 2 tbsp (24g) Swerve brown sugar
- 1 tsp (5g) baking powder
- ¼ tsp (750mg) salt
- ½ tsp (1.5g) cinnamon
- ⅛ tsp (375mg) nutmeg
- 1 tbsp (14g) butter or margarine, at room temperature
- ½ apple, diced into ½-inch (1cm) cubes
- 3 tbsp (45g) nonfat Greek yogurt
- 2 tbsp (15g) Swerve powdered sugar

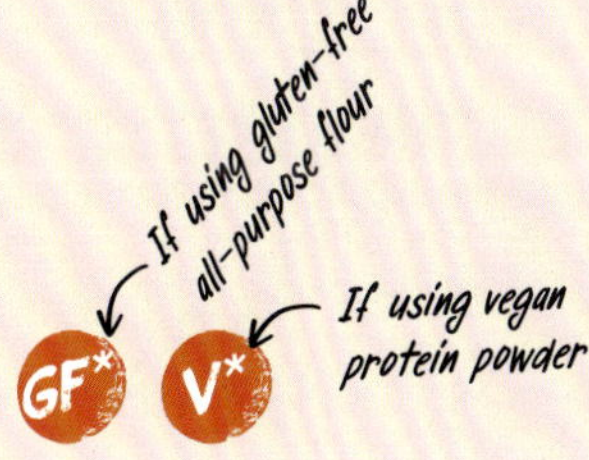

makes 2 fritters / 2 servings

NUTRITION (PER SERVING)

265 calories	**3g** fat
16g protein	**44g** net carbs

Fritter? Hardly know her. One of the many things that keep me up at night is my inner turmoil over whether a fritter is a donut or not. It's still up for debate, but one thing for certain is that this fritter recipe ignites the fire within me usually reserved for donuts. When shaping your fritters, resist the urge to pack the dough tightly—this isn't a snowball fight. Overworking the dough will make the fritters dense and tough, so embrace the imperfect shape and leave some air pockets for that light, tender texture. The more rustic, the better—after all, nobody's ever been impressed by perfect symmetry.

1. If using the oven, preheat it to 375°F (190°C) and line a baking sheet with parchment paper. If using the air fryer, spray the bottom of the air fryer basket with cooking spray.
2. To a large bowl, add the flour, protein powder, brown sugar, baking powder, salt, cinnamon, nutmeg, and butter. Mix until the mixture resembles a wet sand.
3. Add the apple and toss until evenly coated.
4. Add the Greek yogurt. Using your hands, combine the ingredients and form 2 fritters in your desired shape and size. If too wet, add more flour; if too dry, add more Greek yogurt. The fritters should hold their shape.
5. Transfer the fritters to either the prepared baking sheet or the air fryer basket, depending on your chosen method.
6. Air fry at 375°F (190°C) for 12 to 15 minutes or bake for 20 to 25 minutes. You can test with a toothpick to ensure the middle is cooked through.
7. To make the fritter glaze, to a small bowl, add the powdered sugar and ½ tablespoon (7ml) water and stir to combine.
8. Drizzle the glaze over the cooked fritters and serve!

CHOCOLATE PEANUT-BUTTER PROTEIN BARK

- 1 cup (230g) nonfat Greek yogurt
- 1 scoop (31g) protein powder (chocolate peanut butter preferred)
- ¼ cup (26g) PB2 Powdered Peanut Butter
- ½ cup (120ml) low-fat coconut milk
- ½ tbsp (6g) Stevia sweetener
- 2 tbsp (13g) chocolate PB2 Powdered Peanut Butter (optional)

All bark and no bite . . . until you get a taste, and you'll be one-biting your way through the whole tray like Pac-Man on a world record run. To get that perfect balance of creamy and firm, make sure to spread the mixture evenly—too thick and it'll take forever to freeze, too thin and it'll break apart when you try to cut it. Around ¼ inch to ½ inch (5mm to 1cm) in thickness does the trick. If you want to switch things up, try swirling in melted dark chocolate, chopped nuts (if you have the macros), or a pinch of sea salt before freezing for extra texture and flavor. When cutting, let it sit out for a couple of minutes to soften slightly—unless you enjoy chipping a tooth on your dessert.

1. Line a 9 x 13-inch (23 x 33cm) baking sheet with parchment paper.
2. To a medium mixing bowl, add the Greek yogurt, protein powder, PB2 Powdered Peanut Butter, coconut milk, and Stevia and stir to combine well.
3. Onto the prepared baking sheet, pour the mixture and use a spatula to spread the evenly.
4. In a small bowl, mix the chocolate PB2 Powdered Peanut Butter (if using) with 2 tablespoons (30ml) water and drizzle it on top of the protein mixture.
5. Place the baking sheet in the freezer and wait until firm, about 6 hours.
6. For the best results, let the bark sit out for a few minutes before cutting into squares, then serve.
7. Leftover bars can be stored in a container between layers of parchment paper.

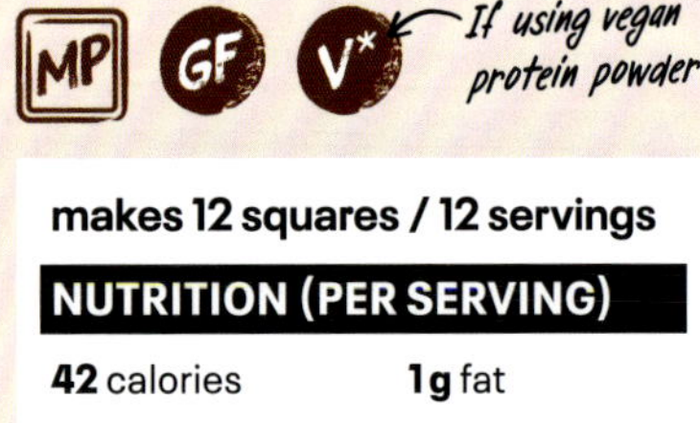

makes 12 squares / 12 servings

NUTRITION (PER SERVING)

42 calories | **1g** fat
6g protein | **2g** net carbs

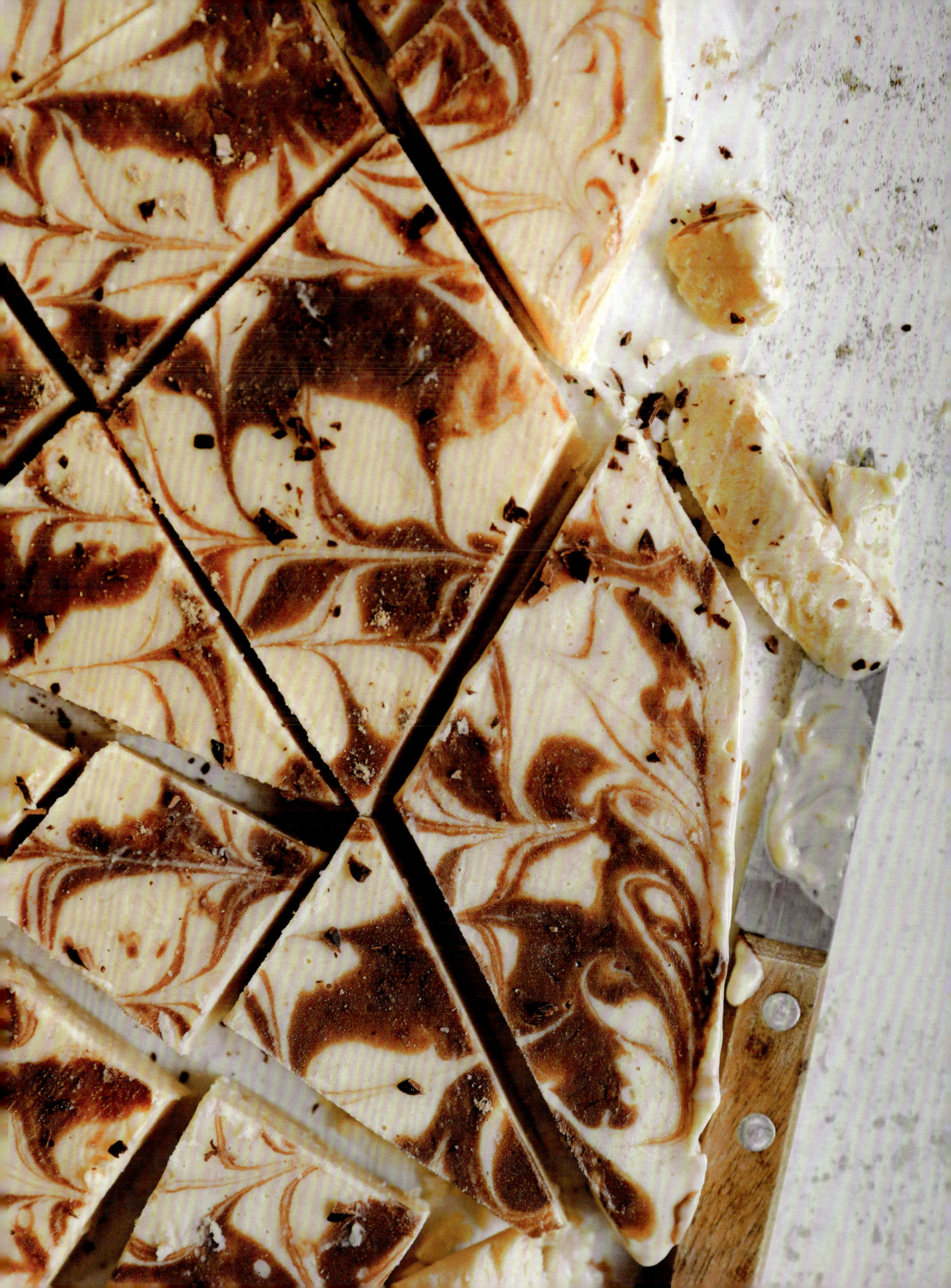

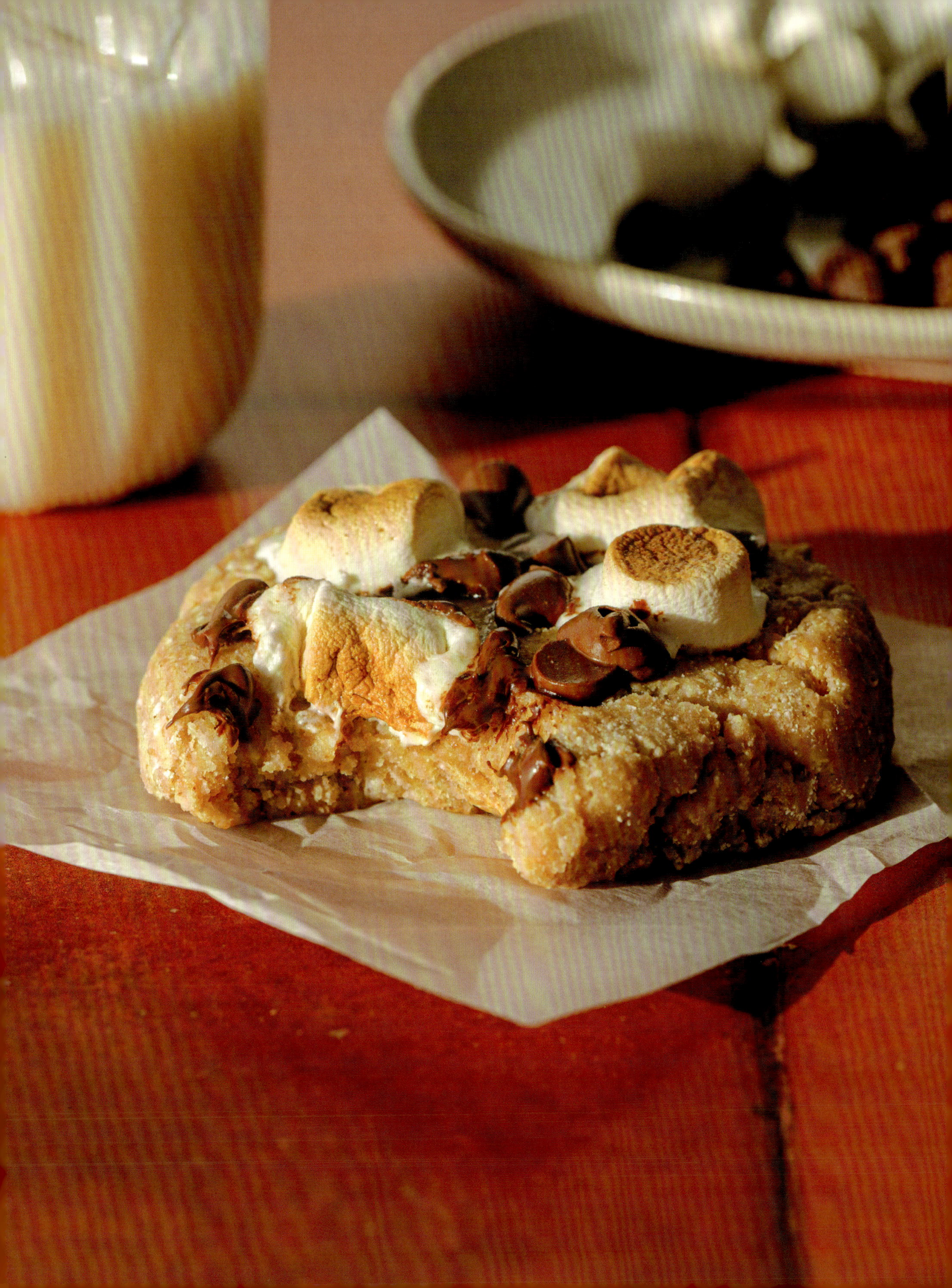

S'MORES PROTEIN COOKIES

¾ cup (88g) oat flour
1 scoop (31g) vanilla protein powder
6½ tsp (16g) coconut flour
1 tsp (5g) baking powder
2 tbsp (32g) peanut butter
6 tbsp (90ml) Silk unsweetened cashew milk
¼ cup (60g) nonfat Greek yogurt
2 tsp (4g) erythritol
3½ tbsp (35g) semisweet chocolate chips
¾ oz (20g) mini marshmallows

Healthy desserts are a lot like open relationships. We're not trying to replace the one we love; we're just trying to make room for even more. If you don't have oat flour on hand, don't panic—just toss regular oats into a blender, and blend until they turn into a fine powder. The texture won't be quite as smooth as store-bought oat flour, but it gets the job done. Fair warning: This dough is stickier and less moldable than traditional cookie dough, and you may start doubting everything as you try to shape them. But trust the process—once they bake up golden with gooey marshmallows and melted chocolate, you'll forget you ever questioned me.

1. Preheat the oven to 350°F (180°C). Line a small baking sheet with parchment paper.
2. In a medium mixing bowl, combine the oat flour, protein powder, coconut flour, baking powder, peanut butter, cashew milk, Greek yogurt, and erythritol. Stir with a mixing spoon until the mixture forms a smooth dough.
3. Onto the prepared baking sheet, spoon the dough into 4 equal cookies, shaping into your desired cookie form using the back of the spoon.
4. Over the top of each cookie, sprinkle the chocolate chips and marshmallows.
5. Bake for 11 to 13 minutes, or until the edges are lightly golden and the marshmallows are slightly melted.
6. Remove the cookies from the oven and allow them to cool on the baking sheet for 5 minutes before serving.

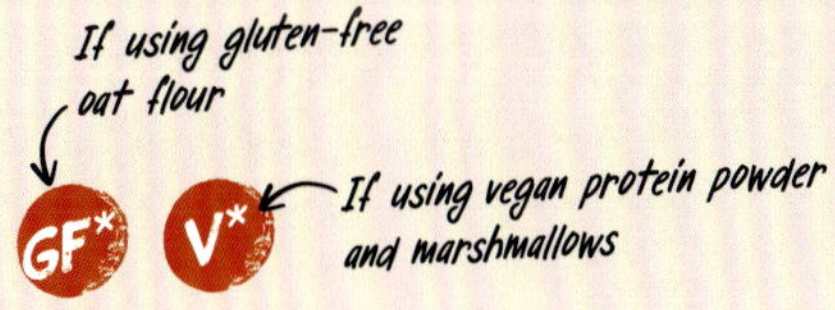

makes 4 cookies / 4 servings

NUTRITION (PER SERVING)

252 calories — **9g** fat
12g protein — **29g** net carbs

PUMPKIN PROTEIN MOUSSE CAKE

- 3¼ tbsp (50g) egg whites
- ½ tsp (2.5ml) vanilla extract
- ¼ cup (60ml) Silk unsweetened cashew milk
- ½ cup (120ml) canned pumpkin purée
- 5½ tsp (14g) coconut flour
- ½ tsp (2.5g) baking powder
- ½ tsp (1.5g) cinnamon
- 1 scoop (31g) protein powder of choice
- 1½ tbsp (25.2g) almond butter
- ¾ cup (175g) nonfat Greek yogurt
- ½ medium apple, cubed
- Drizzle of sugar-free maple syrup

When it comes to protein cakes, sometimes the only thing harder to get down comes after a double dose of Viagra, because they can be very dry. But this pumpkin cake is so moist, even the weatherman will say it's raining. If you'd rather have this in an easier grab-and-go format, you can also turn this recipe into muffins—just divide the batter evenly between 4 muffin cups, and bake for 12 to 15 minutes instead. Feel free to customize the mix-ins too. Stir in chocolate chips or chopped pecans for some crunch, or add raisins if you want a little extra sweetness.

1. Preheat the oven to 350°F (180°C). Line the bottom and sides of an 8½ x 4½-inch (21.5 x 11cm) loaf pan with parchment paper.
2. To a medium mixing bowl, add the egg whites, vanilla extract, cashew milk, and pumpkin purée. Whisk until combined.
3. To a separate medium mixing bowl, add the coconut flour, baking powder, cinnamon, and protein powder. Stir together to combine.
4. Pour the dry ingredients into the bowl with the wet ingredients and mix until well combined into a thick cake batter.
5. Into the lined loaf pan, pour the batter and bake for 15 to 20 minutes, until the top begins to brown and the inside is cooked through. To test if the cake is done, insert a toothpick into the center and check if it comes out clean. Remove from the oven and let it cool for 5 minutes.
6. Carefully remove the cake from the pan by inverting the pan onto a wire rack or plate. As a substitute for icing, spread the almond butter over the top. Top with the Greek yogurt, apple, and maple syrup.

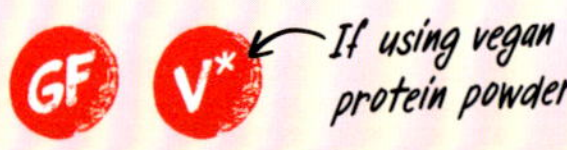

makes 1 cake / 4 servings

NUTRITION (PER SERVING)

132 Calories	**3.75g** fat
13.5g protein	**11.25g** net carbs

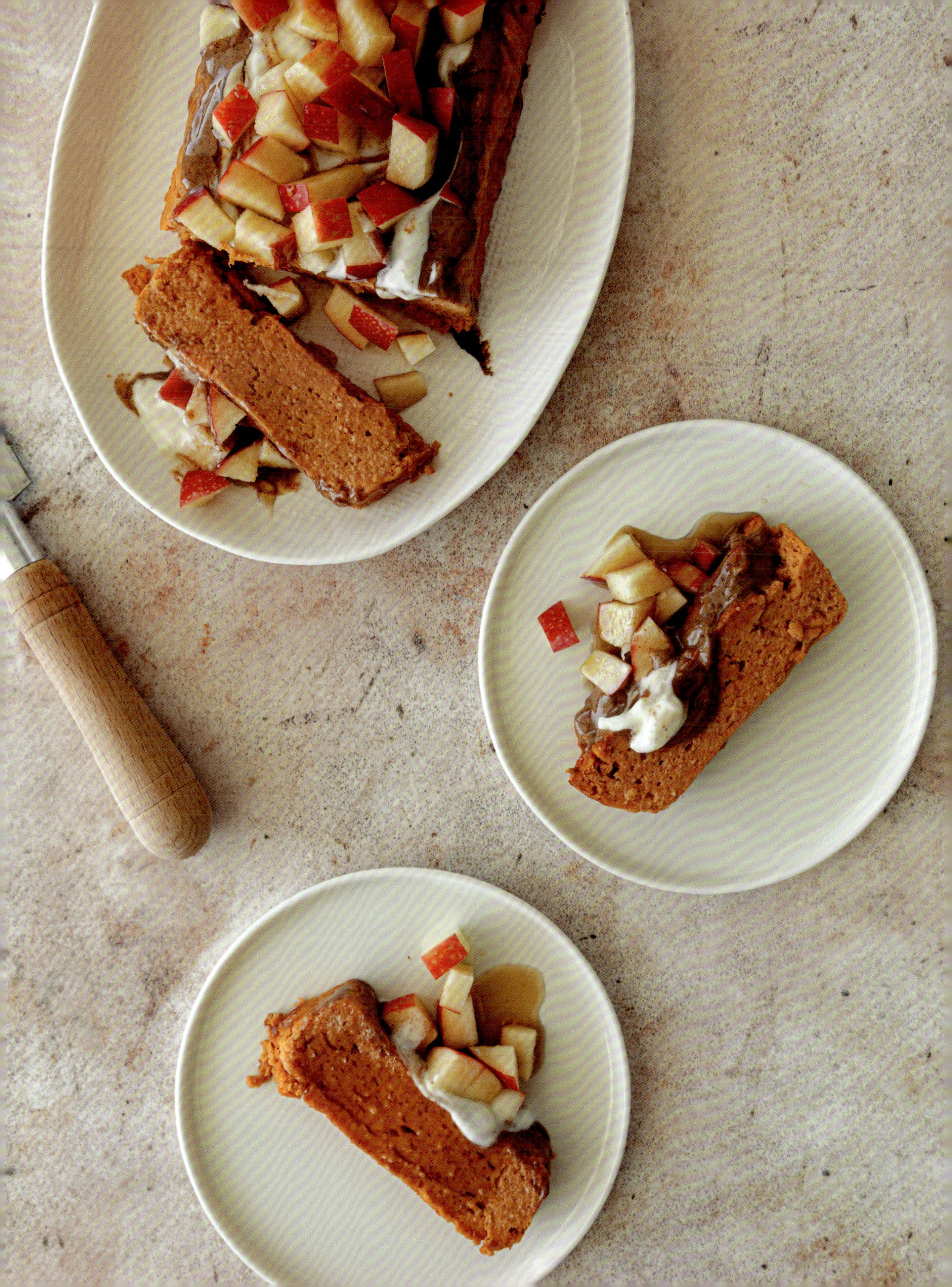

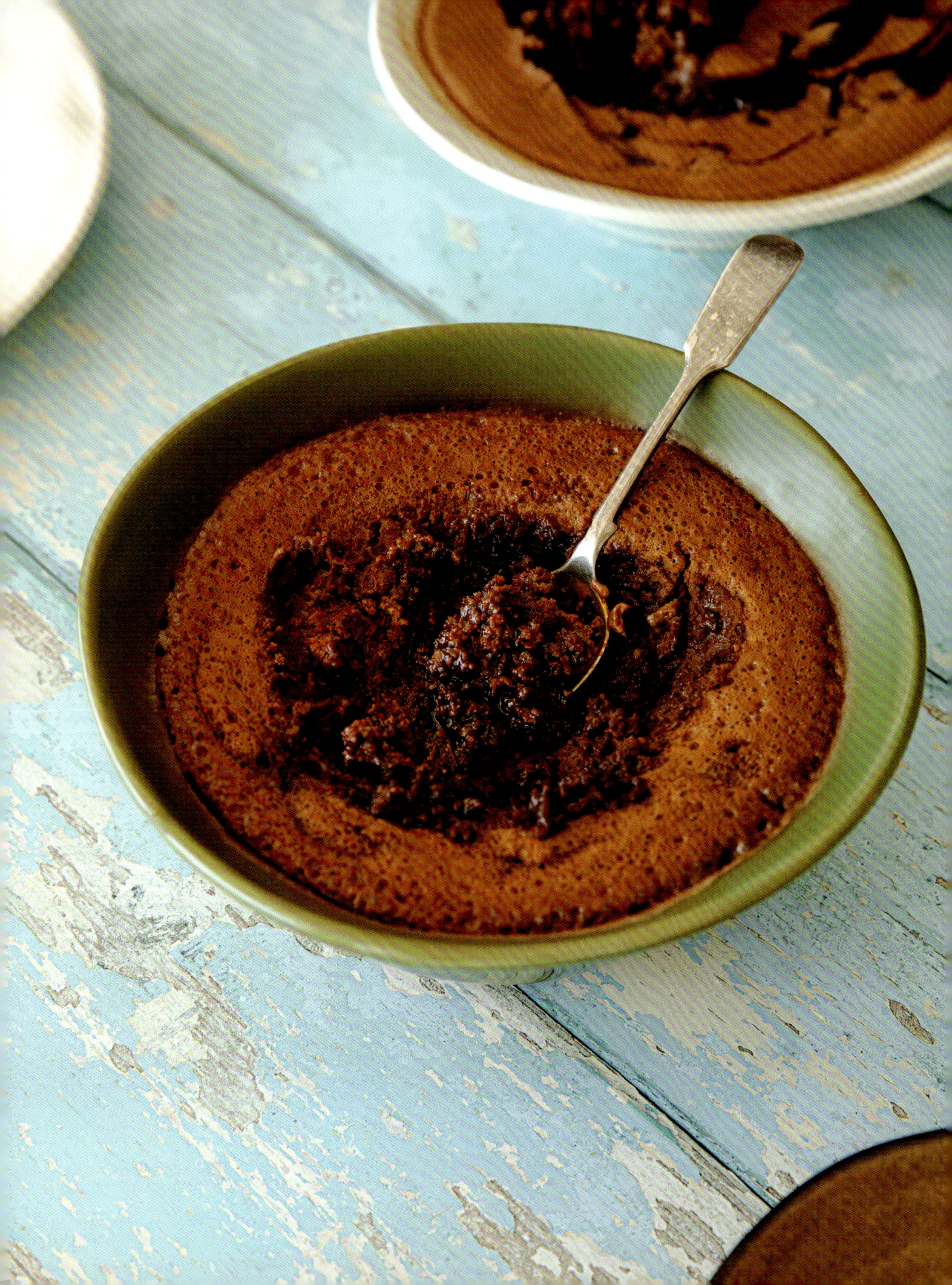

DARK DESIRE CHOCOLATE OAT CAKE

- 1 cup (80g) oats
- 1 scoop (31g) chocolate protein powder
- 5 tsp (10g) cocoa powder
- 2 tbsp (12g) erythritol
- ¼ tsp (1.25g) baking powder
- 1½ tsp (5g) sugar-free chocolate pudding mix
- 1¼ cup (300ml) Silk chocolate almond milk
- 2 tsp (14g) sugar-free chocolate syrup
- 1½ tbsp (14g) chocolate chips

This is my only dark desire I can share with you without getting myself arrested, but luckily, this chocolate oat cake will satisfy all of yours. Even better, it takes less than 10 minutes from start to finish, making it the perfect solution for when you're craving something rich but don't have the patience to bake an entire cake. The microwave does all the work, leaving you with a spongy top and a gooey molten center—because nothing should be dry when it comes to chocolate cake. Bruce Bogtrotter would be proud, and thankfully, you don't have to eat this one under Miss Trunchbull's watchful eye.

1. Spray a medium microwave-safe soup bowl with nonstick cooking spray. Set aside.
2. To a blender, add the oats, protein powder, cocoa powder, erythritol, baking powder, pudding mix, chocolate almond milk, and half (7g) of the chocolate syrup. Blend on medium speed until a smooth batter is formed and there are no clumps.
3. Pour the batter into the greased bowl. Add the chocolate chips and the remaining chocolate syrup and use a knife to swirl them into the batter.
4. Microwave on high in 30-second intervals for 2 to 2½ minutes, keeping watch to ensure the batter does not spill over the bowl.
5. Remove from the microwave and let sit for 5 minutes, until the cake cools, leaving a spongy top and a gooey middle.

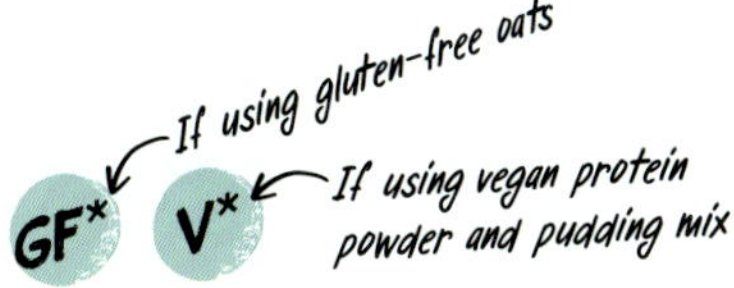

makes 1 cake / 1 serving

NUTRITION (PER SERVING)

607 calories	**15g** fat
40g protein	**78g** net carbs

ANABOLIC "SPREADAROO" COOKIES

2½ cups (575g) nonfat Greek yogurt
1 egg
6¼ tbsp (75g) erythritol
⅔ cup (80g) almond flour
1 scoop (31g) whey-casein blend vanilla protein powder
½ tsp (2.5ml) vanilla extract
Pinch of salt
½ oz (16g) fat-free, sugar-free vanilla pudding mix
1 tbsp (8g) low-calorie powdered sugar
1 tsp (4g) sprinkles (optional)

If you grew up in the golden era of snack packs, you already know what this is about. Inspired by the legendary Dunkaroos, these cookies are made to be dunked straight into the creamy vanilla icing, just like the classic childhood treat. But if you're feeling a little more refined (or just don't want to risk getting icing on your fingers), you can spread it on top like a frosted cookie. Fresh out the oven, they're soft and chewy, but if you let them sit overnight, they firm up and become snappy—perfect for dunking.

1. Preheat the oven to 375°F (190°C). Line a 12 x 16-inch (30 x 40cm) baking sheet with parchment paper.
2. In a medium bowl, combine about ⅓ (about 190g) of the Greek yogurt, the egg, erythritol, almond flour, protein powder, vanilla extract, and salt. With a spatula, mix until the ingredients form a smooth, runny batter.
3. Onto the prepared baking sheet, spoon the batter to create 16 evenly sized cookies about 2 inches (5cm) in diameter.
4. Bake on the middle rack for 15 minutes or until the cookies expand and the surfaces begin to lose their glossy sheen.
5. Set the oven to broil and broil the cookies for 1 to 3 minutes, or until the tops are lightly browned and the edges are golden. Keep a close eye to prevent burning. Remove them from the oven and let the cookies cool on the baking sheet for at least 20 minutes.
6. In a small bowl, combine the remaining 385g Greek yogurt, the pudding mix, powdered sugar, and sprinkles (if using). With a spoon, stir until a thick, smooth icing is formed.
7. Once the cookies have cooled completely, either dip each cookie into the icing or spread the icing evenly over the tops of the cookies.
8. Store leftover cookies and icing in sealed containers in the fridge for up to 5 days.

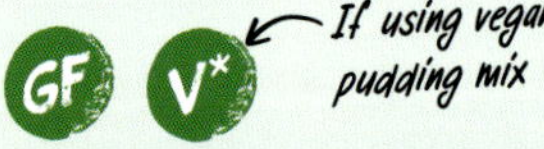

makes 16 cookies / 4 servings

NUTRITION (PER SERVING)

256 calories	**13g** fat
33.5g protein	**10.4g** net carbs

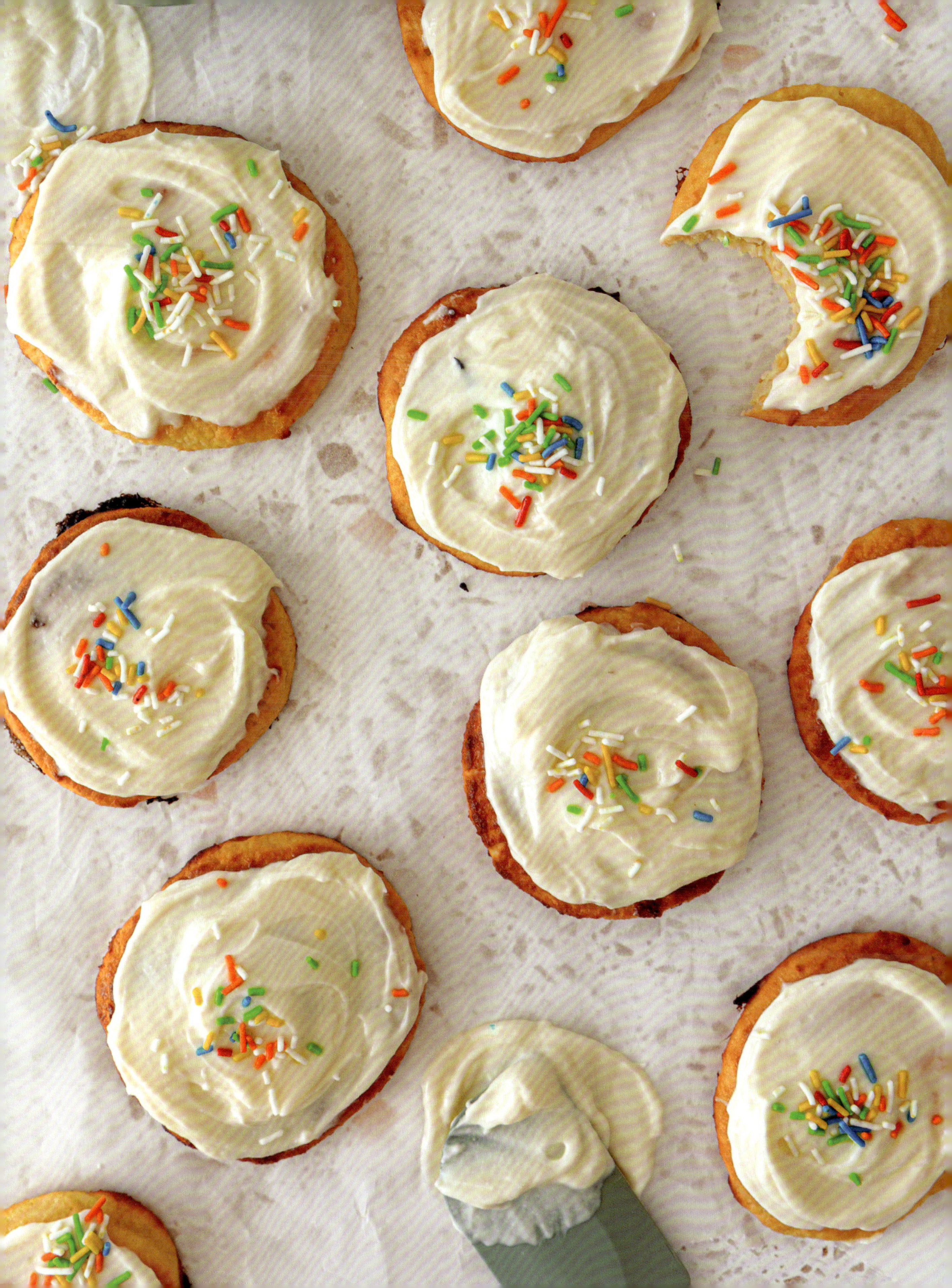

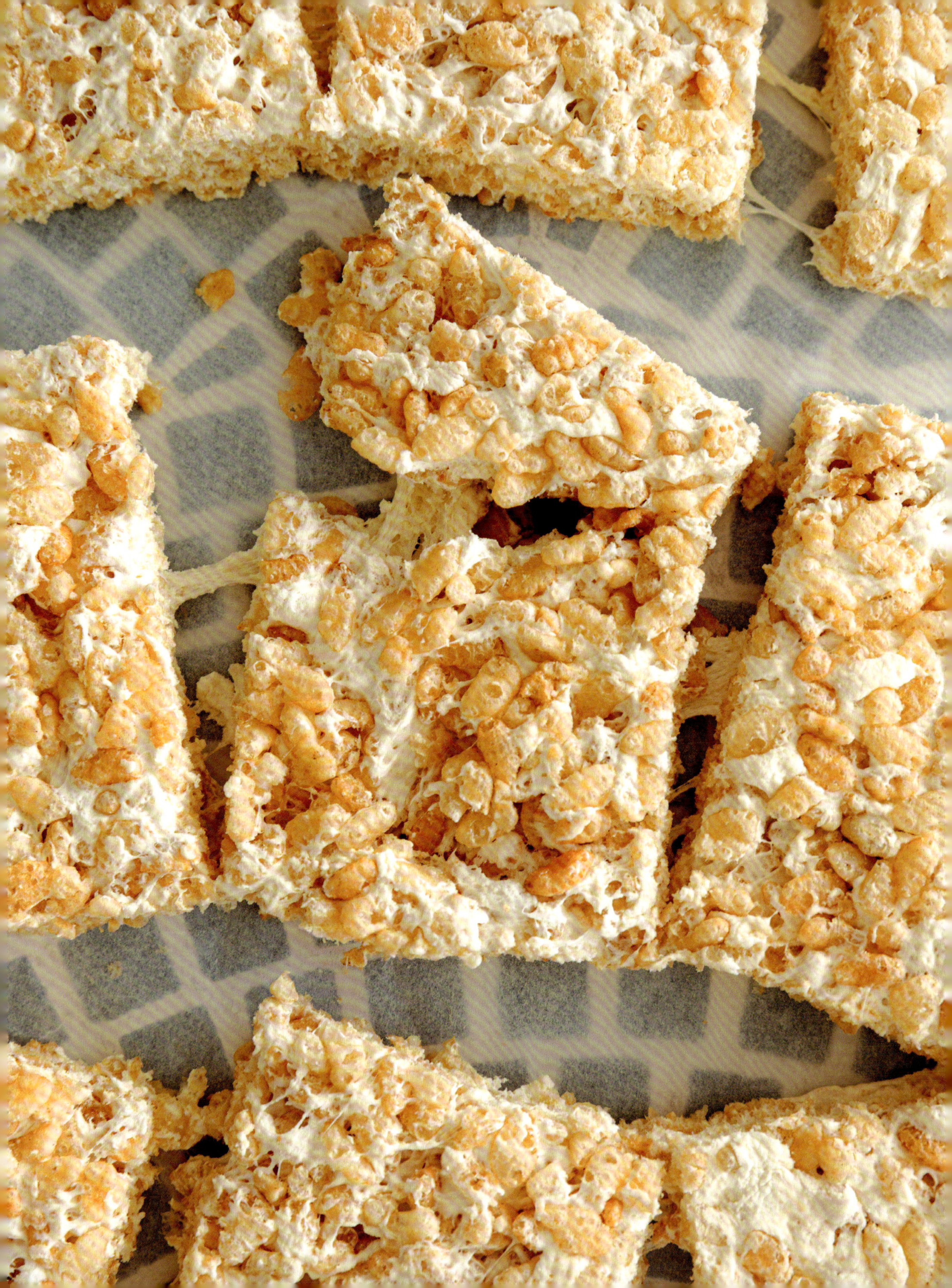

PROTEIN CRISPY RICE SQUARES

2 tbsp (30ml) coconut oil
5½ oz (150g) sugar-free marshmallows
½ cup (80g) casein-whey blend protein powder, flavor of your choosing
2½ cups (68g) crispy rice cereal

Snap, crackle, pop . . . and pump? These protein-packed crispy rice squares upgrade the childhood classic without sacrificing the chewy, crunchy nostalgia. Whether you stick to the OG vanilla marshmallow flavor or experiment with chocolate, peanut butter, or even cinnamon protein powder, these treats are fully customizable. For extra mix-ins, try adding coconut flakes, mini chocolate chips, or a drizzle of melted nut butter on top. For meal prep, store these squares in an airtight container at room temperature for up to 3 days. Just don't expect them to last that long.

1. Line an 8 x 8-inch (20 x 20cm) cake pan with parchment paper.
2. Heat a large saucepan over low heat and add the coconut oil and marshmallows. Stir consistently for 3 to 4 minutes, until melted and combined.
3. Remove the saucepan from the heat and add the protein powder, stirring it in while still hot, until combined.
4. Into the saucepan, pour the cereal and stir together for 2 to 3 minutes, until the cereal is fully coated. This will take time.
5. Scoop the mixture into the cake pan. With your fingers or a spatula, press it flat. Let cool for 10 minutes or until firm.

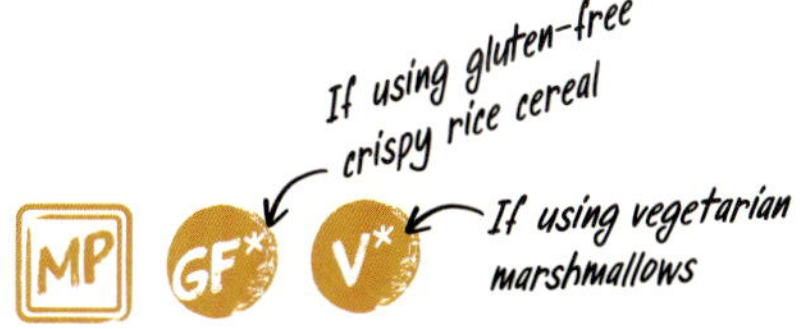

makes 6 squares / 6 servings

NUTRITION (PER SERVING)

207 calories	**5g** fat
10g protein	**30.5g** net carbs

BLUEBERRY COTTAGE-CHEESE PROTEIN CHEESECAKE BOWL

⅓ cup (45g) frozen blueberries
1 tbsp (10g) vanilla protein powder
¼ package (7g) sugar-free cheesecake pudding mix
½ tbsp (3g) erythritol
¾ cup (187.5g) low-fat cottage cheese
1 wedge (16.7g) Laughing Cow Light cheese
6 tbsp (90g) nonfat Greek yogurt
2 tbsp (30ml) Silk unsweetened cashew milk
1 tbsp (15ml) lemon juice
½ tsp (2.5ml) vanilla extract
Pinch of salt
4 tbsp (21g) crushed graham crackers

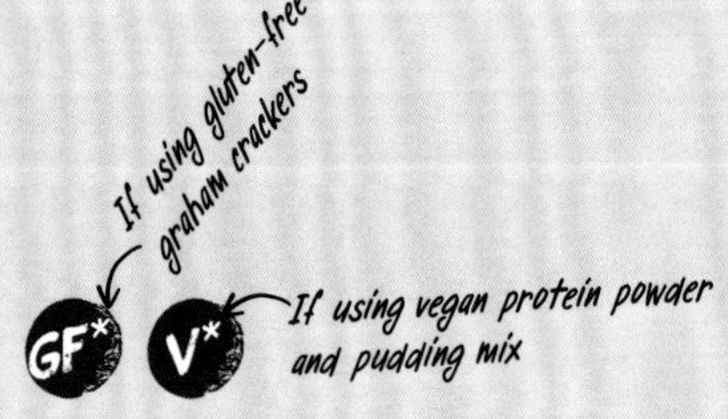

makes 1 cheesecake bowl / 1 serving

NUTRITION (PER SERVING)

395 calories
6g fat
42g protein
43g net carbs

Some recipes make enough to feed an entire family. This one? Just you. Because some things in life are meant to be shared, but this cheesecake isn't one of them. Laughing Cow Light cheese works amazingly well here, adding a smooth, creamy texture without the heaviness of traditional cheesecake ingredients. It blends well with the cottage cheese and Greek yogurt, making the batter extra luscious. Swap out the blueberries for strawberries, raspberries, or diced peaches, or take things in a completely different direction with chopped pretzels, dark chocolate chips, or a swirl of peanut butter for a salty-sweet contrast. Want it even thicker? Let it set in the fridge overnight for an even more authentic cheesecake texture.

1. In a small microwave-safe bowl, place the blueberries and microwave on high for 45 seconds. Set aside to cool.
2. To a blender, add the protein powder, pudding mix, erythritol, cottage cheese, Laughing Cow cheese, Greek yogurt, cashew milk, lemon juice, vanilla extract, and salt and mix on the low speed until all the ingredients combine into a thick batter.
3. To a medium bowl, add the batter and fold in the blueberries. Place the bowl in the fridge for 20 minutes to allow the cheesecake to set.
4. Remove the mixture from the fridge and top with the graham crackers for a much-needed mouth feel.

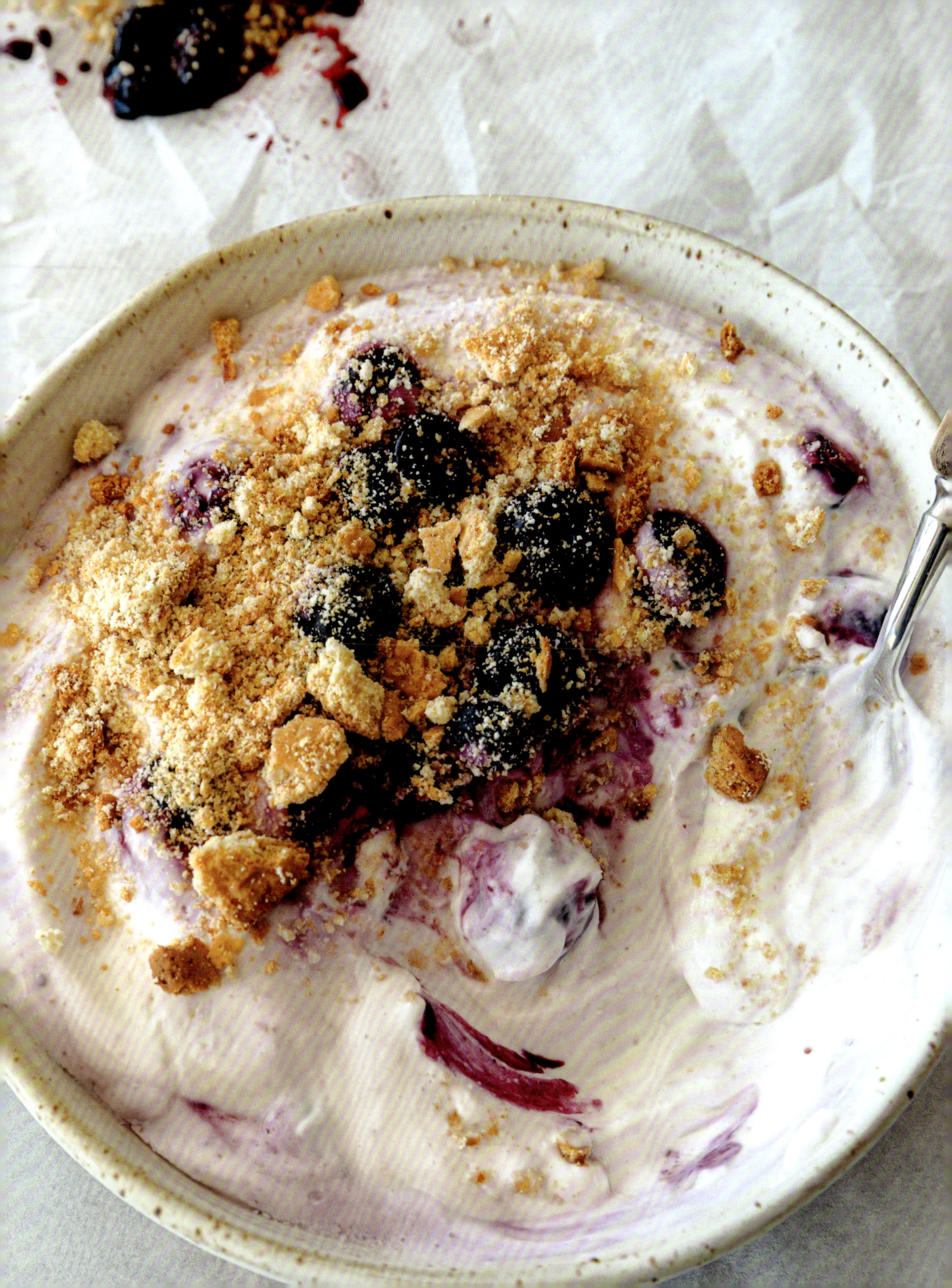

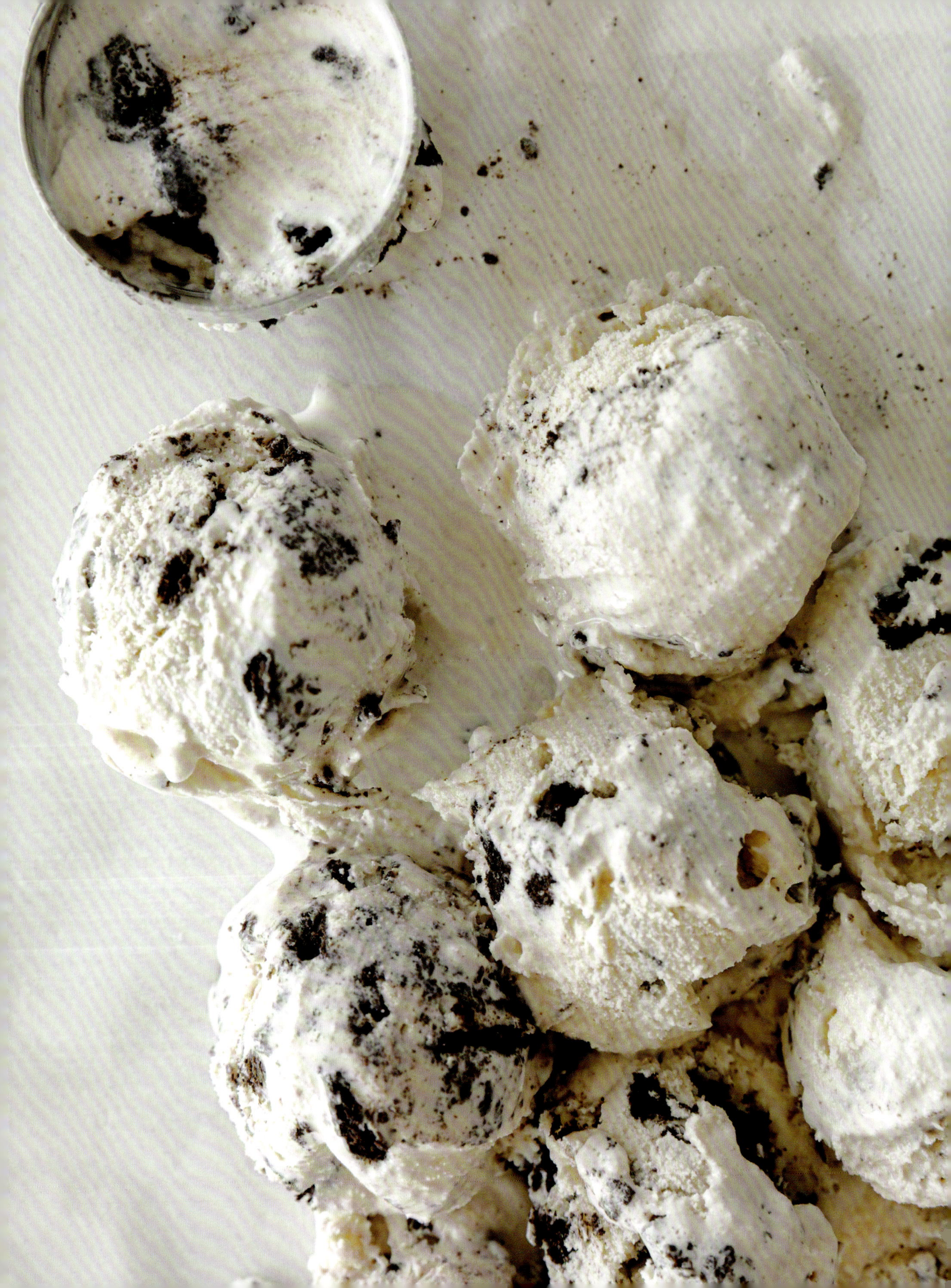

NO-CHURN VANILLA-PROTEIN ICE CREAM

- 4 cups (1L) Cool Whip Light, frozen (sugar-free or low-fat are good alternatives)
- 2 tsp (10ml) vanilla extract
- 2 scoops (62g) vanilla protein powder
- ½ cup (48g) erythritol
- 12fl oz (354ml) can 2% partly skimmed evaporated milk
- Pinch of salt
- Desired mix-ins (optional)

Nothing says nostalgia like Cool Whip. Every Thanksgiving at my Nana and Grandpa's house, pumpkin pie wasn't complete without a towering, borderline excessive dollop of the stuff. But Cool Whip isn't just a holiday indulgence—it's the key to this ultra-light, protein-packed ice cream. Unlike regular whipped cream, Cool Whip stays stable when frozen, giving the ice cream a smooth, scoopable texture without the need for an ice-cream machine. This base is a blank canvas, so go wild with your mix-ins. Crushed Oreos, drizzled chocolate syrup, chopped nuts, or fresh fruit all take it in different directions. Just don't skimp on the Cool Whip—it's what makes this recipe work. Store the ice cream in an airtight container in the freezer for up to 2 weeks. If it gets too firm, let it sit at room temperature for 5 to 10 minutes before scooping.

1. Remove the Cool Whip from the freezer and let thaw for 20 minutes.
2. To a medium mixing bowl, add the Cool Whip, vanilla extract, protein powder, erythritol, evaporated milk, and salt, and stir together for 1 to 2 minutes, until smooth and combined.
3. Into a large sealable container (I use the empty Cool Whip container), pour the mixture and place it in the freezer for 30 minutes, or until the ice cream thickens.
4. Remove the ice cream from the freezer and fold in your desired mix-ins. Reseal the ice cream and return it to the freezer for at least 2 hours, or until the ice cream solidifies.

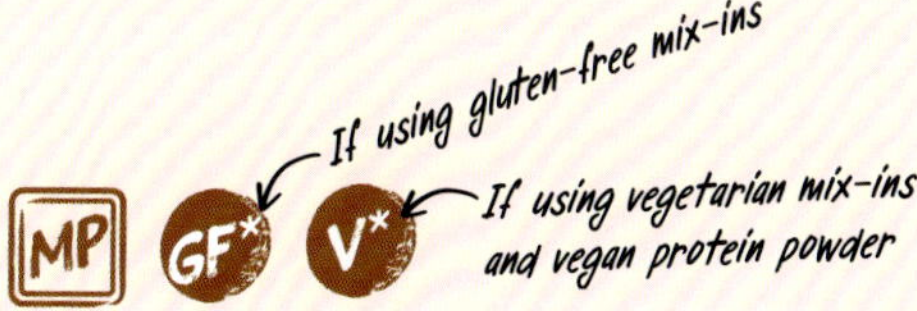

makes 5 servings

NUTRITION (PER SERVING)

323 calories	**16.6g** fat
14.8g protein	**28.6g** net carbs

RASPBERRY CHOCOLATE PROTEIN BLONDIES

½ cup (80g) vanilla protein powder
6 tbsp (45g) oat flour
5½ tsp (14g) coconut flour
½ tsp (2.5g) baking soda
10 tbsp (60g) erythritol
¼ tsp (750mg) salt
1 tsp (5ml) vanilla extract
7 tbsp (113g) almond butter
½ cup (120g) egg whites
1½ cups (350ml) Silk unsweetened cashew milk
½ tsp (2.5ml) vanilla butter extract (optional)
½ cup (70g) frozen raspberries
¼ cup (40g) sugar-free chocolate chips

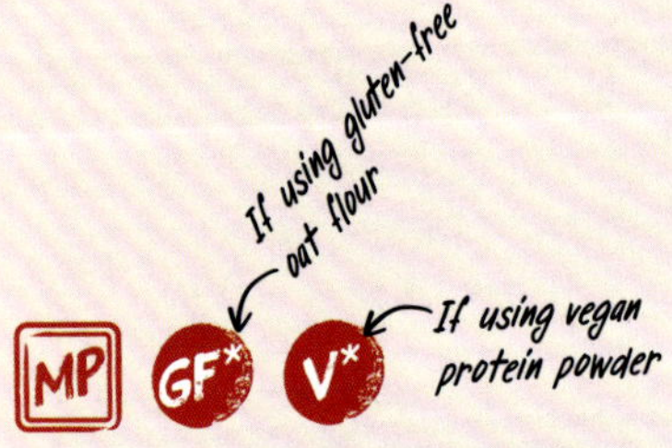

makes 12 squares / 6 servings

NUTRITION (PER SERVING)

160 calories	**4.5g** fat
15g protein	**14.5g** net carbs

They may be blond, but they're far from dumb—these protein-packed blondies are as smart as they are delicious. Overmixing, though? Now that would be a dumb move. Stir just until combined to keep them soft and tender—overworking the batter will make them dense and dry, and nobody wants that. If you're after that classic, buttery bakery-style flavor, don't skip the vanilla butter extract. It adds an extra layer of richness that makes these taste even more indulgent. For meal prep or leftovers, store in an airtight container at room temperature for up to 3 days, or in the fridge for up to a week. If you want to keep them longer, freeze for up to 3 months, and thaw at room temp before enjoying.

1. Preheat the oven to 325°F (160°C). Line an 8 x 8-inch (20 x 20cm) cake pan with parchment paper and spray the parchment paper with nonstick cooking spray.
2. To a medium mixing bowl, add the protein powder, oat flour, coconut flour, baking soda, erythritol, and salt and mix until evenly combined.
3. To a separate medium mixing bowl, add the vanilla extract, almond butter, egg whites, cashew milk, and vanilla butter extract (if using) and mix.
4. Pour the wet mixture into the dry ingredients and stir together for 1 to 2 minutes until a thick, smooth batter forms.
5. Gently fold in the raspberries and chocolate chips, being mindful not to overmix.
6. Into the prepared cake pan, pour the batter and bake for 25 minutes, until the top is golden and the center is set.
7. Remove from the oven and let sit for 10 minutes before cutting and enjoying!

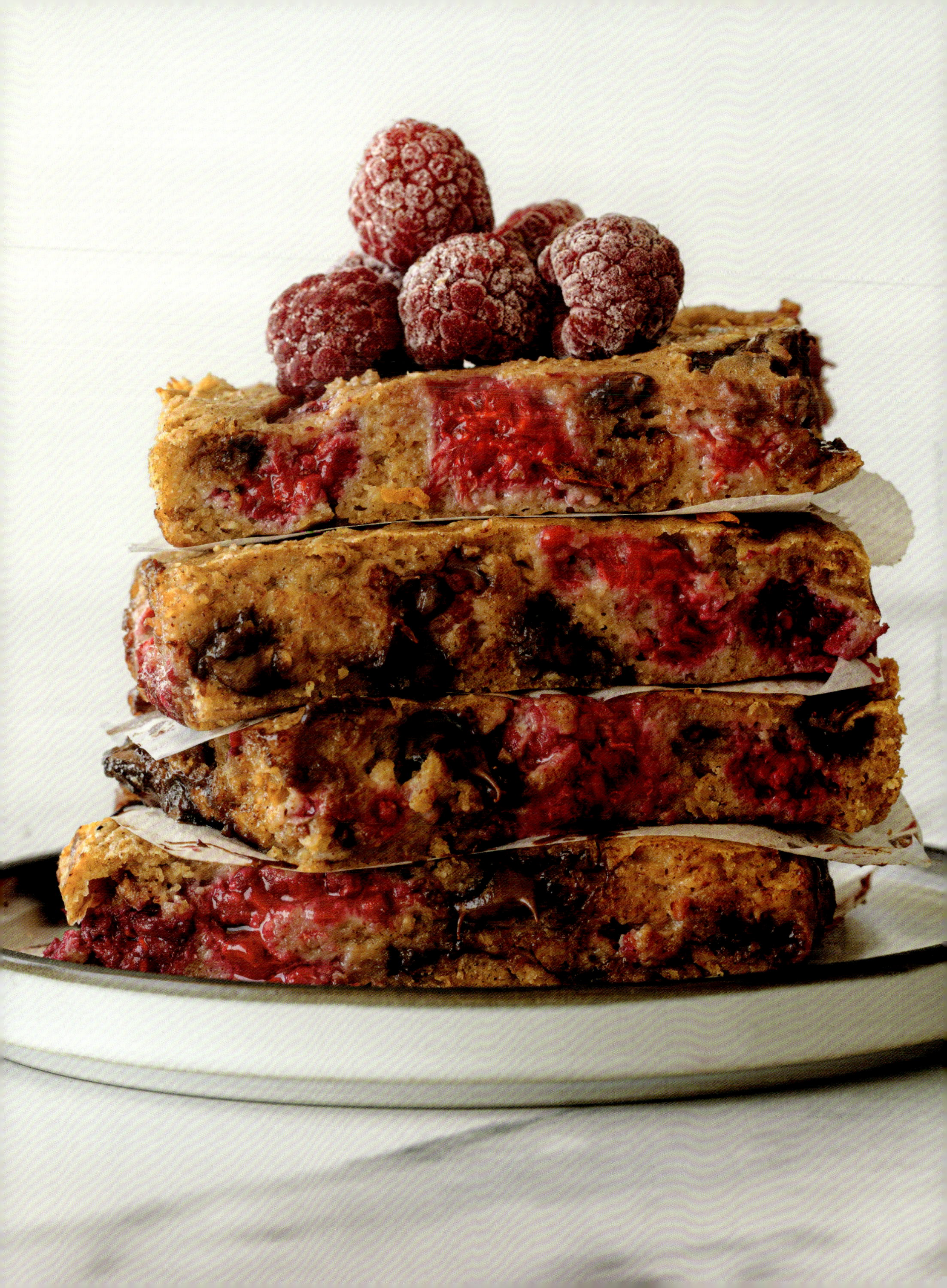

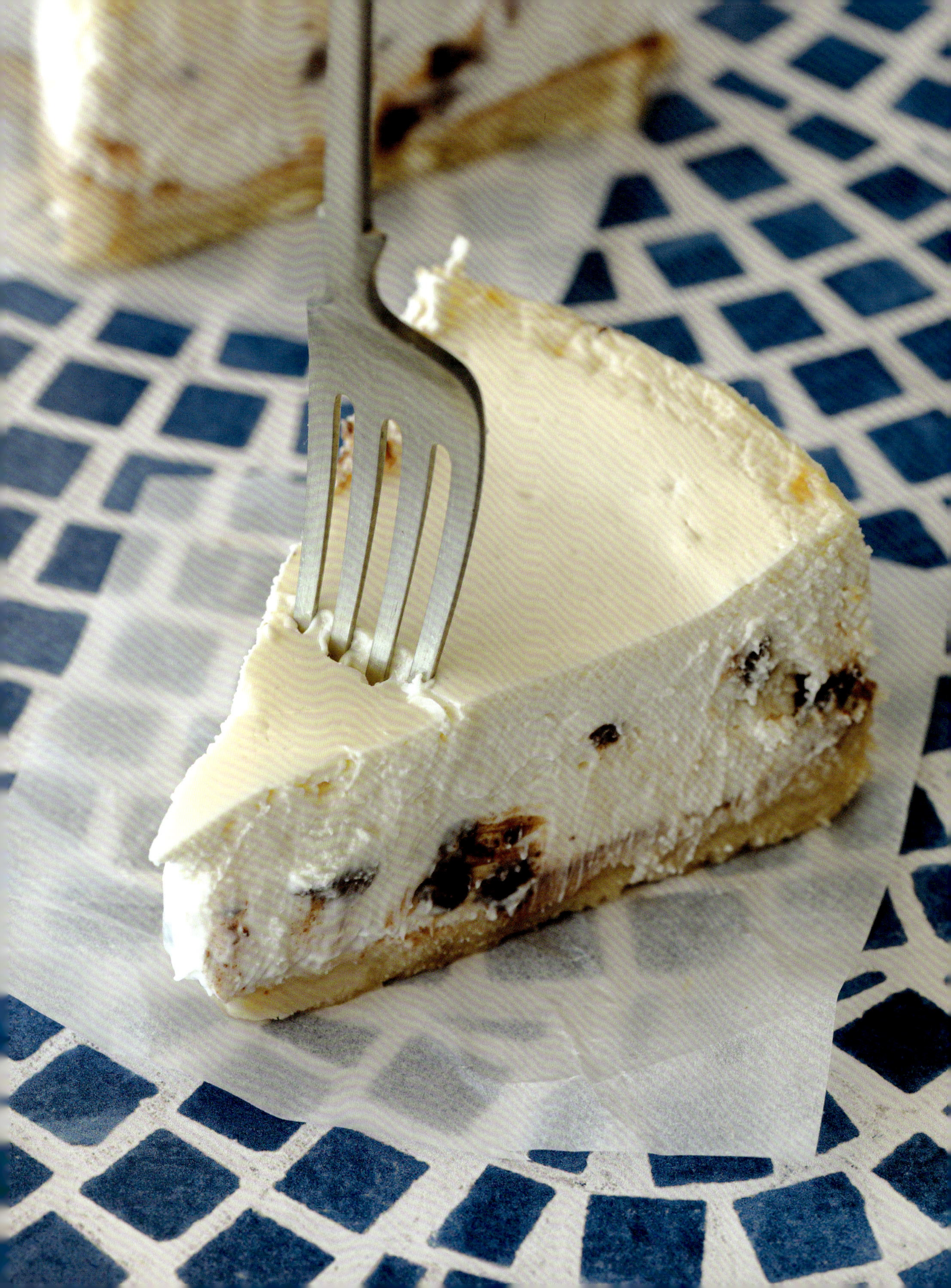

CHOCOLATE-CHIP PROTEIN CHEESECAKE

5½ tbsp (84g) coconut oil, melted
1⅔ cups (200g) almond flour
2 cups (460g) nonfat Greek yogurt
2¾ cups (680g) light cream cheese
1 scoop (31g) vanilla protein powder
1⅓ cups (130g) erythritol
2 tsp (10ml) vanilla extract
7½ tbsp (75g) semisweet chocolate chips

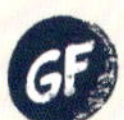
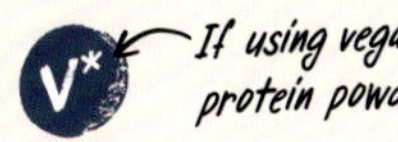

makes 1 cake / 12 servings

NUTRITION (PER SERVING)

360 calories **27.5g** fat
15g protein **12.5g** net carbs

This cheesecake is so thick, it just got verified on Instagram. The trick to getting that smooth texture? A water bath. Keeping a pan of water in the oven adds moisture, which helps prevent cracking and keeps the filling ultra creamy. You'll also need a springform pan for this recipe. Unlike a regular cake pan, a springform pan has sides that can be unclipped and removed, making it much easier to get the cheesecake out without ruining the crust. If you try to bake this in a regular pan, good luck getting that first slice out in one piece. To store, keep it covered in the fridge for up to 5 days or freeze individual slices for up to 3 months. If frozen, let a slice thaw in the fridge overnight before serving.

1. Preheat the oven to 350°F (180°C).
2. In a medium mixing bowl, combine the melted coconut oil with the almond flour. Mix until the texture resembles wet sand.
3. To the bottom of a 9-inch (23cm) springform pan, press in the almond-flour mixture to form the crust. Bake on the middle rack for 15 minutes, or until the crust is firm and golden. Leave the oven on.
4. In a large blender, combine the Greek yogurt, cream cheese, protein powder, erythritol, and vanilla extract. Blend until the mixture forms a smooth filling.
5. Add the chocolate chips. Using a spatula or large spoon, gently fold them in until evenly distributed.
6. Pour the filling over the crust, spreading it evenly across the surface.
7. Fill a medium cake pan two-thirds with water and place it on the bottom rack of the oven. Leave the pan of water in the oven for the entire baking time. This will add moisture during the baking process. Remove the pan only once the oven has cooled completely.
8. Bake on the middle rack for 50 minutes, or until the edges are slightly golden brown and the center still jiggles when gently shaken.
9. Turn off the oven, leaving the cheesecake inside for an additional 10 minutes. This will allow it to set slightly before being removed from the oven.
10. Transfer the cheesecake to the counter and let it cool for at least 20 minutes. Place it in the fridge for 4 to 6 hours to firm up and set completely.
11. Once chilled, carefully remove the ring from the springform pan. Slice the cheesecake into 12 pieces and serve. Enjoy!

PROTEIN WHOOPIE PIE

- ½ cup (60g) pastry flour
- 7½ tbsp (45g) whey-casein blend chocolate protein powder
- 4 tbsp (48g) erythritol
- 6 tbsp plus 6 tsp (40g) cocoa powder
- ½ tsp (2.5g) baking soda
- 1½ cups (345g) nonfat Greek yogurt
- ½ cup (120ml) Silk unsweetened cashew milk
- 2½ tbsp (42g) almond butter
- 1 tsp (5ml) vanilla extract
- ⅓ cup (84g) light cream cheese, room temperature
- 2 scoops (62g) whey-casein vanilla protein powder

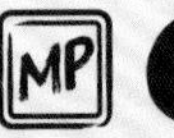

V

makes 6 pies / 6 servings

NUTRITION (PER SERVING)

246 calories	**9.5g** fat
24.5g protein	**16g** net carbs

A whoopie cushion might be an immature prank, but these whoopie pies are a grown-up move. They are packed with protein, taste like dessert, and won't leave you questioning your life choices. Just remember to chill the batter before baking, or you'll end up with something more like a protein frisbee than a soft, fluffy cake. For meal prep, store them in an airtight container in the fridge for up to 5 days. If you prefer a firmer texture, eat them straight from the fridge. If you want them softer, let them sit at room temp for a few minutes before biting in.

1. To a medium mixing bowl, add the pastry flour, chocolate protein powder, erythritol, cocoa powder, and baking soda and mix until well combined.
2. To a large mixing bowl, add about ⅔ (1 cup / 230g) of the Greek Yogurt, about ¾ (about ⅓ cup / 90ml) of the cashew milk, the almond butter, and vanilla extract, and stir together.
3. Pour the dry mixture into the wet mixture and stir together for 1 to 2 minutes, until a smooth batter is formed.
4. Place the batter in the fridge for 20 minutes, or until it chills and slightly thickens.
5. Preheat the oven to 350°F (180°C). Line a large baking sheet with parchment paper.
6. In a small mixing bowl, combine the remaining 115g Greek Yogurt, remaining 30 ml cashew milk, the cream cheese, and vanilla protein powder and stir for 1 to 2 minutes, until there are no clumps. Place the mixture in the fridge for at least 30 minutes.
7. On the prepared baking sheet, spoon the chocolate batter into 12 even cookies. With the back of the spoon, flatten them slightly.
8. Bake for 12 minutes. Remove them from the oven and let them sit for at least 20 minutes, or until completely cool.
9. Remove the vanilla filling from the fridge. On the flat side of half of the cookies, spread a thick layer of the filling until all the filling is used. Create cookie sandwiches by placing another cookie on top of the vanilla filling.

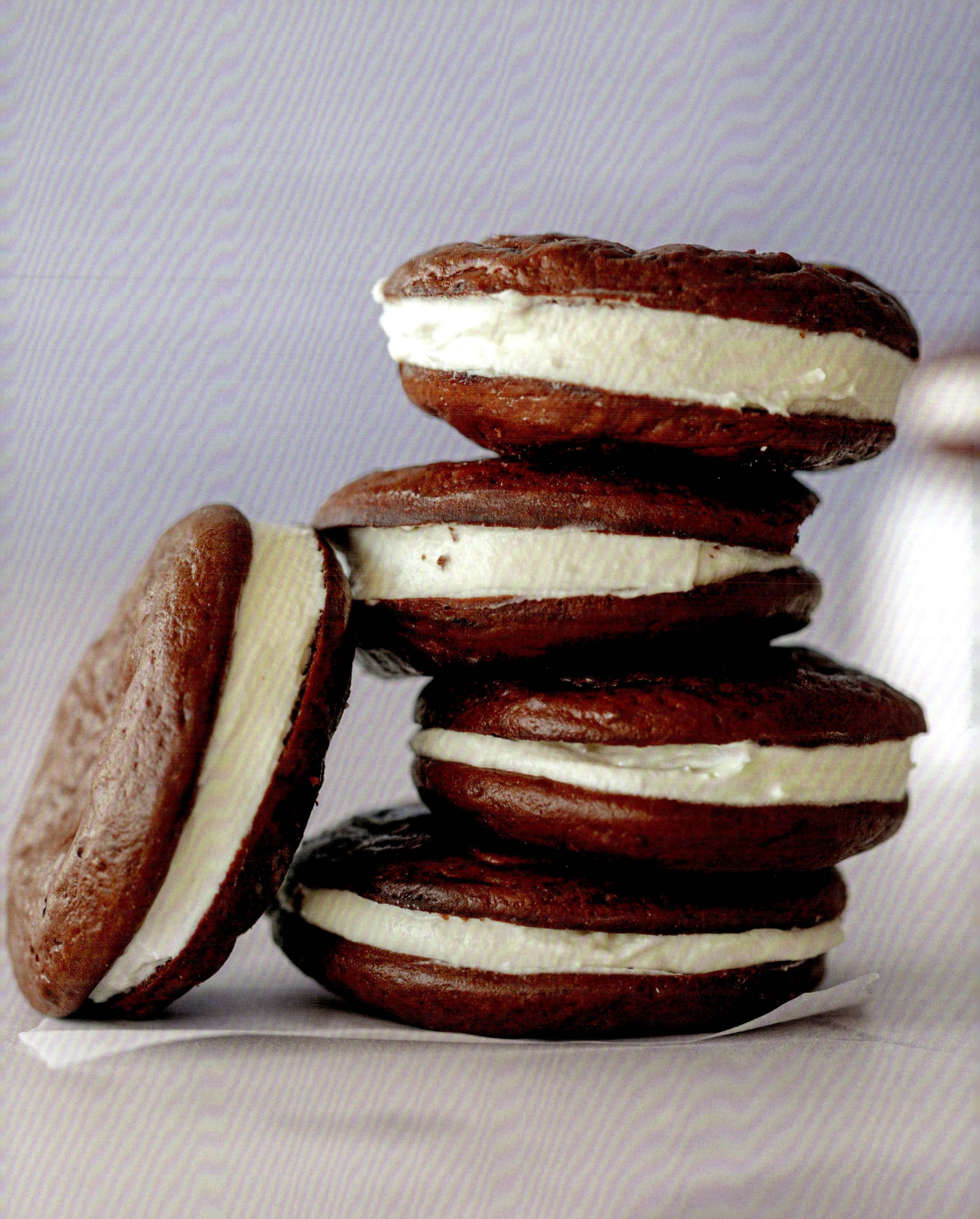

DIETARY CONSIDERATIONS

Please note that the dietary information provided in this book is intended for general informational purposes only. It is not a substitute for professional medical advice, diagnosis, or treatment. Always seek the guidance of your physician or other qualified health provider with any questions you may have regarding your health or a medical condition. Never disregard professional medical advice or delay in seeking it because of something you have read in this book. **Always verify ingredients.**

KEY	
GF	Gluten free
GF*	Easily made gluten free
V	Vegetarian
V*	Easily made vegetarian
V+	Vegan

Wake and Bake • Breakfast Bakes		
Ham and Cheddar Omelet Roll Up		
Breakfast Stuffed Peppers	GF	
Savory Oats with Tempeh "Bacon"	GF*	V
Italian Baked Eggs	GF	V
Healthy Fried Chicken and Waffles with Mustard Syrup		
Turkey-Sausage Breakfast Casserole	GF*	
Breakfast Pizza	GF*	
Savory Quinoa Egg Breakfast Muffins	GF	V
Egg Turkey-Bacon Muffins	GF	
Shredded Potato-Wrapped Quiches	GF	
Egg-White Vegetable Frittata	GF*	V*
Protein Coffee Muffins	GF	V*
Chocolate-Chip Protein Muffins	GF	V*
Cottage-Cheese Protein Bagels		V*
French Toast Protein Bagels		V*
Protein Banana Bread		V*

Morning Quickies • Traditional Brekkies		
Breakfast Quesadilla		V
Vegan Maca Bowl	GF	V+
PB&J Protein Pancake	GF	V*
Lemon-Ricotta Protein Crepes	GF	V*
Breakfast Burritos with Homemade Sweet-Potato Wraps		V*
Healthy Sausage and Egg McWills		
Zucchini Hashbrowns	GF	V*
Chocolate Protein Pancake	GF	V*
3-Minute Breakfast Sandwich		
Protein Waffles	GF	V*
Microwave Breakfast Bowl		
Chocolate Peanut Butter No-Bake Energy Balls	GF*	V*
PB&J Protein Roll Up	GF*	V*
Breakfast Toast 3 Ways:		
Autumn on Toast	GF*	V+
Katie's Sweet Cottage Cheese Toast	GF*	V
Ricotta Be Kiddin' Me Spread	GF*	V

Afternoon Delights • Lunchtime Indulgences		
Spicy Crispy Chicken Sandwiches		
Curried Chicken Lettuce Wraps	GF	
Pecan Chicken Salad	GF	
Asian Mango Chicken Pita		
Grilled Vegetable Salad	GF	V
Savory Sweet-Potato Chicken and Waffle	GF*	
BBQ Pulled Chicken Sliders		
Ricotta-Stuffed Healthy Peppers	GF*	
Tuna Burger with Pineapple Bun	GF	
Steak Taco Salad	GF	
Turkey Meatball Subs	GF*	
White Bean and Artichoke Flatbread	GF*	V+*
Shawarma Chicken	GF	
Tofu Veggie Scramble	GF*	V

Bite Me, Baby • Appetizers		
Zucchini Boats	GF	
Butternut Squash Fritters	GF	V
Quick-Bake Falafel	GF*	V+
Mexican Twice-Baked Stuffed Sweet Potato	GF	
Cauliflower and Leek Soup	GF	V+
Enhanced Twice-Baked Potato	GF	V
Chicken Summer Rolls	GF	
Buffalo Cauliflower Bites	GF	V
Warm Root-Vegetable Salad	GF	
Healthy Caesar Salad	GF	
Tuna-Stuffed Avocados	GF	
Anabolic Spinach Artichoke Dip with Pita Chips		V*
Pineapple Salsa	GF	V+
Chicken Potstickers		

Feeding the Family • Mains		
Khichri and Air-Fried Tofu		V+
Cabbage and Chicken Stir Fry	GF*	
One-Pot Hearty Vegetable Chicken Stew	GF	
One-Pot Deconstructed Lasagna	GF*	
Stuffed Chicken Breast with Spinach, Sun-Dried Tomato, and Ricotta Filling	GF	
Mexican Lasagna		
Chicken Parmesan Bake with Quinoa	GF*	
Budget-Friendly Chili	GF	
Coconut Chicken Curry		
Chicken Cauliflower Fried Rice	GF*	
Cauliflower-Rice Arancini with Turkey Sausage	GF*	
Healthy Pad Thai	GF*	
Cottage-Cheese Fettuccini Alfredo	GF*	
Creamy Tarragon Shrimp Pasta	GF*	

Cheat Codes • Fake the Takeout		
Anabolic Pizza		
Anabolic Shepherd's Pie	GF*	
Cheeseburger Spring Rolls with Thousand Island Dip		
Chicken Nuggies	GF	
Animal-Style Fries	GF*	V
Crispy Cheese Chicken Cups		
Healthier Baked Mac and Cheese	GF*	V
Protein Scalloped Potatoes	GF*	V
Fried Zucchini Chips with Marinara Dip	GF*	V*
Crispy Fried PB&J Sandwich	GF*	V
Pizza Casserole	GF*	
Curry Chicken Tenders with Greek-Yogurt Dip		
Blended Creamy Vanilla-Protein Iced Coffee	GF	V*

Happy Endings • Delectable Desserts		
Greek Yogurt Ice Pops	GF	V*
Handheld Apple Pies		V
Microwave Apple Pie	GF*	V
Protein Apple Fritters	GF*	V*
Chocolate Peanut-Butter Protein Bark	GF	V*
S'mores Protein Cookies	GF*	V*
Pumpkin Protein Mousse Cake	GF	V*
Dark Desire Chocolate Oat Cake	GF*	V*
Anabolic "Spreadaroo" Cookies	GF	V*
Protein Crispy Rice Squares	GF*	V*
Blueberry Cottage-Cheese Protein Cheesecake Bowl	GF*	V*
No-Churn Vanilla-Protein Ice Cream	GF*	V*
Raspberry Chocolate Protein Blondies	GF*	V*
Chocolate-Chip Protein Cheesecake	GF	V*
Protein Whoopie Pie		V

ACKNOWLEDGMENTS

They say that no man is an island and I couldn't agree more. As I've grown in my career, I've been lucky to have the support of so many people, and I'd like to take a few minutes to give my thanks.

To Victoria, this cookbook truly wouldn't have happened without you. You work so hard behind the scenes, and you protect me from getting screwed by my contracts. Your big sister energy is strong. Thanks for having my back.

To Anna and the DK team, thank you for taking a chance on me. The day I got that first email from you guys was a big "pinch me" moment. Your excitement and positivity are infectious. I can never thank you enough for the tireless hard work and time that you put into this.

To Charles, you're the coffee to my donuts when it comes to getting creative. It's rare to know someone with a sense of humor as weird as mine. You bring a unique voice to your work, and I appreciate how you're always innovative and do things with a twist.

To Leonora, your food photography is incredible. You turn every single dish into a work of art. You've been a huge part of this whole process, and you've really brought this cookbook to life.

To Kaitlyn, you are my oasis in the desert. When I'm stressed and anxious, you ground me in the present. You believe in me even on days when I don't believe in myself, and you are always there for me with a smile on your face. I love you so much.

To Clemence, your illustrations brought so much life to this cookbook—you were even able to capture Ollie perfectly! Thank you for sharing your talent.

To Dad, without you in my life, I would basically fall apart. You selflessly give so much of your time to me and my career in order to make me as successful as I can be. You are a constant source of support, and I am so grateful for all that you do. It means the world.

To Mum, my #1 cheerleader since day one, you make sure that no matter what I do, big or small, I'm proud of it. You're always willing to costar in my videos, and you've supported my crazy YouTube life, no questions asked. I'm so lucky I won the egg race.

To Josh, your incredible skill, attention to detail, and passion makes me happy every day that you are part of my team. You bring great energy and always instill confidence in me that my latest video will be something I'm proud of.

To Grandma, our mall and coffee dates will forever be special to me, as will your amazing soup and curries. As a white kid, I can confidently say that I can handle spicy food thanks to you. Nothing will ever beat your keema!

To Patrick, my hype man in the gym and on set! You always bring a positive energy with you and motivate me with our heart-to-hearts. I love being in the company of someone as talented as you, and respect that you'll do anything for the shot.

To Yianni, thank you for making me look like alive when I was deep in a cut. You absolutely nailed the cover photo and lifestyle shots. I'm already plotting how to trick you into working with me again.

To Ollie, we started this together, and thinking of you is what motivates me to keep pushing forward. I hope you're eating lots of Honey Dip Timbits up there. Miss you, bro; I'll always be your cameraman.

To Lizabee, the other Tenny sister. My eating challenge training started nice and young, thanks to you and the macaroni at the Blue Lagoon. Thanks for being an amazing sister and a great friend.

To my subscribers, this cookbook is for you. I have the best community on YouTube. You radiate positivity and enthusiasm, and it inspires me to keep hustling. I am humbled by how many of you are on this ride with me and am deeply thankful that you have stuck around to watch me grow and evolve.

—Will

A

allspice, Shawarma Chicken, 118
almond butter
- Pumpkin Protein Mousse Cake, 232
- Raspberry Chocolate Protein Blondies, 244

almond flour
- Anabolic "Spreadaroo" Cookies, 236
- Chocolate-Chip Protein Cheesecake, 247
- Chocolate-Chip Protein Muffins, 50
- Microwave Apple Pie, 224
- Protein Coffee Muffins, 49

almond milk, Savory Oats with Tempeh "Bacon," 30
apple
- Handheld Apple Pies, 223
- Microwave Apple Pie, 224
- Protein Apple Fritters, 227
- Pumpkin Protein Mousse Cake, 232
- apple sauce, unsweetened, Chocolate-Chip Protein Muffins, 50

artichoke hearts
- Anabolic Spinach Artichoke Dip with Pita Chips, 149
- White Bean and Artichoke Flatbread, 117

asparagus, Grilled Vegetable Salad, 102
avocado
- Chicken Summer Rolls, 138
- Savory Sweet-Potato Chicken and Waffle, 105
- Tofu Veggie Scramble, 121
- Tuna Burger with Pineapple Bun, 110
- Tuna-Stuffed Avocados, 146

B

banana
- PB&J Protein Pancake, 66
- Protein Banana Bread, 57

barley, Khichri and Air-Fried Tofu, 158
basil
- Anabolic Pizza, 190
- Fried Zucchini Chips with Marinara Dip, 206
- Turkey Meatball Subs, 114
- White Bean and Artichoke Flatbread, 117

beans, black
- Budget-Friendly Chili, 173
- Mexican Lasagna, 169

beans, red kidney, Budget-Friendly Chili, 173
beans, white, White Bean and Artichoke Flatbread, 117
bean sprouts, Asian Mango Chicken Pita, 101
beef, eye of round, Steak Taco Salad, 113
beef, ground
- Budget-Friendly Chili, 173
- Cheeseburger Spring Rolls with Thousand Island Dip, 194

bell pepper
- Breakfast Quesadilla, 62
- Breakfast Stuffed Peppers, 29
- Creamy Tarragon Shrimp Pasta, 185
- One-Pot Deconstructed Lasagna, 165
- Ricotta-Stuffed Healthy Peppers, 109
- Tofu Veggie Scramble, 121

blueberries, frozen
- Blueberry Cottage-Cheese Protein Cheesecake Bowl, 240
- Greek Yogurt Ice Pops, 220
- Katie's Sweet Cottage-Cheese Toast, 89

broccoli
- Egg-White Vegetable Frittata, 46
- Healthy Pad Thai, 181

brown sugar, Swerve
- Autumn on Toast, 88
- French Toast Protein Bagels, 54
- Handheld Apple Pies, 223
- Microwave Apple Pie, 224
- Protein Apple Fritters, 227
- Protein Banana Bread, 57

buttermilk
- Healthy Fried Chicken and Waffles with Mustard Syrup, 34
- Spicy Crispy Chicken Sandwiches, 94

butternut squash
- Butternut Squash Fritters, 129
- Coconut Chicken Curry, 174
- One-Pot Hearty Vegetable Chicken Stew, 162
- Warm Root-Vegetable Salad, 142

C

cabbage, green
- Cabbage and Chicken Stir Fry, 161
- Chicken Potstickers, 153

cabbage, red, BBQ Pulled Chicken Sliders, 106
cashew milk
- Autumn on Toast, 88
- Blended Creamy Vanilla-Protein Iced Coffee, 214
- Blueberry Cottage-Cheese Protein Cheesecake Bowl, 240
- Chocolate Protein Pancakes, 77
- Cottage-Cheese Fettuccini Alfredo, 182
- Ham and Cheddar Omelet Roll Up, 26
- Healthier Baked Mac and Cheese, 202
- Lemon-Ricotta Protein Crepes, 69
- Microwave Breakfast Bowl, 82
- PB&J Protein Roll Up, 86
- Protein Banana Bread, 57
- Protein Coffee Muffins, 49
- Pumpkin Protein Mousse Cake, 232
- Raspberry Chocolate Protein Blondies, 244
- S'mores Protein Cookies, 231
- Vegan Maca Bowl, 65

cashews, Buffalo Cauliflower Bites, 141
cauliflower
- Anabolic Shepherd's Pie, 193
- Buffalo Cauliflower Bites, 141
- Cauliflower and Leek Soup, 134
- Healthier Baked Mac and Cheese, 202

cauliflower rice
- Cauliflower-Rice Arancini with Turkey Sausage, 178
- Chicken Cauliflower Fried Rice, 177
- Ricotta-Stuffed Healthy Peppers, 109

cayenne
- Chicken Nuggies, 197
- Shawarma Chicken, 118

celery
- Cauliflower and Leek Soup, 134
- Pecan Chicken Salad, 98

cheddar
- 3-Minute Breakfast Sandwich, 78
- Breakfast Quesadilla, 62
- Breakfast Stuffed Peppers, 29
- Cheeseburger Spring Rolls with Thousand Island Dip, 194
- Ham and Cheddar Omelet Roll Up, 26
- Mexican Lasagna, 169
- Microwave Breakfast Bowl, 82
- Savory Quinoa Egg Breakfast Muffins, 41

cheddar, low-fat
- Animal-Style Fries, 198
- Healthier Baked Mac and Cheese, 202
- Healthy Sausage and Egg McWills, 73

chicken, ground
- Anabolic Shepherd's Pie, 193
- Chicken Nuggies, 197
- Chicken Potstickers, 153
- Mexican Lasagna, 169
- One-Pot Hearty Vegetable Chicken Stew, 162

chicken bacon, Healthy Caesar Salad, 145
chicken breast
- BBQ Pulled Chicken Sliders, 106
- Cabbage and Chicken Stir Fry, 161
- Chicken Parmesan Bake with Quinoa, 170
- Chicken Summer Rolls, 138
- Coconut Chicken Curry, 174
- Crispy Cheese Chicken Cups, 201
- Curried Chicken Lettuce Wraps, 97
- Curry Chicken Tenders with Greek-Yogurt Dip, 213
- Healthy Fried Chicken and Waffles with Mustard Syrup, 34
- Mexican Twice-Baked Stuffed Sweet Potato, 133
- Microwave Breakfast Bowl, 82
- Pecan Chicken Salad, 98
- Savory Sweet-Potato Chicken and Waffle, 105
- Shawarma Chicken, 118
- Spicy Crispy Chicken Sandwiches, 94
- Stuffed Chicken Breast with Spinach, Sun-Dried Tomato and Ricotta Filling, 166

chicken breast, rotisserie
- Asian Mango Chicken Pita, 101
- Chicken Cauliflower Fried Rice, 177

chicken stock
- Anabolic Shepherd's Pie, 193
- Chicken Parmesan Bake with Quinoa, 170
- Healthy Fried Chicken and Waffles with Mustard Syrup, 34

chickpeas, Quick-Bake Falafel, 130
chili flakes, Ricotta Be Kiddin' Me Spread, 89
chili powder, Chicken Nuggies, 197
chives
- 3-Minute Breakfast Sandwich, 78
- Breakfast Stuffed Peppers, 29
- Butternut Squash Fritters, 129
- Curry Chicken Tenders with Greek-Yogurt Dip, 213

chocolate almond milk, Dark Desire Chocolate Oat Cake, 235
chocolate chips

Chocolate-Chip Protein Muffins, 50
Dark Desire Chocolate Oat Cake, 235
S'mores Protein Cookies, 231
cilantro
Asian Mango Chicken Pita, 101
Breakfast Quesadilla, 62
Khichri and Air-Fried Tofu, 158
Mexican Twice-Baked Stuffed Sweet Potato, 133
Pineapple Salsa, 150
cinnamon
Autumn on Toast, 88
French Toast Protein Bagels, 54
Handheld Apple Pies, 223
PB&J Protein Roll Up, 86
Protein Banana Bread, 57
Pumpkin Protein Mousse Cake, 232
Shawarma Chicken, 118
clove, ground, Autumn on Toast, 88
cocoa powder
Chocolate Protein Pancakes, 77
Dark Desire Chocolate Oat Cake, 235
coconut flour
Breakfast Pizza, 38
Butternut Squash Fritters, 129
Chocolate Protein Pancakes, 77
Healthy Fried Chicken and Waffles with Mustard Syrup, 34
Protein Waffles, 81
Pumpkin Protein Mousse Cake, 232
Raspberry Chocolate Protein Blondies, 244
S'mores Protein Cookies, 231
coconut milk
Chocolate Peanut-Butter Protein Bark, 228
Coconut Chicken Curry, 174
coconut yogurt, Savory Oats with Tempeh "Bacon," 30
coffee, brewed, Blended Creamy Vanilla-Protein Iced Coffee, 214
Cool Whip Light, No-Churn Vanilla-Protein Ice Cream, 243
corn, Mexican Lasagna, 169
cornflakes
Crispy Fried PB&J Sandwich, 209
Healthy Fried Chicken and Waffles with Mustard Syrup, 34
cottage cheese
Blueberry Cottage-Cheese Protein Cheesecake Bowl, 240
Cottage-Cheese Fettuccini Alfredo, 182
Cottage-Cheese Protein Bagels, 53
Katie's Sweet Cottage-Cheese Toast, 89
Pizza Casserole, 210
Protein Scalloped Potatoes, 205
Protein Waffles, 81
cream
Blended Creamy Vanilla-Protein Iced Coffee, 214
Cottage-Cheese Fettuccini Alfredo, 182
Creamy Tarragon Shrimp Pasta, 185
cream cheese
Chocolate-Chip Protein Cheesecake, 247
Crispy Cheese Chicken Cups, 201
crispy rice cereal, Protein Crispy Rice Squares, 239
cucumber
Chicken Summer Rolls, 138
Curry Chicken Tenders with Greek-Yogurt Dip, 213
Steak Taco Salad, 113
cumin
Curry Chicken Tenders with Greek-Yogurt Dip, 213
Shawarma Chicken, 118
Tofu Veggie Scramble, 121
curry powder
Curry Chicken Tenders with Greek-Yogurt Dip, 213
Shawarma Chicken, 118

D

daikon, Warm Root-Vegetable Salad, 142
Dijon mustard, Pecan Chicken Salad, 98
dill, fresh, Pecan Chicken Salad, 98
dumpling wrappers, Chicken Potstickers, 153

E

eggs
3-Minute Breakfast Sandwich, 78
Anabolic "Spreadaroo" Cookies, 236
Breakfast Burritos with Homemade Sweet-Potato Wraps, 70
Breakfast Pizza, 38
Breakfast Quesadilla, 62
Breakfast Stuffed Peppers, 29
Butternut Squash Fritters, 129
Chicken Cauliflower Fried Rice, 177
Chicken Nuggies, 197
Egg Turkey-Bacon Muffins, 42
Fried Zucchini Chips with Marinara Dip, 206
Ham and Cheddar Omelet Roll Up, 26
Italian Baked Eggs, 33
Lemon-Ricotta Protein Crepes, 69
Microwave Breakfast Bowl, 82
PB&J Protein Pancake, 66
Protein Banana Bread, 57
Savory Quinoa Egg Breakfast Muffins, 41
Shredded Potato-Wrapped Quiche, 45
Turkey-Sausage Breakfast Casserole, 37
Zucchini Hashbrowns, 74
egg whites
Breakfast Burritos with Homemade Sweet-Potato Wraps, 70
Breakfast Pizza, 38
Chicken Nuggies, 197
Chicken Parmesan Bake with Quinoa, 170
Cottage-Cheese Protein Bagels, 53
Crispy Fried PB&J Sandwich, 209
Egg-White Vegetable Frittata, 46
Healthy Sausage and Egg McWills, 73
PB&J Protein Roll Up, 86
Protein Waffles, 81
Pumpkin Protein Mousse Cake, 232
Raspberry Chocolate Protein Blondies, 244
Savory Sweet-Potato Chicken and Waffle, 105
eggplant, Coconut Chicken Curry, 174
endive, Grilled Vegetable Salad, 102

F

fennel, BBQ Pulled Chicken Sliders, 106
feta, Steak Taco Salad, 113
fettuccini, Cottage-Cheese Fettuccini Alfredo, 182
Frank's RedHot Original, Buffalo Cauliflower Bites, 141

G

garlic cloves
Chicken Potstickers, 153
Cottage-Cheese Fettuccini Alfredo, 182
Creamy Tarragon Shrimp Pasta, 185
Crispy Cheese Chicken Cups, 201
Pizza Casserole, 210
Protein Scalloped Potatoes, 205
Ricotta Be Kiddin' Me Spread, 89
Tofu Veggie Scramble, 121
garlic powder
Animal-Style Fries, 198
Chicken Nuggles, 197
Cottage-Cheese Fettuccini Alfredo, 182
Creamy Tarragon Shrimp Pasta, 185
Fried Zucchini Chips with Marinara Dip, 206
Shawarma Chicken, 118
Tofu Veggie Scramble, 121
ginger
Autumn on Toast, 88
Cabbage and Chicken Stir Fry, 161
Chicken Potstickers, 153
Healthy Pad Thai, 181
Khichri and Air-Fried Tofu, 158
goat cheese, Grilled Vegetable Salad, 102
grainy mustard
Grilled Vegetable Salad, 102
Healthy Fried Chicken and Waffles with Mustard Syrup, 34
Greek yogurt
Anabolic Pizza, 190
Anabolic Shepherd's Pie, 193
Anabolic Spinach Artichoke Dip with Pita Chips, 149
Anabolic "Spreadaroo" Cookies, 236
Animal-Style Fries, 198
Blueberry Cottage-Cheese Protein Cheesecake Bowl, 240
Breakfast Pizza, 38
Breakfast Quesadilla, 62
Chocolate-Chip Protein Cheesecake, 247
Chocolate Peanut-Butter Protein Bark, 228
Chocolate Protein Pancakes, 77
Cottage-Cheese Protein Bagels, 53
Curried Chicken Lettuce Wraps, 97
Curry Chicken Tenders with Greek-Yogurt Dip, 213
Enhanced Twice-Baked Potato, 137
French Toast Protein Bagels, 54
Greek Yogurt Ice Pops, 220
Healthy Caesar Salad, 145
Pecan Chicken Salad, 98
Protein Apple Fritters, 227
Protein Banana Bread, 57

Protein Coffee Muffins, 49
Protein Scalloped Potatoes, 205
Pumpkin Protein Mousse Cake, 232
Shawarma Chicken, 118
S'mores Protein Cookies, 231
Steak Taco Salad, 113
green onion
Cabbage and Chicken Stir Fry, 161
Chicken Potstickers, 153
Enhanced Twice-Baked Potato, 137
Ham and Cheddar Omelet Roll Up, 26
Mexican Lasagna, 169
green peas, Chicken Cauliflower Fried Rice, 177
green pepper, Pizza Casserole, 210

H

half-and-half
Blended Creamy Vanilla-Protein Iced Coffee, 214
Cottage-Cheese Fettuccini Alfredo, 182
Creamy Tarragon Shrimp Pasta, 185
ham
3-Minute Breakfast Sandwich, 78
Ham and Cheddar Omelet Roll Up, 26
honey, Katie's Sweet Cottage-Cheese Toast, 89

J

jalapeño
Mexican Twice-Baked Stuffed Sweet Potato, 133
Pineapple Salsa, 150
Tuna Burger with Pineapple Bun, 110

K

kale, Tofu Veggie Scramble, 121
kimchi, Tuna Burger with Pineapple Bun, 110
kiwi, Vegan Maca Bowl, 65

L

leek
Cauliflower and Leek Soup, 134
Coconut Chicken Curry, 174
lemon
Blueberry Cottage-Cheese Protein Cheesecake Bowl, 240
Handheld Apple Pies, 223
Healthy Caesar Salad, 145
Katie's Sweet Cottage-Cheese Toast, 89
Lemon-Ricotta Protein Crepes, 69
Pineapple Salsa, 150
Quick-Bake Falafel, 130
Ricotta Be Kiddin' Me Spread, 89
lentils, Khichri and Air-Fried Tofu, 158
lime, Curry Chicken Tenders with Greek-Yogurt Dip, 213

M

maca powder, Vegan Maca Bowl, 65
mango
Asian Mango Chicken Pita, 101
Greek Yogurt Ice Pops, 220
maple syrup, Autumn on Toast, 88
mayonnaise, Pecan Chicken Salad, 98
mozzarella
Anabolic Pizza, 190
Anabolic Spinach Artichoke Dip with Pita Chips, 149
Breakfast Burritos with Homemade Sweet-Potato Wraps, 70
Breakfast Pizza, 38
Cauliflower-Rice Arancini with Turkey Sausage, 178
Egg-White Vegetable Frittata, 46
Italian Baked Eggs, 33
One-Pot Deconstructed Lasagna, 165
Pizza Casserole, 210
Ricotta-Stuffed Healthy Peppers, 109
Turkey Meatball Subs, 114
Turkey-Sausage Breakfast Casserole, 37
mushrooms
Anabolic Shepherd's Pie, 193
Breakfast Burritos with Homemade Sweet-Potato Wraps, 70
Chicken Parmesan Bake with Quinoa, 170
One-Pot Deconstructed Lasagna, 165
Pizza Casserole, 210
Tuna Burger with Pineapple Bun, 110

N

nutmeg, ground, Autumn on Toast, 88

O

oat flour
Raspberry Chocolate Protein Blondies, 244
S'mores Protein Cookies, 231
oats
Chocolate Peanut-Butter No Bake Energy Balls, 85
Dark Desire Chocolate Oat Cake, 235
Microwave Apple Pie, 224
Savory Oats with Tempeh "Bacon," 30
onion
Anabolic Shepherd's Pie, 193
Animal-Style Fries, 198
Breakfast Burritos with Homemade Sweet-Potato Wraps, 70
Breakfast Quesadilla, 62
Budget-Friendly Chili, 173
Chicken Parmesan Bake with Quinoa, 170
Creamy Tarragon Shrimp Pasta, 185
Crispy Cheese Chicken Cups, 201
One-Pot Deconstructed Lasagna, 165
Pizza Casserole, 210
Ricotta-Stuffed Healthy Peppers, 109
onion powder
Animal-Style Fries, 198
Chicken Nuggies, 197
Shawarma Chicken, 118
oregano, Pizza Casserole, 210

P

paprika, Animal-Style Fries, 198
Parmesan
Anabolic Spinach Artichoke Dip with Pita Chips, 149
Chicken Nuggies, 197
Cottage-Cheese Fettuccini Alfredo, 182
Creamy Tarragon Shrimp Pasta, 185
Crispy Cheese Chicken Cups, 201
Fried Zucchini Chips with Marinara Dip, 206
One-Pot Deconstructed Lasagna, 165
Zucchini Hashbrowns, 74
parsley, Quick-Bake Falafel, 130
pasta
Cottage-Cheese Fettuccini Alfredo, 182
One-Pot Deconstructed Lasagna, 165
Pizza Casserole, 210
pastry sheets, Crispy Cheese Chicken Cups, 201
PB2 Powdered Peanut Butter
Chocolate-Chip Protein Muffins, 50
Chocolate Peanut Butter No-Bake Energy Balls, 85
Chocolate Peanut-Butter Protein Bark, 228
Crispy Fried PB&J Sandwich, 209
Healthy Pad Thai, 181
PB&J Protein Pancake, 66
PB&J Protein Roll Up, 86
peanut butter
PB&J Protein Roll Up, 86
S'mores Protein Cookies, 231
pecans, Pecan Chicken Salad, 98
pickle
BBQ Pulled Chicken Sliders, 106
Spicy Crispy Chicken Sandwiches, 94
pineapple
Anabolic Pizza, 190
Cabbage and Chicken Stir Fry, 161
Pineapple Salsa, 150
Tuna Burger with Pineapple Bun, 110
portobello mushroom, Grilled Vegetable Salad, 102
potato
Animal-Style Fries, 198
Enhanced Twice-Baked Potato, 137
Protein Scalloped Potatoes, 205
Shredded Potato-Wrapped Quiche, 45
Tofu Veggie Scramble, 121
potato buns, BBQ Pulled Chicken Sliders, 106
powdered sugar, low-calorie, Anabolic "Spreadaroo" Cookies, 236
powdered sugar, Swerve, Protein Apple Fritters, 227
protein pancake mix, PB&J Protein Roll Up, 86
protein powder
Anabolic "Spreadaroo" Cookies, 236
Blended Creamy Vanilla-Protein Iced Coffee, 214
Blueberry Cottage-Cheese Protein Cheesecake Bowl, 240
Chocolate-Chip Protein Cheesecake, 247
Chocolate-Chip Protein Muffins, 50
Chocolate Peanut-Butter Protein Bark, 228
Chocolate Protein Pancakes, 77
Cottage-Cheese Protein Bagels, 53
Dark Desire Chocolate Oat Cake, 235
French Toast Protein Bagels, 54
Greek Yogurt Ice Pops, 220
No-Churn Vanilla-Protein Ice Cream, 243
PB&J Protein Pancake, 66
PB&J Protein Roll Up, 86
Protein Apple Fritters, 227
Protein Banana Bread, 57
Protein Coffee Muffins, 49
Protein Crispy Rice Squares, 239
Protein Waffles, 81
Pumpkin Protein Mousse Cake, 232

Raspberry Chocolate Protein Blondies, 244
S'mores Protein Cookies, 231
protein powder, vegan, Vegan Maca Bowl, 65
puff pastry dough, Handheld Apple Pies, 223
pumpkin purée
Autumn on Toast, 88
Pumpkin Protein Mousse Cake, 232

Q

quinoa
Chicken Parmesan Bake with Quinoa, 170
Savory Quinoa Egg Breakfast Muffins, 41
Vegan Maca Bowl, 65

R

radicchio, Grilled Vegetable Salad, 102
raisins
Curried Chicken Lettuce Wraps, 97
French Toast Protein Bagels, 54
raspberries, frozen, Raspberry Chocolate Protein Blondies, 244
rice noodles, Healthy Pad Thai, 181
rice paper, Chicken Summer Rolls, 138
rice vinegar, Healthy Pad Thai, 181
ricotta
Lemon-Ricotta Protein Crepes, 69
One-Pot Deconstructed Lasagna, 165
Ricotta Be Kiddin' Me Spread, 89
Stuffed Chicken Breast with Spinach, Sun-Dried Tomato and Ricotta Filling, 166
rosemary, fresh, Anabolic Shepherd's Pie, 193
rutabaga
One-Pot Hearty Vegetable Chicken Stew, 162
Warm Root-Vegetable Salad, 142

S

sage, fresh, Butternut Squash Fritters, 129
semisweet chocolate chips, Chocolate-Chip Protein Cheesecake, 247
sprinkles, Anabolic "Spreadaroo" Cookies, 236
sesame oil
Healthy Pad Thai, 181
Khichri and Air-Fried Tofu, 158
shallot, Cauliflower and Leek Soup, 134
shrimp
Cottage-Cheese Fettuccini Alfredo, 182
Creamy Tarragon Shrimp Pasta, 185
Healthy Pad Thai, 181
soy sauce
Chicken Cauliflower Fried Rice, 177
Chicken Potstickers, 153
Healthy Pad Thai, 181
Tofu Veggie Scramble, 121
spinach, fresh
Creamy Tarragon Shrimp Pasta, 185
Italian Baked Eggs, 33
Ricotta-Stuffed Healthy Peppers, 109
Savory Sweet-Potato Chicken and Waffle, 105
Steak Taco Salad, 113
Warm Root-Vegetable Salad, 142
spinach, frozen
Anabolic Spinach Artichoke Dip with Pita Chips, 149
Savory Quinoa Egg Breakfast Muffins, 41
Shredded Potato-Wrapped Quiche, 45
Stuffed Chicken Breast with Spinach, Sun-Dried Tomato and Ricotta Filling, 166
spring mix, Chicken Summer Rolls, 138
Stevia
Handheld Apple Pies, 223
Lemon-Ricotta Protein Crepes, 69
strawberries, frozen, PB&J Protein Pancake, 66
sun-dried tomato, Stuffed Chicken Breast with Spinach, Sun-Dried Tomato and Ricotta Filling, 166
sweet potato
Breakfast Burritos with Homemade Sweet-Potato Wraps, 70
Healthy Fried Chicken and Waffles with Mustard Syrup, 34
Mexican Twice-Baked Stuffed Sweet Potato, 133
Savory Sweet-Potato Chicken and Waffle, 105

T

tahini, Quick-Bake Falafel, 130
tarragon, Creamy Tarragon Shrimp Pasta, 185
tempeh, Savory Oats with Tempeh "Bacon," 30
tofu, extra firm, Khichri and Air-Fried Tofu, 158
tofu, firm, Tofu Veggie Scramble, 121
tomatoes, canned, diced, Budget-Friendly Chili, 173
tomatoes, canned, whole
Cauliflower-Rice Arancini with Turkey Sausage, 178
Creamy Tarragon Shrimp Pasta, 185
Italian Baked Eggs, 33
tomatoes, strained
Anabolic Pizza, 190
Chicken Parmesan Bake with Quinoa, 170
Fried Zucchini Chips with Marinara Dip, 206
Ricotta-Stuffed Healthy Peppers, 109
Turkey Meatball Subs, 114
tomato paste
BBQ Pulled Chicken Sliders, 106
Budget-Friendly Chili, 173
tomato sauce
One-Pot Deconstructed Lasagna, 165
Pizza Casserole, 210
tortilla
Breakfast Quesadilla, 62
Mexican Lasagna, 169
White Bean and Artichoke Flatbread, 117
tuna, canned, Tuna-Stuffed Avocados, 146
tuna steak, Tuna Burger with Pineapple Bun, 110
turkey, ground
One-Pot Deconstructed Lasagna, 165
Pizza Casserole, 210
Ricotta-Stuffed Healthy Peppers, 109
Turkey Meatball Subs, 114
turkey bacon
Breakfast Pizza, 38
Breakfast Stuffed Peppers, 29
Egg Turkey-Bacon Muffins, 42
Shredded Potato-Wrapped Quiche, 45
turkey pepperoni, Pizza Casserole, 210
turkey sausage
Cauliflower-Rice Arancini with Turkey Sausage, 178
Healthy Sausage and Egg McWills, 73
Turkey-Sausage Breakfast Casserole, 37
Zucchini Boats, 126
turmeric
Shawarma Chicken, 118
Tofu Veggie Scramble, 121
turnip, One-Pot Hearty Vegetable Chicken Stew, 162

V

vanilla butter extract, Raspberry Chocolate Protein Blondies, 244
vanilla extract
Anabolic "Spreadaroo" Cookies, 236
Blueberry Cottage-Cheese Protein Cheesecake Bowl, 240
Chocolate-Chip Protein Cheesecake, 247
Crispy Fried PB&J Sandwich, 209
French Toast Protein Bagels, 54
Lemon-Ricotta Protein Crepes, 69
No-Churn Vanilla-Protein Ice Cream, 243
Protein Banana Bread, 57
Pumpkin Protein Mousse Cake, 232
Raspberry Chocolate Protein Blondies, 244
vegetable broth
Buffalo Cauliflower Bites, 141
Cauliflower and Leek Soup, 134
Coconut Chicken Curry, 174
vinegar, apple cider
BBQ Pulled Chicken Sliders, 106
Healthy Fried Chicken and Waffles with Mustard Syrup, 34
vinegar, balsamic
BBQ Pulled Chicken Sliders, 106
Grilled Vegetable Salad, 102
vinegar, white, Buffalo Cauliflower Bites, 141
vinegar, white wine, Pecan Chicken Salad, 98

Z

zucchini
Anabolic Shepherd's Pie, 193
Coconut Chicken Curry, 174
Fried Zucchini Chips with Marinara Dip, 206
Grilled Vegetable Salad, 102
Healthy Pad Thai, 181
One-Pot Hearty Vegetable Chicken Stew, 162
Steak Taco Salad, 113
Turkey Meatball Subs, 114
Warm Root-Vegetable Salad, 142
Zucchini Boats, 126
Zucchini Hashbrowns, 74

ABOUT THE AUTHOR

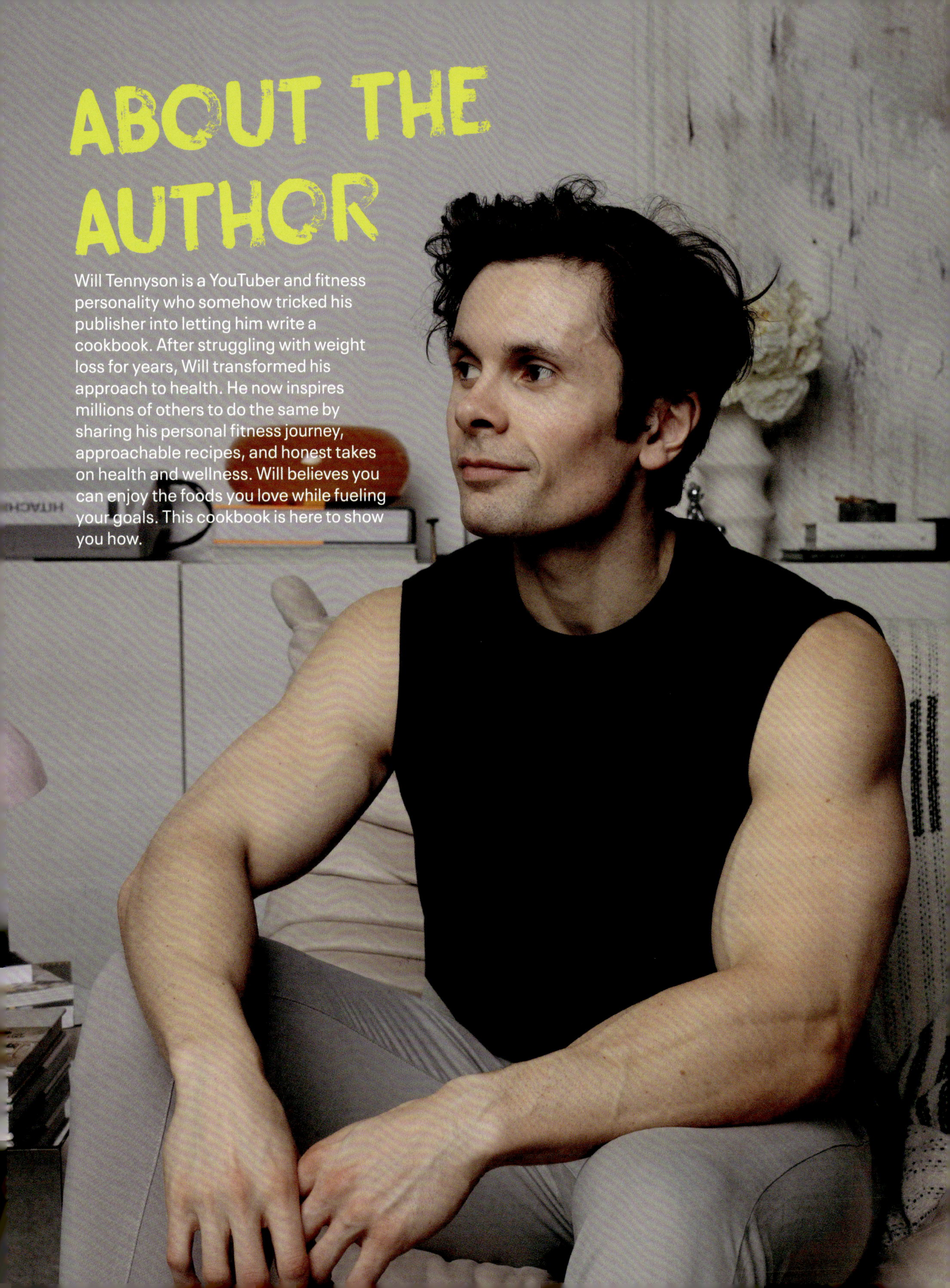

Will Tennyson is a YouTuber and fitness personality who somehow tricked his publisher into letting him write a cookbook. After struggling with weight loss for years, Will transformed his approach to health. He now inspires millions of others to do the same by sharing his personal fitness journey, approachable recipes, and honest takes on health and wellness. Will believes you can enjoy the foods you love while fueling your goals. This cookbook is here to show you how.